The Crimean Doctors
VOLUME TWO

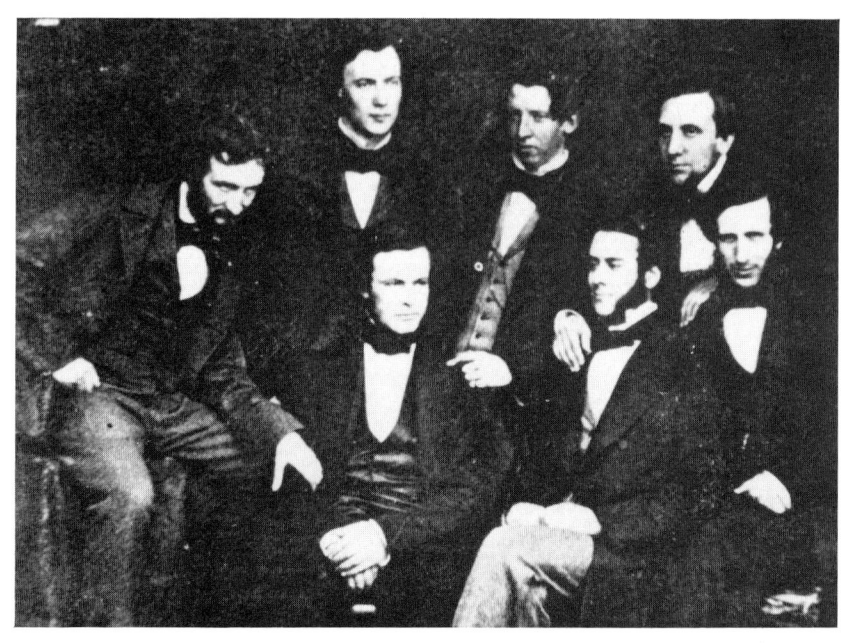

House officers at Edinburgh Royal Infirmary (early 1854).
Standing: John Kirk, George Pringle, Patrick Heron Watson.
Sitting: John Beddoe, Joseph Lister, David Christison, Alexander Struthers.
Christison, Struthers and Watson joined the army as assistant-surgeons; Pringle served in hospital transports and Beddoe and Kirk as civil surgeons. Lister, a Quaker, did not serve.

THE CRIMEAN DOCTORS

A History of the British Medical Services in the Crimean War

VOLUME TWO

JOHN SHEPHERD

'Unlicked cubs and old bears'
Florence Nightingale

published for the
Department of History
University of Liverpool

LIVERPOOL UNIVERSITY PRESS
1991

Liverpool Historical Studies, no. 7
General Editor: P. E. H. Hair

Published in Great Britain, 1991
by the Liverpool University Press,
Senate House, PO Box 147, Liverpool, L69 3BX

Copyright © 1991 by John Shepherd

British Library Cataloguing in Publication Data are available

ISBN (Vol. 1): 0 85323 107 9
ISBN (Vol. 2): 0 85323 167 2
ISBN (Set): 0 85323 177 X

Printed in the European Community
at The Bath Press, Avon, United Kingdom

CONTENTS

Volume II

CHAPTER X   **The Scutari hospitals (January to March 1855)**   **341**

The medical conditions treated **343** - medical staffing **351** - contemporary descriptions **356** - medical casualties **361** - Miss Nightingale, the nurses, and the chef **362**

CHAPTER XI   **Commissions and Committees (1854 - 1855)**   **373**

The First Commission **374** - the Roebuck Committee **381** - the Sanitary Commission **395** - the Supplies Commission **401** - the Pathology Commission **405**

CHAPTER XII   **The Civil Surgeons and the Civil Hospitals (1855 - 1856)**   **412**

Smyrna Civil Hospital: doctors and nurses **421** - the prefabricated hospital at Renkioi **435** - conclusions **445**

CHAPTER XIII   **The Final Months of the Siege of Sebastopol (April to September 1855)**   **452**

The Fall of Sebastopol **452** - the medical circumstances of the siege **456** - medical conditions (diseases) **463** - surgical conditions and war wounds **468** - the doctors in the front line **484** - the Naval Brigade (April-September 1855) **492** - Miss Nightingale visits the Crimea **498** - nurses and other women in the Crimea **502** - the death of Lord Raglan **509**

CHAPTER XIV The Scutari Hospitals (April 1855 to June 1856)   517

The final period (April to September 1855) **517** - Miss Nightingale and the nurses **522** - the later period (October 1855 to June 1856) **526** - Miss Nightingale and the nurses and orderlies **531** - conclusion **535**

CHAPTER XV The Navy in the Baltic and Black Seas (1855-1856)   539

The Baltic Fleet 1855 **539** - diseases and surgery **540** - medical staffing **541** - the Black Sea Fleet 1855-1856 **542** -diseases and surgery **544** - medical staffing **548** - the Naval Hospital at Therapia **549** - the total naval casualties (1854-1855) **554**

CHAPTER XVI The Turkish Contingent   559

The Turkish military hospitals **562**

CHAPTER XVII Stalemate and Withdrawal from the Crimea (October 1855 to July 1856)   572

Medical and surgical conditions **573** - the Crimean Medical Society **581** - the later visits of Miss Nightingale to the Crimea **587**

CHAPTER XVIII Epilogue: Post War Consequences   591

Mortality of armies and doctors **591** - the post-war Sanitary Commission and its results **592** - clinical lessons of the war **597** - the Medical Services in later wars **602** - post-war careers **605** - the Naval Medical Service after the war **611** - Miss Nightingale **614** - conclusion **618**

SOURCES   **625**

APPENDICES   **640**

INDEXES   **651**

ILLUSTRATIONS   after **662**

CHAPTER X

THE SCUTARI HOSPITALS
(JANUARY TO MARCH, 1855)

The activities and the expansion of the base hospitals in Scutari up to December 1854 have been described in Chapter VI, and an account has been given in Chapter VIII of Miss Nightingale's influence on the hospitals by the introduction of nurses and by her early reforms. As in the Crimea, between January and March 1855 a major crisis had to be faced. The mortality rates in the hospitals (i.e. the ratio of deaths to admissions) were now to reach the highest levels experienced throughout the war, as shown in Table 1 below.

Table 1

Admissions to Scutari Hospitals
(January to March 1855)

	Admissions	Deaths	
January	4,761	1,393	(29%)
February	2,688	1,386	(52%)
March	2,833	575	(20%)
Totals	10,282	3,354	(33%)

These figures are derived from tables in which the statistics of the main hospitals (the General, the Barrack and Koulali) are combined for January, but separate ones are given for Koulali in February and March.[1] Koulali was not functioning fully until the end of January and in that month it is unlikely that more than 300 patients were admitted. But a comparison for February and March between the two larger hospitals on the one hand and Koulali on the other, reveals that the mortality rates were almost equal. The mortality on passage from Balaclava to Scutari in this period is shown in Table 2.[2]

Table 2

Deaths in Hospital Transports
(January to March 1855)

	Patients conveyed	Deaths
January	2,877	239 (8%)
February	2,328	43 (2%)
March	1,200	6 (0.5%)
Totals:	6,415	288 (4%)

The worst figures were recorded for the transport 'Shooting Star', which took on 130 patients at Balaclava, of which 47 died in transit. The voyage lasted from 7 to 20 January, and the disembarkation of casualties was not begun until 24 January and not completed for another three days. In such circumstances the conditions on board must have been appalling, with all stores exhausted. The delays in landing patients must have been due to lack of beds in the hospitals. The mortality rates indicate a great improvement in the hospital transport service by February.

As the previous tables show, the proportion of patients at Scutari coming from the war front in the Crimea varied.

Table 3

Proportion of Admissions to Scutari Hospitals
from the Crimea
(January to March 1855)

	Total Admissions to Scutari	Cases from the Crimea
January	4,761	2,877 (60%)
February	2,688	2,328 (87%)
March	2,833	1,200 (43%)
Totals:	10,282	6,405 (62%)

In Table 3 a balance of 38 per cent of non-Crimea admissions to the hospitals during the three months must be accounted for by cases from the large army camps in the vicinity in which reserves were accommodated while in transit, by cases landed from the transports arriving from England (in which the sickness rate was often high), and by the sick of all grades of hospital staff. Exact figures from the Scutari and Gallipoli camps cannot be calculated, but in the autumn these camps were often overcrowded, unhygienic, and in close contact with the disease-ridden Turkish population. It is difficult to explain the low percentage of cases admitted from local sources in February (13 per cent).

To accommodate this heavy load, in January there were approximately 4,400 beds in the base hospitals. Cantlie calculates the distribution of beds as follows:[3]

General Hospital	968
Barrack Hospital	1,704
Huts in the Barrack Hospital Compound	530
Hyder Pasha Hospital (mainly convalescent)	444
Koulali Hospital and Barracks	748
Total	4,394

The Haidar (or Hyder) Pasha Hospital is often referred to as the Palace Hospital (the so-called Hareem Hospital was a rather flimsy annexe of the Palace Hospital and was burnt down in February). A variable number of convalescents was transferred to the hulks and to Abydos; and there was also a constant transfer of patients to convalescent hospitals established in Malta and Corfu, or direct to England, according to the availability of sea transport. Not until April was the first Civil Hospital, at Smyrna, in full operation.

It follows that in January and February there were many occasions when the General and the Barrack Hospitals had all available beds occupied, and when additional patients had to be accommodated on mattresses or palliasses in the wards and corridors. Smith deserves some credit for his earlier insistence that 5,000 beds should be made available for the winter. In the Crimean campaign the consequences of overcrowding were exceptionally serious, accounting for much cross-infection, inadequate patient care, and a very high mortality. Under this pressure, in February the total of beds available in the main hospitals was increased by 600.[4]

In the home press it was frequently suggested that the overcrowding and the death rates in the hospitals were much greater than those stated above. Newspaper correspondents tended to report exceptional weekly figures, not always from reliable sources, when the death-rate was excessive or when the overcrowding was temporarily at a very high level. However, throughout the war and thereafter, Miss Nightingale questioned the official mortality rates. As in November 1854 she continued to quote figures derived from the burial records. After the war, when she was interrogated by the Commissions in 1857, she gave a total of 3,042 deaths in the General and Barrack Hospitals from January to March 1855.[5] The official figure, as quoted above, was 3,334, but this included at least 436 deaths in Koulali Hospital. Miss Nightingale may therefore have slightly exaggerated the total in the first three months of 1855. (The methods by which she finally calculated the hospital death rates are not at all clear and it is very likely that the Commissioners were rather bewildered by her reasoning). For this critical phase we have therefore little choice but to accept the figures of admissions and deaths provided officially after the war. There are admittedly gaps in the records. The derived totals take no account of the number of admissions carried forward from one month to another. There is no way of calculating the average stay in hospital. But from the number of beds available it is clear that many patients were in hospital for long periods, often only to die there of their original disease or injury, or of infection acquired in hospital.

THE MEDICAL CONDITIONS TREATED

The Scutari hospitals treated almost exclusively medical conditions, bowel diseases and fever accounting for more than half.

The figures for BOWEL DISEASES are these.

Table 4

Admissions to Scutari Hospitals for Bowel Diseases
(January to March 1855)

	Admissions	Deaths
January	1,468	841 (57%)
February	837	571 (68%)
March	691	220 (32%)
Totals	2,996	1,632 (55%)

Not only were 29 per cent of the hospital admissions in this period listed under the headings of Diarrhoea and Dysentery, but these diseases accounted for 49 per cent of the deaths.[6] The former figure represents approximately the proportion of bowel disorders among the causes of sickness in the Crimea. The mortality rates are higher in the Scutari hospitals than in the regimental hospitals because the most intractable cases were sent to the former. Moreover, many deaths from bowel disorders occurred in patients admitted originally with a different diagnosis on admission, since fatal bowel infection was often picked up in the base hospital. The crowded beds, the general lack of hygiene, the absence of even the most rudimentary nursing precautions against cross-infection, the debilitated state of the patients, and the poor diet combined to favour the spread of infective bowel conditions, particularly the bacillary dysenteries. The significant fall in hospital admissions in March was directly related to the fall in the incidence of bowel diseases in the regiments. That the mortality was halved in March is most likely attributable to the control of overcrowding, to improved hygiene, to better standards of cooking and diet, and to better nursing care.

The medical treatment of bowel conditions differed little from that used in the regimental hospitals. But some of the more useful palliative medicines such as opium were more readily available, and in the wards for which Miss Nightingale had set up extra-diet kitchens, the patients were better nourished. The young Acting Assistant-Surgeon, Robert Bakewell[7], was one of the few, other than Pyemont Smith, to record details of the treatment of bowel conditions. Bakewell noted that almost all the soldiers admitted to the Scutari hospitals from the Crimea had some form of dysentery. "I might sum up my account by saying that everything was tried and that nothing succeeded. At least I can say that I never cured a case, and I never saw a case cured." Bakewell acknowledged the benefit of opium symptomatically. He tried all forms of treatment, astringents, castor oil, cod-liver oil and ipecacuanha. More unusual was his use of silver nitrate enemata which he claimed had been successful in India, acting, he suggested, "by allaying the irritability of the rectum."[8] In some wards individual medical officers succeeded in establishing strict rules which cut down cross-infection, but segregation of the patients with infective types of bowel disease was never complete.

FEVER accounted for 25 per cent of the hospital admissions, being listed under the headings Quotidian Intermittent, Common Continuous, Remittent, Typhus and Typhoid. This was a different classification from that adopted in the regimental lists and even more confusing. Fevers accounted for 18 per cent of the deaths in this period.

Table 5

Admissions to Scutari Hospitals for Fevers
(January to March 1855)

	Admissions	Deaths
January	704	152 (22%)
February	900	278 (31%)
March	983	164 (17%)
Totals:	2,587	594 (23%)

While in March in the regimental hospitals the mortality from fevers had doubled, in the base hospitals it was halved. This supports the suggestion that virulent fevers broke out in the Crimea in March, and that patients died quickly, and so were not sent to Scutari. The fall in the mortality rate in March in the base hospitals may be explained partly by the general improvements. The medical treatment of fevers was little different from that used in the camps. The environment in the base hospitals was marginally more conducive to recovery, in terms of warmth and shelter. Some of those acutely ill had the chance of receiving good nursing. The contagious nature of many of the fevers led to much cross-infection. A degree of segregation in special fever wards was established, but at the peak of overcrowding these precautions were not very successful. The high rates of morbidity and mortality among the medical and nursing staff in these months were largely due to fevers.

Once more, as with the cases in the regimental hospitals in this period, the precise identification of the fevers is impossible to achieve. It is surprising that disastrous epidemics of typhus did not sweep the overcrowded wards, all the conditions being present to favour such epidemics. The patients arrived from the transports in the clothes they had worn in the Crimea; in the hospitals some were at once given clean shirts but for others there was a long delay before they were washed or given fresh clothes. Sarah Terrot, one of the Sellonite Sisters who came out originally with Miss Nightingale and who worked in the Barrack Hospital, commented in her journal. "The patients brought in during December were in a very bad state - some dying, some in a state of filth no words can describe, miserable skeletons, devoured by lice."[9] Again, in January "one poor fellow neglected by the orderlies because he was dying ... was very dirty, covered with wounds and devoured by lice. I pointed this out to the orderlies, whose only excuse was 'It's not worth while to clean him: he's not long for this world. The men in bed on each side of him told me his state was such that lice swarmed from him to them."[10] There are many other observations of the infested state of the men, in fact it was almost taken for granted. Yet the cases designated Febris Typhus admitted to the base hospitals from January to March totalled only 78 (of which 31 died). The vast majority of fever cases, approximately 90 per cent, were recorded under the heading Febris Continua Communis. This is as indeterminate a title as 'low fever', so commonly used to indicate the cause of death in fever cases.

Less common ailments were rheumatic conditions, diseases of the respiratory tract, and frost-bite.

Table 6

Admissions to Scutari Hospitals for Rheumatic Conditions
(January to March 1855)

	Admissions	Deaths	
January	595	43	(7%)
February	304	64	(21%)
March	417	25	(6%)
Totals:	1,316	132	(10%)

Some 12 per cent of the hospital admissions were listed under Acute RHEUMATISM, Chronic Rheumatism, Lumbago and Joint Diseases, and these conditions accounted for 8 per cent of the deaths. The high admission rate in January was the aftermath of the excessive rain-fall and the damp sleeping conditions in the camps in November and December, while the relatively low mortality in January suggests that these were predominately chronic diseases. Later, in the extremely cold weather, the admission rate fell but the mortality rose. The reason for the increased mortality is uncertain. No details are available of the treatment given to these patients. For the chronic conditions transfer to a warmer climate would have offered the greatest benefit.

Table 7

Admissions to the Scutari Hospitals for Diseases of the Respiratory Tract
(January to March 1855)

	Admissions	Deaths	
January	338	31	(9%)
February	140	64	(45%)
March	212	29	(14%)
Totals	690	124	(18%)

Almost 7 per cent of the hospital admissions were listed under Pleuritis, Pneumonia, Haemoptysis, Pulmonary Phthisis, Acute Catarrh, Chronic Catarrh, Bronchitis, Dyspnoea, and Asthma; and these RESPIRATORY DISEASES accounted for 4 per cent of the deaths. The high mortality in February was most likely associated with the overcrowded state of the wards and to the poor physical condition of most patients at this time. Pneumonia contributed largely to the total death rate from respiratory tract disease. In the three months there were 20 cases of pulmonary tuberculosis admitted, of which 14 died. The medical management of these cases was little different from that given in the regimental hospitals. The more seriously ill, such as those with pneumonia or acute bronchitis, may have had the advantage of special diets, but until the nurse/patient ratio improved they lacked the benefit of good nursing in salubrious surroundings, the main essentials to recovery.

Table 8

Admissions to the Scutari Hospitals for Frost-Bite (Gelatio)
(January to March 1855)

	Admissions	Deaths	
January	249	53	(21%)
February	288	139	(48%)
March	121	65	(53%)
Totals	658	257	(39%)

Some 6 per cent of the hospital admissions were listed under FROST-BITE, and deaths from the effects of this condition accounted for 8 per cent of the total deaths. Many of these patients were very ill, often suffering from severe infections of frost-bitten feet. Some had already had amputations and inevitably the stumps were grossly septic. The number requiring late amputation is uncertain. These were patients in very poor condition, often with scurvy and always with severe infection. The high death rate in February and March was due in many instances to acquired infection from the fevers or bowel diseases so rife in the wards. Some unfortunate men lingered on for weeks, while for those that did survive, healing was slow and convalescence greatly prolonged. Pyemont Smith gives a description of seven cases of frost-bite under his care, of which four died.[11]

Only four cases of cholera were recorded as having been admitted in these three months and all died.[12] OTHER MEDICAL CONDITIONS, infrequent or rare, appear sporadically on the lists, the diagnoses being similar to those recorded in the regimental tables. A fairly large number of admissions was listed under the heading Unknown. Of a total of 919, in January 861 were recorded, in February 58, and in March none. Of these 244 died (26 per cent of the group). The cases were almost certainly medical but of uncertain diagnosis, or were of patients with multiple conditions in which it was difficult to state a primary condition. This general heading is to be found in the Scutari tables between August 1854 and February 1855, but not thereafter. It may be that instructions were given in February that a specific diagnosis on admission and a specific cause of death should be given in every case. This increases doubts about the accuracy of diagnosis in so many cases and reflects the weakness of the nosological tables generally, aspects of the medical situation so strongly criticised by Miss Nightingale. With the limitations of clinical methods of diagnosis and the almost complete lack of laboratory aids it was surely a retrograde policy to pretend that no cases were admitted in which diagnosis was obscure. It was not until later, largely on Miss Nightingale's recommendations, that facilities for post-mortem examinations were established. Prior to this, few autopsies were performed in the Scutari hospitals, whereas if more had been done, a cause of death would in some cases have been more accurately defined.

Only 3 per cent of the admissions during the three months were related to WAR WOUNDS, subdivided as Vulnus Sclopitorum and Vulnus Incisum.[13] Of a total admission in these categories of 262, there were 197 in January, 35 in February and 30 in March. The total mortality was 88 (34 per cent). These figures reflect the small number of such cases requiring transfer from the regimental hospitals. The death rate was not excessive. The number of secondary amputations performed is uncertain, but such operations always carried a high mortality rate even in the best conditions. The risks of death from infective conditions acquired in the wards was high. The operating conditions were still primitive and all wounds were septic before the casualties reached Scutari. The numbers of wounded requiring surgery were so small that any analysis is valueless, and in fact details of these cases are very scanty. The number of general surgical conditions admitted was very small. The incidence of abscesses and other minor septic conditions was much less than in the regimental hospitals. The necessity for amputation in some cases of frost-bite has been mentioned already. As in the Crimea the hospital doctors had to deal with relatively few surgical problems, once the Inkerman casualties had been cleared. When the intensive assaults on Sebastopol began again in the late spring the numbers of wounded reaching Scutari again climbed.

The high admission rates and mortality rates cited above indicate the challenge which faced the hospital doctors at Scutari. It was not only the dilapidated state of the buildings converted for hospital use and their general unsuitability for this purpose which accounted for many of the problems, but also the weak hospital organisation. When Menzies, in April 1854, had to plan the general hospitals he wrote to Smith asking for the regulations which should be applied. Smith searched the records as far back as the Peninsular War but found nothing helpful. The only general hospital at home of any note was at Fort Pitt, and this, compared with the Scutari hospitals, was small. Accordingly, Menzies had to follow the rules which were applied to regimental hospitals, the administration of which was very different to that suitable for large hospitals. Chaos in matters of staffing, supplies, and in essential services such as kitchens, laundry and the like was the result. It took a long time to correct these administrative defects. The army doctors were all brought up on the regimental system, under the military discipline of their commanding officers, and similarly, but unsuitably, in a general hospital a senior medical officer found himself with a field officer (of lower rank) in overall command. That the high command had a low opinion of general hospitals as opposed to regimental hospitals was all too apparent from their reluctance to do much to ensure that any improvement to the system was given adequate support. Raglan and his staff officers patently saw general hospitals as a necessary temporary evil.

During the winter the home newspapers regaled their readers with accounts of the Scutari hospitals. **The Times** was determined to put much of the blame for the bad management of the hospitals on Smith and his staff in London, but Hall also came under severe criticism, as the senior medical officer in the East. The medical press did not blame the doctors but saw more clearly that the faults lay in the army organisation, in the neglect of medical affairs for so many years, and in the failure to have improved the supply and commissariat system since the time of the Peninsular Wars. The Director-General was exonerated from the charge of neglect in his preparations.

When **The Times** refused to publish a letter from a young army doctor defending the mode of treatment at Scutari, he sent his letter to the **Medical Times and Gazette** and the Editor printed it in full.[14] The letter-writer was Acting Assistant-Surgeon Bakewell who signed himself as "one of the medical staff at Scutari". A leader in **The Times** had charged the Scutari doctors with incompetence in their treatment of dysentery and fever, claiming that "the sick who have come down with dysentery and fever have almost all died". This, Bakewell insisted, was a very exaggerated statement. **The Times** had also presented the following argument.

> The medical men, French, English and Perote [i.e. of Pera] who practise in the Capital [Constantinople] are of the opinion that the English doctors are killing their patients at Scutari with a wrong-headed adherence to a mode of practice, which if successful anywhere is certainly not adapted to the climate of Constantinople. The sick who come into the Hospital are treated with stimulants: wine, brandy and ammonia are given as tonics, as the Medical Staff assert the disease to be the effect of weakness and exhaustion. On the other hand the Medical men of the Capital avoid the use of stimulants, and look upon dysentery as inflammation, to be allayed by low diet and in some cases by leeching.[15]

Bakewell pointed out that the Staff Surgeons had mostly served in India and were well experienced in the management of dysentery, and he denied that all cases were treated with stimulants. He affirmed - "The treatment is not confined to one particular plan but necessarily varies with the previous health, and present state of the patient ... The patients who die within the first twenty-four hours after arriving at Scutari are those who on admission are in a state of extreme prostration ... They die not from the use of stimulants, but in spite of their use." This young man had shown some courage in refuting the accusations in **The Times**. It may be that his seniors thought the intervention presumptuous, but they might have shown appreciation that someone was prepared to defend them publicly. Later Bakewell was to incur severe censure for a less tactful letter which was sent to **The Times** and on this occasion accepted for publication.

Koulali Hospital was at times criticised even more severely than the Barrack Hospital. In fact during February and March the mortality rates at Koulali were no worse than those in the two larger hospitals. Koulali originally received convalescent patients from the main hospitals but increasingly took admissions straight from the transports. The mortality of patients with bowel diseases was only half that in the Barrack and the General Hospitals, but the mortality from fevers was twice as great. Reports reached England that conditions in Koulali were very bad and that the mortality rates were exceptionally high. These reports were exaggerated. It has already been noted that the building was very unsuitable for conversion to a hospital. In consequence sanitation, ventilation, heating, and kitchen arrangements were defective. Hall does not seem to have taken much interest in Koulali for he makes no mention of it in his diary or his letters. Cumming, who was in overall charge in Scutari, referred to Koulali only once in his letters to Hall - "Koulali going strong". The establishment was quite large, with about 750 beds. Heron Watson worked for several weeks at Koulali. Of the doctors' accommodation he wrote - "They are more like condemned cells than quarters for men who spend the rest of their time in the wards full of patients suffering from contagious disease". He had charge of two wards, containing about 120 medical patients. His ward round started at 9 a.m. and lasted until 4 p.m., and he made a two-hour visit in the evening. Of the fever epidemic, which was at its worst in March, he recorded - "The fever here is horrible in its virulence owing in great measure to the way they crowd the patients together - only 11/2 feet between beds". He did not have a high opinion of the nurses, "Sisters of Charity under Miss Stanley who promise to do, but don't and can't perform". He had to tend sick nurses, "often ill and malingering". Thwarted of opportunities to operate and bored with tedious medical duties, he was greatly relieved when he was drafted to the Crimea after five months at Koulali.[16]

Some of the nurses at Koulali published their impressions of the hospital. Miss Taylor recorded that initially there were only five doctors under one Staff-Surgeon. She confirmed that most of the cases were medical and gave her own diagnosis for the fever cases, "dysentery turned to a malignant type of low spotted fever". There is, in fact, evidence that a true typhus was more common in Koulali than elsewhere. Some of the doctors, including Watson, and some of the nurses suffered from this condition. Miss Taylor had a good opinion of the doctors - "During a year's residence among them the writer and all her companions never experienced from any surgeon other than assistance and gentlemanly treatment".[17] The medical staff at Koulali changed frequently during the winter. Staff-Surgeon Nicholas O'Connor[18] was in charge in the winter. Apart from Watson little is known of the junior doctors. There are references to a Dr. Temple[19], "assiduous in cases of sickness".

MEDICAL STAFFING

Menzies was in overall charge of the Scutari Hospitals from June 1854 to 2 January, 1855. Forrest, who succeeded him, resigned two weeks later; thereafter Lawson and Cruikshank, by virtue of their seniority, were in command for short periods, until Cumming took over completely. Menzies had not proved very successful, but had been faced with great difficulties. By 21 December, 1854, he was exhausted. He wrote to Hall - "My health is giving way under recent attacks of renal complaints and having since been affected with bronchitis and now scarcely able to leave my quarters ... I ask for a Board".[20] In his last weeks before he was invalided home Menzies' management must have been increasingly ineffective. His successor, Forrest, proved a broken reed. After only two days he wrote to Hall - "I feel confident I shall break down"[21]; and later he wrote - "I am sorry I find I must divert to England for a change of climate as I am quite unfit to carry on duty here. Lawson and others seem to think there is serious disease of the kidney going on and I daresay they are right".[22] He too was invalided. In evidence later to the Roebuck Committee, Smith was rather vague as to who was in charge after Menzies left.

> Dr. Menzies ... ceased to have charge on the 1st or 2nd of January, 1855. Dr. Forrest succeeded him, and performed the duties for probably about ten days or a fortnight, when he was taken ill with inflammation of the liver, and was laid up and Mr. Cruikshank then succeeded Dr. Forrest. The witness did not know whether there was an interim of a day or two during which Dr. Lawson had charge, but it was not more than a day or two, when Dr. Cumming, having concluded the work in which he had been employed, namely, the Commission, assumed the duty.[23]

The situation was very confused. It does seem that Lawson exerted authority for a short period until Cumming took over. Cumming wrote to Hall on 3 February indicating that his work on the Commission was completed, and he continued in charge until 1 October, 1855.

These changes during January must have been very unsettling, and hardly conducive to smooth running of the hospitals at this difficult period. As already recorded,

Cumming, although at first engaged on his duties with the Commission, had often overruled the decisions of Menzies by the exertion of his superior rank. In the evidence he gave to the Roebuck Committee the Director-General indicated that the base hospital appointments were made by Hall, with the agreement of the Commander-in-Chief. But he pointed out that,

> supposing a medical man was at the head of the hospitals and another who was his superior arrived ... the latter would, ipso facto, have taken direction of the hospitals. If anything like system was wanted in any department this must be allowed, unless some regulation existed to the contrary ... He urgently recommended the despatch of Dr. Cumming, who would not be interfered with by any senior officer arriving: his rank put him in that position, in which there was very little chance of him being superseded.[24]

Smith had selected Cumming to serve on the Commission but had intended that he should soon take charge of the Scutari Hospitals, whereas the Duke of Newcastle had decided that Cumming should not assume his duties as Principal Medical Officer until he had completed his work on the Commission. It may seem in retrospect that Hall can be blamed for much of the confusion over the senior appointments at Scutari, but he was in a difficult position. He felt he had to get the approval of the Director-General for new appointments, and communications to London were very slow. He had also to deal with undercurrents of jealousy and intrigue. Concerning promotions or appointments, some of his senior officers communicated directly to Smith, while others wrote to Herbert or other influential persons. In addition, Miss Nightingale was sending a constant flow of opinions and information to Herbert concerning the senior doctors at Scutari. Hall's failure to re-visit the base hospitals after October 1854 did not strengthen his position. Had he done so he would have been better able to assess the ability or otherwise of the medical officers there, and he would have been more aware of the mounting problems.

There were difficulties enough in January other than the frequent changes in the medical command. The increasing sick rate among all grades of doctors created many problems. **The Times** correspondent summed up this situation late in January.

> While every day's experience makes the want of superior medical officers more severely felt the crowded state of the hospitals, the increasing prevalence of infectious fever, and the increasing severity of their labours, are rapidly diminishing the number of those available for duty. Dr. Forrest is the third Deputy-Inspector obliged to go home on sick leave and the number of officers

> holding that rank now in the East is quite inadequate for the present requirements of the service ... the want of First-Class Surgeons is equally felt. Dr. McIlree[25] is too unwell for duty. Dr. O'Connor[26] at Kulalee will immediately have more patients under his care than he can possibly look after. At the Barrack Hospital there is scarcely a single Second-Class Surgeon left for some have been taken away to duty in the sick transports and of the few left behind Dr. Summers[27] is very ill and Dr. Newton[28] I regret to say is dead ... When I arrived here early in November the maximum number of deaths scarcely exceeded twenty a day; now it is nearly three times as high. At that time the proportion of sick and wounded was about equal; now the former vastly preponderate ... Men no longer come down newly attacked and presenting symptoms favourable for a cure; they arrive exhausted with chronic disease firmly rooted in their broken constitutions, and almost all beyond the chances of successful treatment.[29]

In February Cumming had the assistance of Deputy Inspectors-General McGrigor, Lawson and Cruikshank. McGrigor continued in charge of the Barrack Hospital, while Lawson and Cruikshank were presumably engaged in general administrative duties in the whole area. Relations between Cumming and McGrigor were not friendly, possibly because of the latter's premature promotion through Miss Nightingale's influence. Cumming reported to Hall that, on a recent inspection, "McGrigor's division was in the worst order". Later following a quarrel between McGrigor and a civilian doctor, Cumming stated that "McGrigor is an ass". When Lawson was transferred to Scutari he was under a cloud because of his involvement in the 'Avon' case. Hall however had confidence in him, and Cumming also gave him support, considering that Lawson had been treated with unjustifiable harshness by Raglan and by the press. Miss Nightingale did not view Lawson's attachment to Scutari with much favour as she saw in this the power of the medical department (and of Hall in particular) to protect those who had (in her opinion) failed in their duty, and to cover up incompetence on the part of senior medical officers. Such undercurrents contributed to a lack of confidence among the senior medical staff, and equally to a public lack of confidence in them. Lawson and Cruikshank remained in Scutari until the end of the war, but McGrigor died at Scutari in November 1855.

From January to March the number of medical officers attached to the Scutari hospitals fluctuated greatly because of sickness and death. But the total available was almost double that in October 1854. The number of staff surgeons is uncertain, but the junior doctors, originally made up almost entirely by regulars, were now augmented by newly joined assistant-surgeons with full commissions, or by those with acting rank. Most of these, however, were recently qualified and inexperienced. Many of the temporary acting officers came straight from their teaching schools, including a small group from Edinburgh sponsored by Professors Simpson and Syme. Because of frequent staff changes the doctors were frequently switched from one ward or division to another, or from one hospital to another. The new recruits, particularly the young volunteers, constantly pressed for transfer to regiments in the front line. In consequence there was a lack of continuity of medical care, which was not conducive to efficiency.

Major Sillery had been appointed Commandant of the Scutari Hospitals in June 1854. He remained in this post until February 1855, when he was replaced by Lord William Paulet. Cantlie says of Sillery that he "appears to have been completely paralysed in his attempts to govern the hospitals under his orders".[30] He had had no previous experience of hospital management and showed little initiative, dealing only with minor matters and being ready to pass major problems to others. Miss Nightingale had a very low opinion of him, receiving little cooperation in her efforts to improve conditions in the hospitals. Yet Lord Paulet, a Brigadier-General and a much more experienced general officer, was not much of an improvement. Of him Miss Nightingale wrote - "Lord Wm. Paulet is appalled at the view of evils he has no idea what to do with ... and then he shuts his eyes and hopes when he opens them he shall see something else".[31] Wealthy and well-connected, Paulet spent more time socialising with Lady Stratford than applying himself to his duties. The Commandant had authority to spend money locally to meet emergencies but neither Sillery nor Paulet exercised these powers. It was not until the autumn of 1855 that an efficient and cooperative Commandant, General Storks, replaced Paulet.

Meanwhile the gross ineptitude of the Purveyor and his staff continued as a source of constant irritation to the medical staff and as the cause of much hardship to the patients. Wreford, who had taken over from the inept Ward, served in the winter months. He had apparently shown some ability in assisting the Director-General to prepare the list of medical stores, equipment and drugs to be sent out on the outbreak of war.[32] But although the amended regulations concerning the duties and responsibilities of the Purveyor gave Menzies more authority over Wreford than he had had over Ward, Wreford proved obstructive and unimaginative, and he too was wedded to the concept that it was his duty to save money. When Miss Nightingale left England she was told that the Purveyor would supply her with all her needs, but she was soon disillusioned. She found Wreford uncooperative, partly because he did not know what was held in his stores, and it was with great reluctance that he issued anything on the requisition of Miss Nightingale or of the doctors. He discouraged local purchase of urgent material, although authorised to do this in emergency. In December Miss Nightingale wrote to Herbert to recommend that an intelligent young man, Mr. Rogers of the Purveyor's staff, should be put in charge.[33] Instead the War Office sent out a senior official, Mr. Milton, to "supervise" Wreford. Milton made no impact and the muddle continued to add to all the other difficulties of the situation. In her letters to Herbert, Miss Nightingale constantly made derisory criticisms of the Purveyor's department, and advised that the whole organisation should be scrapped and re-planned. She had written of "Messrs. Wreford, Ward, and Reade [the Apothecary], veterans of the Spanish War, coming to me for a moment's solace, trembling under responsibility and afraid of informality".[34] Menzies had tried to get rid of Ward but failed, and in general he had little success in dealing with the deplorable weaknesses of the Purveyor's department. Reade, the Apothecary, had died in November, leaving his department in a disorganised state.[35] He was an obstinate exponent of the out-of-date supply system inherited from the Napoleonic Wars, and saw it as his duty to economise even in the most dire emergency. Although a new Chief Apothecary was not appointed until February, there was a great improvement when medicines could at last be requisitioned by the medical officers without the necessity of the form being countersigned by the medical officer in charge.[36]

CONTEMPORARY DESCRIPTIONS

At the beginning of January 1855, the Reverend J.E. Sabin, the Chief Chaplain, reported favourably on improvements.

> A walk through our vast corridors, crowded as they are in every part, fills me with lively satisfaction, for I see how much has been done, and how rapidly, for the welfare of our Soldiers. One corridor alone contains 225 beds, every one occupied and the wards leading out of the same corridor contain 313 beds. The whole of this corridor has been repaved, and every ward had new floors within the last month, and now it is occupied from end to end. Surgeries are built on the wide stair-cases, boilers for hot water are erected at intervals, stoves are constantly kept burning in each ward and down the corridor which, to lessen the cold, is divided by wooden partitions: large tin baths are standing at the corners and entrances and ready for use, and every man has a wooden bedstead and a comfortable bed and bedding.[37]

At first sight this report suggests that much had been done to improve the hospitals by the end of December. But there is no confirmation that new floors had been laid in all the wards, or that the corridors had been repaved in the greater part of the hospitals. Both in the Barrack and the General Hospitals there were still gross defects of sanitation, related to the poor drainage system and poor ventilation. Such basic problems were not to be corrected until the Commission headed by Dr. Sutherland arrived, since it was powerful enough to ensure that its recommendations were carried out effectively. If in parts of the hospitals some progress had been made to create safer and more comfortable conditions for the patients, such minor gains were partly dissipated by two new factors in the winter months. First, the extreme cold created considerable problems. In the effort to conserve heat from the limited number of open stoves, windows were kept closed, thus causing an uncomfortable, smoky atmosphere conducive to the spread of infections. Secondly, the gross overcrowding which built up in January and February greatly aggravated the deleterious effects of bad sanitation and ventilation. To many observers the hospitals now appeared to have come near to a complete breakdown.

In addition to the reports from the philanthropists, M.P.s and newspaper correspondents, other reports from visitors to the hospitals at this time are available. Most observers brought out the full horror of the situation in their letters or in their published reminiscences. An anonymous author was struck "by the unbroken silence, like a catacomb", and by the uniformly "sombre and distressing appearance of the patients".[38] He suggested that at the entrance to each hospital there should be inscribed, "All hope abandon ye who enter here". Of Miss Nightingale he commented - "How can coarse, ruder man appreciate the purer, holier, motives that impel a woman in the full employment of earthly blessings to risk life and health in increasing strife with death in every shape ... It is her name and her story that later generations will delight to honour." An American, a Mr. MacNamara (apparently a non-medical), visited both British and French hospitals. He commented on the latter as "airy, light and clean ... as good as any in New York or London".. Of the Scutari hospitals he had this to say - "How widely different were affairs in the English Hospitals". He had praise only for Miss Nightingale - "An amiable and highly intelligent-looking lady, of some thirty summers, delicate in form and prepossessing in her appearance ... Until her providential interposition the hospitals had been without the commonest preparation for the reception and care of the thousands of sick and wounded".[39]

For the period between January and March there are few reports from civilian doctors who had visited the hospitals. Dr. Pyemont Smith, whose clinical reports have already been mentioned, was in charge of three wards and one corridor in the Barrack Hospital. He attributed the high January mortality of his patients (most of them with bowel conditions) to the extreme cold, but he did not mention overcrowding as a significant factor.[40] In official and private reports to Hall, and in their evidence to the various Commissions, the senior medical officers provided a number of observations on the situation. Inevitably their views were influenced by the fact that any adverse report might reflect on their own competence. Cumming wrote to Hall complaining of the shortage of medical staff, of the high sickness rate among the doctors, of the inadequacies of the Purveyor, and of problems relating to the nursing staff, but made few comments on the general defects of the hospitals. He was more concerned with transmitting his personal opinions about his colleagues and with discussing whether or not they should be promoted. He was concerned also with his own prospects, for on 17 March he applied for leave, telling Hall "I am completely done", but also expressing his hopes regarding promotion - "You may give London hopes of a step". However he was not allowed leave, so that he wrote plaintively to Hall at a later date - "I envy your constitution. I am quite used up."[41] Cumming's letters reveal the exhausted state of some of the senior medical staff and their defeatist attitudes.

Few junior commissioned medical officers published contemporary accounts of the hospitals during the winter, and few wrote reminiscences. The favourable verdict of Assistant-Surgeon Taylor has been quoted in Chapter VI. It does not appear that he was on the medical staff at Scutari, but merely visited the hospitals briefly while convalescing from an illness in the Crimea. The early impressions of Assistant-Surgeon Heron Watson, unlike most of his Edinburgh contemporaries a commissioned medical officer, have also been recorded in Chapter VI. He continued to write home with frank and often sweeping criticisms. When he was first commissioned in December 1854, he had been sent for three weeks to Fort Pitt Hospital at Chatham. Of the senior medical officers there he wrote - "they don't even trust you as a gentleman and contrive as much as possible to approximate your state to that of slavery. We are in fact men under authority." At Scutari too he disliked various of his superiors - "Hope Lawson will be recalled". Later, when moved to Koulali, he complained - "Only objection is the society". This rather critical and at times snobbish attitude was held by only a minority of the volunteers, whether commissioned or temporary. Watson was an ambitious and opinionated young man, but in his letters he was perhaps merely letting off steam. Like his Edinburgh friend, MacKenzie, he had hoped to gain surgical experience by serving in the East, and he too had an eye on the forthcoming vacancy for the Chair of Military Surgery. After he arrived at Scutari he was at times very depressed - "in low spirits - no mistake could be greater than coming out". Later he wrote - "Advice to people coming out - don't let them ever think of doing so unless they can give up every comfort and all privacy of home ... for unless they have friends no one will help them". In his reports, which did not go beyond his family, he criticised adversely not only his medical colleagues but also the nursing staff. In February he commented on the policy of sending out civilian doctors. "Government sending out a set of wretched incapables of civilians - civilians no good - either young and inexperienced or old egotistical fools." He viewed the meddlesome interference in hospital affairs by Lady Stratford with distaste, and despised those who were at her beck and call. "Freeth, the C. of E. chaplain, insists in having the guard present arms to him! Trots after Lady Stratford - to carry her reticule." Watson's letters are full of concern at the illnesses, often fatal, of his medical contemporaries and friends. He frequently refers to his prospects on demobilisation. The advancement of Joseph Lister on the surgical staff of the Edinburgh Infirmary rankled - as a Quaker Lister had stayed at home. Watson applied for an assistant surgeon's post, confiding to his parents - "Should such a thing as an odious comparison have to be made by my friends between Joseph and myself, it is that I am altogether a pupil of the Edinburgh School, that Lister has been in no respect". A month later he was seeking support for an application for the Chair of Military Surgery. He was tempted to resign from the army but, to his credit, did not do so. At the end of January Watson was transferred to Koulali Hospital and his experiences there have been described.[42]

Of the acting assistant-surgeons, Bakewell was one of the few whose opinions were publicised in the home press. In the letter he sent to **The Times** on 22 March (as noted above), he drew attention to the shortage of medical officers in the hospitals which still persisted at the end of the winter.

> The great want is more medical officers. The present staff is dreadfully overworked. Although the number of patients to each officer is not apparently very large, yet, for the serious and extremely complicated nature of the cases, we have more than we can properly attend to. I have between 80 and 90; a friend of mine has 150 ... It is simply impossible to give each case the attention it merits.

Of the sickness rate amongst the doctors he wrote -

> Of fifteen medical officers attached at Kullalie two or three days ago ten were sick, one of whom has since died. All these had caught their illness in the discharge of their duty ... I know of instances where medical officers have risen from a sick bed when so much enfeebled that they could hardly stand, and have dragged themselves to the bedsides of their patients, though themselves as ill as most of those they attended. Soldiers have told me of a Medical Officer dropping down exhausted in the hospital. A few days ago

at Kullalie, in consequence of the great sickness amongst the staff, one officer had for a short period to take charge of four hundred patients. What is the consequence? The mortality rate among the Medical men fearful, and of those who recover many go home with shattered health and enfeebled constitution.

By late March Bakewell was able to give a good report on the hospital food.

The hospital at Scutari is now profusely supplied with all food and luxuries for the sick. I venture to affirm there is no hospital in London in which so many extras are ordered and given. The number of fowls, eggs, jellies etc. used daily would provide a very strong remonstrance from the governors of any civil hospital if ordered by their medical officers. The bread supplied is far better than that which the officers commonly receive, the wine and porter are excellent, the meat is of the best quality the country can afford.[43]

The regimental medical officers in the Crimea at first heard rumours and then confirmation from eye-witnesses that all was not well with the hospitals in Scutari. They were aware that the mortality in the hospital transports was excessive. George Lawson wrote in January - "Vessels crowded with sick and wounded are being sent away daily to Scutari, many are invalided home, but few return again to the Crimea after they have been sent away".[44] Many regimental doctors were reluctant to send their patients to Scutari, since officers and men alike began to regard transfer to the base hospitals almost as a death sentence. While the younger doctors at Scutari clamoured to join the regiments at the front there were some regimental doctors who sought to be moved to the base hospitals, either as a relief from the strain of conditions in the Crimea, or in the hope of gaining wider medical experience. George Lawson learned at the end of December that Forrest, the P.M.O. of his Division, was shortly to go to Scutari to take charge. Lawson had a high opinion of Forrest.

It requires a man of good capabilities to take charge. Had he been there before there would never have been a complaint against the place ... He has kindly promised to have me removed there, but this I am obliged to keep to myself, as it requires some management to be sent down. I shall first get sent down to Scutari with wounded and sick, and he will detain me there and give me, I have asked of him, one of the surgical wards."[45]

But Lawson's hope was not fulfilled. There were no doubt others who tried to get to Scutari, but as the winter progressed few could be spared from regimental duties.

CHAPTER X

MEDICAL CASUALTIES

Nine medical officers died in the Scutari Hospitals between January and March 1855. Of these five were on the hospital staffs, two were transferred from the Crimea, and the details of the two others are uncertain. Assistant-Surgeon Alexander Struthers[46] died on 20 January at Scutari. He had been ill with a fever, thought to be typhoid, and developed a parotid abscess from which a rapidly fatal septicaemia developed. He had been a house surgeon in the Royal Infirmary with Lister before volunteering for war service, having been regarded as "a gifted and accomplished student ... the most distinguished among our university's more recent alumni". He had started work at the Barrack Hospital early in November. Heron Watson, his Edinburgh contemporary and close friend, wrote of Struthers that "he overworked himself trying to do justice to his patients and sitting up until 3 in the morning and rising whenever he was called for (which is not ones duty as there is an orderly officer who ought to do it) ... he had indeed won for himself no ordinary laurels here". Greig, another close friend, wrote to Struthers' brother John, with details of Alexander's last days. "At his death bed there were three of his greatest friends ... and at his funeral there were many more who had learned to appreciate his worth since he came out here ... Miss Nightingale I may state was exceedingly kind to him during his illness and latterly visited him often and did all she could for him." Whether or not Miss Nightingale had known of the the letters from Struthers which had caused such a furore in medical circles at home in December 1854, she showed her invariable compassion for a dying young medical officer.

Staff-Surgeon John Newton[47] died at Scutari on 26 January of fever. He came out to Scutari as a staff-surgeon early in November 1854, and later that month did one passage to the Crimea in the hospital transport 'Medway', before working mainly in the Barrack Hospital. Assistant-Surgeon Edmund Wason[48] died on 7 February at Scutari "of typhoid fever". In an obituary it was said that -

> Dr. Wason was untiring in his attention to the sick in the Barrack Hospital. He was one of several Edinburgh surgeons who earned distinction by the mode in which they discharged their laborious duties. Dr. Wason had but shortly

before watched at the bedside of his fellow-labourer and affected friend Dr. Alexander Struthers, whose lot was soon to become his own. He died of an attack of the same typhoid fever.

Dr. Alibert[49] died on 10 February at Koulali "of fever". Since his name does not appear in the army lists or in the list of civil surgeons, he may have been a local practitioner in Constantinople who volunteered to work in the Scutari hospitals. There is a suggestion that he looked after the Russian wounded in Koulali.

Staff-Surgeon John Marshal[50] died at Koulali Hospital on 10 February "of malignant fever". He appears to have come out to the Crimea as a staff surgeon in November, and he became S.M.O. of the Second Division, but was invalided to Scutari shortly before he died. Assistant-Surgeon John Grabham[51] died on 16 February at Scutari "of malignant fever". His regiment, the 71st had just landed at Balaclava when Grabham took ill and was sent to Scutari. Assistant-Surgeon Frederick Macartney[52] died on 12 February, 1855, at Scutari "of fever". As a staff assistant-surgeon at Scutari, he served in the hospital transport 'Andes' in November on one voyage, and otherwise worked mainly in the Barrack Hospital. Assistant-Surgeon George Stewart[53] is reported to have died in Scutari in February and to have been attached to the 33rd Regiment. Staff-Surgeon Michael Jane[54], who died at Scutari on 7 March, came out as a staff surgeon to Scutari in November 1854.

MISS NIGHTINGALE, THE NURSES, AND THE CHEF

Increased by Miss Stanley's party, there were now some 82 nurses serving in the Scutari hospitals under the management of Miss Nightingale. Allocated to specific surgeons and wards throughout the three main hospitals the ratio of nurses to patients was still poor. Miss Taylor at one point found herself with one other nurse responsible for over a thousand sick. From Miss Taylor's account we learn of the duties required of the heterogeneous collection of Sisters, professional nurses, and ladies. A large part of the nurses' work was in relation to the patients' diet. On the daily ward round the surgeon ordered each patient's diet and the requisition had to be countersigned by a senior medical officer. 'Full diet' consisted daily of 1 lb. of meat, 1 lb. of bread, 1 lb. of potatoes, two pints of tea and half a pint of porter. 'Half diet' was half the latter amount. 'Low diet' was a quarter of the full diet. 'Spoon diet' was 1 lb. of bread and two pints of tea daily. For the ill patient these alternatives were sparse and monotonous. The meat was badly cooked. Those on spoon diet were the special care of the nurses and only this group were allowed extras. The extras varied at the whim of the Purveyor, but Miss Nightingale organised the distribution of additional supplies from the special diet kitchens and the stock she had established. There was often much delay before extras, such as "fowls, mutton chops, milk, arrowroot, rice, sago, and lemons for lemonade", were made available. The nurses were aware of the impurity of the water supply and spent much time boiling small quantities on the stoves in the corridors and wards.

The second task with which the nurses were largely concerned was the supply of clean linen. the laundry arrangements were still inadequate but again Miss Nightingale, from her private store and from **The Times** Fund, was able to make up some deficiencies. Bedding and shirts were often in short supply, and the requisition of such essentials was a complicated business. Miss Taylor alleged that some of the doctors were reluctant to order extra diets or extra linen, as they feared they would be accused of extravagance. She commented that, in January, "it was a common thing to find men with sheets and shirts unchanged for weeks. I have opened the collar of a patient's shirt and found it literally lined with vermin."

In addition the nurses had to exert control over the orderlies, who, particularly at night, often neglected their duties. In time some of the nursing staff succeeded in training individual orderlies. Miss Taylor recorded - "Often when one had a good orderly willing to learn, and had trained him into the way of waiting on the sick, he would be sent for to his regiment, his place supplied by another quite unused to hospital work, and with whom the teaching had to begin all over again". There was not much opportunity for the more professional aspects of nursing. Few of the nurses were allowed to dress wounds. It was some time before they were employed on special duty for the care of a patient in a serious condition, but eventually some medical officers allocated nurses to this task, a great comfort to the sick. In due course nurses on special duty were allowed to stay in the ward over-night. The hours were long and the work tedious and exhausting. After a long day the nurses went out for a walk with one of the ladies in charge, but otherwise there was little recreation, and their quarters were crowded and uncomfortable. It was not surprising that the sickness rate was high and that some died. Miss Taylor describes the rooms allocated to those at Koulali in a house overrun with rats. Discipline sometimes broke down and several of the professional nurses had to be sent home for drunkenness or sexual misbehaviour.[55]

Because of the inadequate numbers, the restricted duties they performed, and the relatively small number who were properly trained, the contribution of the nurses towards the recovery of the patients is difficult to measure. It is perhaps most clear that their presence boosted morale and introduced a more caring and humane attitude toward the sick than had ever before been found in a military hospital. The assiduous care, which could only be exerted on some patients, was appreciated by the men and gave them hope in their terrible situation. To even the roughest soldier, unused to any comfort, the nurses appeared as saints.

In this trying period Miss Nightingale toiled without rest at the formidable tasks she had set herself. With all her administrative duties she continued to find time to visit regularly all the wards of the Barrack and the General Hospital. Frequently she herself undertook the nursing of those most seriously ill, or sat for hours at the bedsides of the dying. Countless letters were written to relatives at home, particularly to comfort the bereaved. She continued to fight for improvements in the conditions which prevailed, stirring the authorities into action, cajoling the senior medical officers, and constantly bombarding Herbert and others in high position with her reports, suggestions and criticisms. The nurses were not easy to handle. The religious factions were a constant trouble to Miss Nightingale and although there were some Sisters of Charity who became her close friends and her most reliable assistants, she had, in general, a poor opinion of their nursing abilities. Only a few of the professional nurses proved efficient.

Although by her appointment she was technically in charge of the nursing staff at Koulali she disclaimed all responsibility for this establishment after she had sent Miss Stanley to take charge. It was recorded by Miss Taylor that Miss Nightingale never visited Koulali during the difficult period of February to March. She had developed a low opinion of Miss Stanley's nursing and administrative abilities, and she confided to Herbert her differences with her former friend.

> I have ... by strict subordination to the authorities, and by avoiding all individual actions, introduced a number of arrangements within the regulations of the service, useful on a large scale but not interesting to individual ladies ... This is not so amusing as pottering and messing about with little cookeries of individual beef teas for the poor sufferers, and my ladies do not like it ... Miss Stanley has taken the opposite tack. She may be able to work it at Koulali, if so God speed her, say I more heartily than anyone. I have done everything in my power to speed her, so help me God - though she does not think so ... Privately and to you, I protest most emphatically now, before it is too late, against the Koulali plan, i.e. the lady plan. It ends in nothing but spiritual flirtation between the ladies and the soldiers ... The ladies all quarrel amongst themselves. The medical men all laugh at their helplessness, but like to have them about for the sake of a little female society, which is natural but not our object.[56]

Miss Nightingale saw her strict control of the nurses eroded and she had not forgiven Herbert for sending out Miss Stanley without her prior approval. Behind all this was her recognition that the Roman Catholic nurses were at least as interested in the spiritual care of their patients as in their physical state, and hence, perhaps, not averse to proselytising. It was this aspect which she feared would be greatly criticised at home and which, if allowed to persist, would ruin her plans and influence. At this time Miss Nightingale's friends in England thought she should be freed of any responsibility for Koulali, believing it was a great worry to her. When Herbert resigned, the new Secretary at War, Lord Panmure, was reluctant to separate Koulali from the other hospitals as far as the nursing organisation was concerned, for fear of giving umbrage to Miss Nightingale. This was somewhat ironic as she had already disclaimed any responsibility. In retrospect it may be thought that Miss Nightingale failed in her duty and had mishandled the situation. It does not seem in character for her to have allowed what she saw very clearly as a defective nursing system to continue, but it must be said that her responsibilities in the Barrack and the General Hospitals were so great that she could not be diverted from her determined efforts to establish her strict discipline at these establishments. Later, however, she had no hesitation in extending her authority to the nursing organisation in the Crimea, which in fact was not, at the time, in her contract.

Miss Nightingale had already seen some improvements effected. In the Barrack Hospital work had begun on a new drainage system, on repaving the corridors and reflooring the wards. She knew that much was still to be done in all the hospitals. She had come to depend more and more on MacGrigor to help in her reforms, although there was still resentment in some quarters that she had been instrumental in the promotion of MacGrigor to the rank of Deputy Inspector-General. Her power in such matters was an excuse for hostility from some senior medical officers. Increasingly Bracebridge aggravated the doctors, and this became a matter of concern to Miss Nightingale. Nevertheless she felt that she was gradually overcoming resistance. The distribution of the numerous gifts which now poured into the hospitals from many sources was largely in her hands but she was tactful enough to give the control of these matters to the doctors, much to the chagrin of the nurses. All the work involved in storing and listing these extra supplies fell on Miss Nightingale and the Bracebridges. She would have preferred gifts of money to spend at her discretion, for many items sent were useless and the consignments of food and drink could in some instances be deleterious.

Although with her extra-diet kitchens she had done much to improve some aspects of the hospital diet, she had not been able to do much towards the establishment of more efficient general kitchens. In these reforms she received unexpected help by the arrival of Alexis Soyer, the former chef of the Reform Club.[57] Soyer arrived at Scutari early in March 1855. Miss Nightingale had not been forewarned of his coming but received him in a friendly manner. He at once became an admirer, close friend, and collaborator. When to her sorrow he died in 1858 she wrote of him - "His death is a great disaster. Others have studied cooking for the purpose of gormandizing, some for show, but none but he for the purpose of cooking large quantities of food in the most nutritious manner for great numbers of men. He has no successor."[58] Soyer, a Frenchman, had learned his culinary art in Paris. He decided to come to London in 1830 and after various posts in the great houses of Britain was appointed chef to the Reform Club in 1841, there to become well-known to politicians, the aristocracy and royalty. A flamboyant character, renowned for his wit, his sartorial elegance, and his knowledge of art, he became a leading figure in society. He wrote widely on diet and cooking. In 1851 he published a book, **The Modern House-wife,** and at the time of the Crimean War it was said, "officers being compelled to cook for themselves, have with the aid of Soyer's **Housewife** and their servants, attained a degree of culinary skill which would astonish their friends at home".[59] Soyer had turned his immense energy to philanthropic activities by establishing soup kitchens for the poor of London. During the Irish Famine he was sent to Dublin to establish soup kitchens there, at the request of the Lord Lieutenant of Ireland. In 1846 he gave lectures to ladies on how to make soup for the "hungry poors", and Miss Nightingale first met him when she attended these classes.[60] In 1851 he resigned from the Reform Club and devoted his time to catering for the elaborate banquets which had become frequent in high society. At the time of the Great Exhibition he did not accept a contract to provide refreshments for the thousands of visitors to the Crystal Palace, instead he established a private restaurant nearby for the rich, in Gore House, and this almost rivalled the Exhibition in its furnishing and originality.

Late in 1854 Soyer became aware of the conditions in the hospitals at Scutari. On 16 January, 1855, a letter appeared in **The Times** from a soldier appealing for Soyer's help.[61] To this Soyer responded.

> After carefully perusing the letter of your correspondent ... I perceive that although the kitchens under the superintendence of Miss Nightingale afford much relief, the system of management at the large one in the Barrack Hospital is far from being perfect. I propose offering my services gratuitously, and proceeding direct to Scutari, at my personal expense, to regulate that important department, if the Government will honour me with their confidence, and grant me full power of acting according to my knowledge and experience in such matters.[62]

Lord Panmure accepted this generous offer. Soyer was aware of the inadequacy of the army cooking stoves and before he set out he designed a portable model for use in camp or hospital, much more efficient and more economical of fuel than the existing types. He left England in February, stopping at Paris to inspect the cooking arrangements in the French military hospitals. He broke his journey at Athens and cooked a dish of eggs over his highly efficient spirit stove set up in the Parthenon. This piece of publicity was duly portrayed in the **Illustrated London News.**[63]

As soon as he arrived at Scutari Soyer inspected the antiquated cooking arrangements. In the Barrack Hospital he found only eight usable copper boilers, which with a few tin pots on braziers had to supply some 2,000 patients with three meals daily. The General Hospital had only five working boilers. The meat was issued in the morning but the patients did not get it until the later afternoon, often overcooked or undercooked. In consequence the wastage was considerable. The joints of meat for each ward were tightly tied together, without removing the bones, and often only the ends were properly cooked. Soyer was horrified that the water in which the meat was boiled was thrown away, so he showed the cooks how to use it for the nutritious soup. He found that the orderlies marked the joints for each ward with any old piece of dirty cloth. All these defects Soyer put right very quickly. For the first time salt and pepper, at his instigation, were supplied to season the food while cooking it. Prior to Soyer's visit the cooks were changed frequently and none became efficient; he appointed a sergeant as a permanent overseer. The copper boilers were renovated, ovens were built, and the whole kitchen was replanned. Not least Soyer greatly improved the method of making tea. Previously it was brewed in a copper just emptied of soup. He invented his "Scutari teapot", a large kettle in which there was a filter to hold the tea, a great improvement on a dirty tea-bag. Similar reforms were urgently needed in the General and the Koulali Hospitals and Soyer initiated these as soon as he had dealt with the kitchen at the Barrack Hospital, which he had officially opened in the presence of many eminent medical men and senior army doctors from the Allies. So popular had Soyer become that when he passed through the corridors of the hospital he was cheered by the soldiers. To complete everything a supply of his new stoves arrived, although this was not until late in April.

Having completed his task at Scutari in record time, Soyer later accompanied Miss Nightingale to the Crimea. There he brought order to the cooking arrangements in the hospitals at Balaclava and in the camps, and he stayed in the East until some months after the fall of Sebastopol. He continued to supervise the kitchens in the Scutari hospitals, to instruct the army cooks, and to ensure that the soldiers' rations in the Crimea were well planned. Soyer achieved all this because of his great energy, enthusiasm and personality. There is no hint that the medical officers viewed his reforms unfavourably. It may well be that they were more ready to accept advice from a man, rather than from Miss Nightingale. They knew also that Soyer had been sent out officially and was well known to so many people of influence at home.

When Soyer returned to England in May 1857 (he had broken his journey for a long tour of Europe), he was publicly thanked by Lord Panmure and he had become even more of a celebrity than before. Innumerable banquets were given throughout the country in his honour. The soldiers had been in no doubt concerning the benefits he had brought to them, particularly in the hospitals. He had been loaded with gifts, from the Sultan of Turkey, the British Ambassador in Constantinople and many others, and he had received glowing testimonials from the generals and the medical officers of the Allied Armies. The influence of Soyer on the morale and health of the Army, whether in the Crimea or at Scutari, is incalculable. Cantlie dismisses his achievement in a few lines, but Soyer's rapid and total reform of the cooking arrangements and of the soldiers' diet brought great changes for the better. In previous chapters it has been constantly reiterated that bad cooking and a monotonous, deficient diet were major factors influencing the spread of certain diseases, in lowering the resistance to all conditions, in reducing the stamina and, not least, in lowering the morale of the soldier. If Soyer can scarcely be ranked with Miss Nightingale for his contribution to the welfare of the

SCUTARI HOSPITALS (II)

British soldier, nevertheless the part he played in reforming this particular deficiency in the army organisation should not be forgotten or under-estimated.

NOTES

1. **Med. Surg. Hist.**, 2: after p.480, "General Hospital Returns, I, Hospitals in the Bosphorous".
2. **Med. Surg. Hist.**, 2:468-471, "Return of Vessels which arrived at Scutari".
3. **Cantlie**, 2:128. The 'Compound' was probably temporary accommodation.
4. Ibid., 2:147.
5. **Royal Commission**, 362-370.
6. The various diseases have been discussed in Chapter IX; the source of the statistics is as in note 1 above.
7. Robert Bakewell (1832-?1902); M.R.C.S., L.S.A. 1854; joined as acting assistant-surgeon January 1855; served in the East March - August 1855; dismissed August 1855; M.D. St. Andrews 1856; M.O.H. Trinidad 1868; in New Zealand after 1873. See Chapter XIII for Bakewell's dismissal. After the war Bakewell bombarded the medical journals with material, often controversial.
8. R.H. Bakewell, 'Notes on the diseases most commonly treated at the Scutari Hospitals', **M.T.G.** (1855), 2:441-442.
9. S. Terrot, **Reminiscences of Scutari Hospitals** (London, 1898), 117.
10. Ibid., 91-92.
11. G.P. Smith, 'On Military Medical Practice in the East', **Lancet**, (1855), 2:582.
12. Although there were no serious epidemics of cholera during this period this very low figure is surprising and may be inaccurate.
13. The source of the statistics as note 1 above.
14. **M.T.G.** (1855), 1:395-396.
15. **The Times**, 9.3.1855.
16. 'Heron Watson Letters'.
17. 'A Lady Volunteer', **Eastern Hospitals and English Nurses** (London, 1857). The author was Miss Fanny Taylor, one of Miss Stanley's party of nurses, who worked at Koulali Hospital.
18. Nicholas O'Connor (1815-1856); M.B. Dublin 1834; joined as assistant-surgeon 1839; surgeon 1847; served in the East from October 1854 until death (**Drew**). For O'Connor, see also note 50 to Chapter XVII.
19. 'W. Temple' appears in a list of civil surgeons (in **Med. Surg. Hist.**, 1:524-525) as having served at Scutari in November and December 1854, but Koulali was not opened until January 1855. It is uncertain whether this is the right man.
20. 'Hall/Menzies Letters', 21.12.1854.
21. 'Hall/Forrest Letters', 4.1.1855.
22. Ibid., 23.1.1855.
23. **Ass.Med.J.** (1855), 497.
24. Ibid.
25. John McIlree (1812-1894); joined as assistant-surgeon 1835; surgeon October 1854; served in the East November 1854 - July 1856; retired 1876 as I.G. (**Drew**).
26. For O'Connor, see note 18 above.
27. John Summers (1818-1893); M.D. Edinburgh 1839; joined as assistant-surgeon 1840; surgeon 1853; served in the East November 1854 -December 1855; retired in 1871 as I.G. (**Drew**).
28. For Newton, see note 47 below.

CHAPTER X

29. Quoted in **M.T.G.** (1855), 1:151.
30. **Cantlie**, 2:167.
31. C. Woodham-Smith, **Florence Nightingale, 1820-1910** (London, 1950), 212.
32. **Cantlie**, 2:11.
33. I.B. O'Malley, **Florence Nightingale 1820-1856** (London, 1931), 268.
34. Lord Stanmore, **Sidney Herbert, Lord Herbert of Lea: a memoir** (2 vols., London, 1906), 1:361.
35. **Cantlie**, 2:102.
36. Ibid., 129.
37. **M.T.G.** (1855), 1:75.
38. Anon., **Two months in and about the camp before Sebastopol** (London, 1855), 135-145.
39. - MacNamara, **A trip to the trenches** (London, 1855), 74-77.
40. **Lancet** (1855), 2:510.
41. 'Hall/Cumming Letters', 17.3.1855.
42. 'Heron Watson Letters'.
43. **M.T.G.** (1855), 1:395-396.
44. V. Bonham-Carter, ed., **Surgeon in the Crimea: the experiences of George Lawson described in letters to his family 1854-1855** (London, 1968), 152.
45. Ibid., 112.
46. Alexander Struthers (1830-1855); L.R.C.S.Ed., M.D. Edinburgh 1850; joined as acting assistant-surgeon October 1854; served in the East from October 1854 until death; buried at Scutari (obituaries **M.T.G.** (1855), 1:173; **Monthly J.Med.Sc.** (1855), 1:226). For his death, see also 'Heron Watson Letters' and 'Greig Letters', January, 1855.
47. John Newton (1813-1855); joined as assistant-surgeon 1839; surgeon November 1854; served in the East from November 1854 until death (**Drew**).
48. Edmund Wason (1830-1855); M.D. Edinburgh 1854; joined as assistant-surgeon November 1854; served in the East November 1854 until death; buried at Scutari (obituary **M.T.G.** (1855), 1:223; **Drew**).
49. Alibert's name does not appear on any official list. Referred to as Polish in S. Osborne, **Scutari and its hospitals** (London, 1855), 21.
50. John Marshall (1809-1855); joined as assistant-surgeon 1833; surgeon 1842; served in the East from November 1854 until death (**Drew**).
51. John Grabham (1831-1855); joined as assistant-surgeon November 1854; served in the East January 1855 until death; buried at Scutari (**Drew**).
52. Frederick Macartney (1831-1855); joined as assistant-surgeon November 1854; served in the East November 1854 until death; buried at Scutari (**Drew**).
53. Probably acting assistant-surgeon. Stewart is not in any official list, but his death was noticed in **M.T.G.** (1855), 1:464, and **Medical Directory**, 1856.
54. Michael Jane (1821-1855); joined as assistant-surgeon 1847; surgeon February 1855; served in the East 1854 until death (**Drew**).
55. For Miss Taylor's account, see note 17 above.
56. Woodham-Smith, **Nightingale**, 193-194.
57. A. Soyer, **Soyer's culinary campaign - with the plan of the art of cooking** (London, 1857); H. Morris, **Portrait of a Chef: the life of Alexis Soyer** (Cambridge, 1938).
58. E. Cook, **The life of Florence Nightingale** (2 vols., London, 1913), 1:582.
59. Morris, **Soyer**, 87.
60. O'Malley, **Nightingale**, 129.
61. **The Times**, 16.1.1855.
62. Morris, **Soyer**, 130.
63. **Illustrated London News**, 7.4.1855, with an illustration.

CHAPTER XI

COMMISSIONS AND COMMITTEES (1854-1855)

Any historian of the Crimean doctors must sympathise with the cri-de-coeur of Sir Edward Cook, the biographer of Florence Nightingale.

> Royal Commissions ... when they had finished sitting on the hospitals, began sitting on each other. Enormous piles of Blue-books were accumulated, and in the course of my work I have disturbed much dust upon them. The conduct of every individual concerned was the subject of charge, answer, and countercharge innumerable. Each generation deserves, no doubt, the records of mal-administration which it gets: but one generation need not be punished by having to examine in detail the records of another.[1]

In this chapter four Commissions and one Select Committee are studied, all of which were initiated between November 1854 and April 1855. The Commissions were the First (or Newcastle) Commission, the Sanitary Commission, the Supplies Commission, and the Pathological Commission. The Select Committee was the Roebuck (or Sebastopol) Committee. The evidence to the latter Committee was published during its proceedings (and is here quoted from the **Medical Times and Gazette**): the reports of the four Commissions appeared at varying intervals after the completion of investigations.

The evidence presented to these different bodies was from a wide range of individuals. While that given by the doctors is of great interest and often very informative, the statements of non-medical army officers of all ranks, of civilians of different occupations, and of politicians are also relevant, particularly in respect of their attitudes towards the medical service. In one category is the Committee, often politically motivated and intent on placing blame for mismanagement. In another category are the Commissions - since these during the war went out to the East, to investigate, to make suggestions for improvements, and, in some cases, even to initiate urgent reforms without reference to the home authorities. The reports of all these bodies deserve some attention, for their evidence allows us to re-assess some of the more virulent criticisms of the medical service which had appeared, and continued to appear, in the contemporary press.

THE FIRST COMMISSION

The first of the Commissions was initiated by the Director-General in November 1854. Smith stated in March 1855 -

> When the reports got so current in the newspapers, I felt so astonished at what was there stated that I thought it was desirable to send out a Commission for the purpose of ascertaining how far the assertions in the newspapers were well founded. I asked the sanction of the Duke of Newcastle to do it: he agreed to it and I selected Mr. Cumming from his long experience in the service, and his known integrity of character: I also selected my own professional assistant (Dr. Thomas Spence) in whom I could place every reliance, to tell me the truth, whether it was advantageous to my cause, or disadvantageous to my cause, and along with them was associated Mr. Maxwell, a Barrister, who was able to sift the evidence.

This determination of Smith to discover why things were going wrong shows a responsible attitude. But soon the organisation was taken out of his hands.

> It appeared to the authorities better that the Commission should be purely a Government Commission, independently of the Department altogether: the powers were taken from me by the Duke of Newcastle.[2]

In consequence the Commission reported to the War Office and Smith was not even sent the preliminary report when it was completed in March 1855. The terms of reference of the Commission were to enquire into the condition and wants of the sick and wounded officers and soldiers, the state and condition of the hospital accommodation in Scutari and the Crimea, the state of medical and other hospital staffing, and the adequacy of medical stores, medicines, and comforts for the sick. The Commission was asked to suggest necessary reforms in all these matters.

The two doctors on the Commission reached Scutari in the second week of November 1854. While awaiting Maxwell's arrival Spence went on to Balaclava, where he was drowned during the storm of 14 November. His place was taken by Staff Surgeon Patrick Laing.[3] With considerable energy the Commissioners collected information from many sources, by interviews, by the issue of questionnaires seeking written replies, and by their own observations. Their report, in four sections, and finally printed in June 1855, presented their results, "following the career of the sick or wounded man step by step from the moment that sickness supervenes, or the wound is received, until he leaves our great military hospitals".[4]

The first section concerned the transport of sick and wounded and the medical supplies "on a march or on the field of battle". Comment was made particularly on the shortage of light ambulances, on the incompetence of the aged pensioners in the ambulance corps, and on the need for transport vehicles for medical stores. The second section concerned the conditions in the Crimean hospitals, their staffing, and the supplies of medicine and medical comforts in the field. The Commissioners criticised the regimental hospitals, finding the bell-tents unheated and bedding in short supply. The Balaclava hospital was reported overcrowded. They interviewed Hall and other senior medical officers, the regimental commanders, some regimental medical officers, and some of the sick or wounded. But much of their evidence was derived from a questionnaire circulated, despite an amount of opposition from army officers, to the surgeons of all the regiments in the field. Some doctors were reluctant to criticise or complain, no doubt anxious to avoid giving offence to their commanding officers, but most answered frankly and often made useful suggestions. Assistant-Surgeon Charles White[5] wrote on his form - "As to making any suggestions my being so junior in the Service would render it an act of presumption on my part"; whereas Surgeon Robert Cooper[6] wrote - "I shall not abstain from expressing myself with the utmost degree of candour ... regardless of the consequences".

From a survey of some 40 answers sent in during December 1854 and January 1855, it is clear that at this period many regiments were short of medical officers. In several instances an assistant-surgeon was on his own in charge of a regiment. Surprisingly, all the doctors were satisfied with the orderlies, perhaps because once a soldier was given this task and had proved efficient the commanding officer allowed him to continue in it. All complained of the inadequate bell-tents, of the delay before marquees were provided, and of the deficiencies of bedding and heating. There was little complaint of scarcity of medicines (although the Commission reported a shortage of opium preparations), or of surgical instruments. The standards of cooking, cooking utensils, and the quality of the diet were condemned. The lack of suitable transport for the sick or for medical stores was invariably criticised. Some doctors advanced their criticisms in a forceful manner.

A few staff medical officers were interviewed and one of them, Alexander, sent a long letter to the Commissioners on 15 January, 1855. He affirmed that when his regiments embarked for Varna, the P.M.O. of the Division refused to issue extra stores although large reserves were available. He complained of the shortage of medicines in Bulgaria and that at the landing in the Crimea he was not able to get extra supplies of drugs or equipment. He condemned the lack of transport for the wounded after the battle of the Alma. Of the conditions in the Crimea he wrote -

> The misery and wretchedness of the troops here, but more particularly the sick, are scarcely credible, and require to be seen to be believed - poor sick wretches lying on the ground, with some miserable blankets, in tents that let in rain as if they were sieves, and with no fuel except the miserable brushwood and roots that could be gathered for cooking ... great misery has also been caused from the want of transport for the sick ... I think the Board will perceive that much blame is due somewhere for all the wretchedness and misery that has taken place during the present campaign, and which, in my opinion, could have been so easily prevented.

The evidence given by the regimental surgeons leaves one in no doubt that the majority were caring and compassionate men, deeply concerned with the conditions which prevented them from treating their patients adequately.

On 18 January, Hall made a long statement to the Commissioners. Not surprisingly he found it necessary to defend his own actions. He believed that the medical staffing was adequate, "sufficient for the ordinary purposes, but the present state of things is exceptional". He had recognised that throughout the campaign there had been serious shortages of medical stores but once more complained that he had received no advance notice of embarcation of the army for the Crimea. He gave a rather complacent account of the treatment and evacuation of the wounded after the Alma. "To the best of my knowledge no wounded man was put on board till his wound was dressed." He agreed that medical transport had been deficient but pointed out that he had not been given sufficient of the type of ambulances and wagons he had requested. Other shortages Hall blamed squarely on the purveyors, whether of medicines, medical comforts, tents, or marquees. He told the Commissioners of his difficulties in getting the hospital tents replaced by huts.

The commanding officers of the regiments in the Crimea were sent the same questionnaire as that sent to the doctors. Only 22 replied, usually briefly, because they knew few details of the medical organisation. Some merely approved and countersigned the surgeon's reports. In one case, the 95th Regiment, only the commanding officer sent in a reply, and he did not even give the names of his medical staff. Lieutenant-Colonel West of the 21st Fusiliers began by opiniating that "the miseries endured by our sick I consider to be the usual concomitants of any great enterprise such as we undertake", but he went on to say that "the utter helplessness of our medical department, their total inability to meet the pressing emergencies as they arose, became conspicuously manifest". He blamed the Commissariat for most of the troubles. A few officers made useful comments. Colonel Adams of the 27th Regiment attributed the high sickness rate to "excess of duty", to salt provisions, and to shortages of bedding and clothing. Colonel Walker of the Scots Fusiliers tried to help his regimental surgeon. He had produced for the regimental hospital a discarded pork barrel to serve as an operating table. "I consider something light and portable might be added to the medical chest affording less discomfort to the unhappy victim to be operated on than a pork barrel tub."

A few soldiers described their experiences when sick and wounded. One who suffered a severe shoulder injury complained that he had his arm taken off without chloroform while in the sitting position. But he had survived. Many complained of the uncomfortable journeys to the transports in jolting bullock carts, or in one case, "in an araba drawn by dromedaries". They complained of lack of food, overcrowding, and a shortage of doctors in the hospital transports.

The Commission produced many useful recommendations as a result of this part of their investigation. They recommended that large reserves of medicines and medical comforts should be held at divisional headquarters, sufficient for three months, and that the stores in the regimental hospitals should always be sufficient for two weeks. They considered that the regimental surgeon should be allowed to requisition stores without the approval of the divisional medical officer. They advised that all the men should be inspected daily by the regimental surgeon for the early detection of disease, particularly the effects of frost-bite. However, although they had observed the filthy state of many of the camps they made few comments on the need to improve general standards of hygiene.

The third section of the report concerned the transport of the sick and wounded from Balaclava to Scutari. A questionnaire dealing with such matters as the size of the vessels, the accommodation, the ventilation, the provision of cots and bedding, the water supply, the diet and the cooking, the supplies of medicine and surgical equipment, and the staffing with doctors and orderlies, was sent to a large number of the army medical officers who had served in the transports between October 1854, and January 1855. Deputy-Inspector-General Lawson reported on one voyage he had made in the 'Niagara', and Staff-Surgeon Laing, of the Commission, did a single trip in the 'Cleopatra'. Lawson's report was favourable, but Laing was highly critical of the exhausted state of the patients when they arrived at Balaclava to be transferred to the ships, and of the deficient ventilation in the 'Cleopatra'. The more junior medical officers in some instances were not unduly critical, but most did report shortages of medical staff and orderlies, food, water, medicines and bedding. The Commissioners condemned in particular the unsuitability of the vessels, the overcrowding, the shortage of doctors and orderlies, and the deplorable organisation of both the embarcation and disembarcation of the patients.

The fourth section of the report dealt with the Scutari hospitals. Evidence was sought first from the purveyors Wreford and Ward on the requisition and supply system.

Maxwell was later to report that even after three months of inquiry he still did not know who was responsible for the purveying! Medical officers of all ranks were interviewed. Questioned on various problems, Menzies affirmed that he had asked for numerous improvements in the hospitals but stated that these were not carried out because of shortages of materials and labour. He admitted that he was short of medical staff and orderlies, but claimed that he was never short of medicines, dressings or medical comforts. McGrigor complained of shortages of linen and of difficulty in keeping the Barrack Hospital clean.

Miss Nightingale was first interviewed on 23 December. She gave details of the duties allocated to her nurses, stressing that they were never sent to the wards without there being a request for them from the medical officers. She described how she distributed extras. The Commissioners seemed unduly interested in the amount of port wine given to the patients. Miss Nightingale agreed that some of the men received excessive amounts of spirits or wine and that, not infrequently, the orderlies stole the surplus and became intoxicated. She denied any gross shortage of medical extras but complained of the difficulties of requisition from the purveyor. Of the food supply she said - "We have always had plenty of sugar, rice and biscuits from the Commissariat, and with the exception of about six days, an abundant supply of fresh meat. The quality of the meat, however, has been very frequently inferior." Her statements seem to have been limited by the questions put to her. She refrained from adverse criticism of the medical officers. Whether or not she had the opportunity of expressing her opinions to the Commissioners in private is unknown. It may be suspected that she did not believe that this Commission would have much influence at home. As two of the three members were regular army officers she may have felt that their report would be biassed. She had another opportunity of giving evidence, on 20 February, and described, at some length, the difficulties in establishing an adequate laundry service.

The Commissioners gave a very full report on the Scutari hospitals and this has already been quoted in Chapter VI.

They commented on the unsuitability of soldiers as hospital stewards, ward masters, or orderlies. These posts, in their opinion, should be filled by educated and specially trained personnel, "independent of military power" (and so unlikely to be taken out of their posts at short notice). They advised an increase in the number of medical staff at all levels, and recommended that the doctors should be relieved of excessive administrative duties. They considered that the purveyor's duties were "too numerous and heterogeneous to be performed by one person, and that they might be conveniently distributed". A firm recommendation was made that many of the purveyor's duties should be transferred to the Commissariat, as in the French hospitals.

The Commission finished its task in March. Its work received little publicity. It appears that a preliminary report was sent to the Minister of War very quickly, but little comment was made in parliament about the findings. The medical journals made no mention of the work of the Commission. It cannot be said that the First Commission achieved much. Unfortunately it had no authority to implement reforms, but only to make recommendations. However, one reason why this mission had relatively little influence is that, before its completion, the Sanitary Commission had arrived in the East, armed with much wider powers. In January 1855, John Roebuck, M.P., moved for the establishment of a Parliamentary Committee to enquire into the condition of the Army before Sebastopol. Once established, the Roebuck Committee started its work quickly and its findings were widely publicised, this completely overshadowing the work of the First Commission. On the credit side it must be said that the assiduous enquiries of the First Commission, giving the doctors the opportunity to express their opinions, must have helped them to realise that they were not completely forgotten or neglected. It may also be conjectured that the preliminary draft of the report was seen by many members of the Government and it must have brought home to them the true state of affairs both in the Crimea and in Scutari. It was not until June that the final report of the First Commission, "presented to both Houses of Parliament", was printed.

THE ROEBUCK COMMITTEE

On 26 January, 1855, John Roebuck, a barrister and Independent member for Sheffield, who had served for many years in the House of Commons, moved - "That a Select Committee be appointed to enquire into the condition of our Army before Sevastopol and into the conduct of those Departments of Government whose duty it has been to minister to the Wants of the Army".[7] The motion was approved and this resulted in the fall of Lord Aberdeen's government. The terms of reference could be widely interpreted but it was clear that much of the enquiry would be directed towards the medical services. Without delay a Committee of eleven Members of Parliament was appointed under the chairmanship of Roebuck, who had "appointed himself to the office of public accuser".[8] The ten other Members of Parliament selected included five notable individuals.[9] Sir John Pakington and Edward Ellice had both held Cabinet rank in previous years; General Peel and Colonel Lindsay were both senior army officers; Austen Layard, a close friend of Lord Stratford de Redcliffe, was a distinguished traveller in the East. In view of the medical aspects of the investigation it might have been appropriate to have included a medical Member of Parliament, but this was not done.[10] It was the opinion of Kinglake that the Committee "comprised a good number of wise, sober and painstaking men and, if the Chairman was indeed the accuser ... there were other members to make the tribunal work justly in a patient search after truth".[11] Yet there were misgivings in some quarters as to the desirability of creating such a committee. Kinglake noted that some observers feared

> that the inquest perhaps might result in fierce, passionate demonstrations and vindictive impeachments more likely to generate distracting troubles at home than to enlighten our Government in its task of conducting the war.[12]

It is against this political background that the conduct and findings of the Roebuck Committee must be seen and assessed.

The Roebuck Committee (often referred to as the Sebastopol Committee) began to take evidence on 5 March and continued its work for two months, in all 61 witnesses being called. No member of the Committee was sent abroad and no individual was recalled from the Crimea to give evidence. In consequence the choice of appropriate witnesses was restricted. As far as the services were concerned, witnesses who had been actively involved in the campaign were limited to those who happened to be in England in March or April. These were usually individuals who had been invalided home, who had resigned, or who had been relieved of their posts. Those who had been invalided but still held commissions were all too likely to be guarded in their statements, appreciating that any criticisms might jeopardise their future careers. Those who had resigned or had returned home disgraced were likely to have personal grievances.

Six high-ranking executive officers, all of whom had held important commands in the Crimea, together with three high-ranking home officers, appeared before the Committee. Ten army executive officers between the ranks of captain and lieutenant-colonel were examined, most of whom had served in regiments in the Crimea and been invalided. Only one "other rank" was interviewed, Sergeant Thomas Dawson. Of the army medical officers, the most important witness was Smith, the Director-General. But in addition Menzies, Forrest, and Dumbreck were called, all of whom had been invalided and doubtless were concerned about their future appointments and promotion. Staff-Surgeon Henry Mapleton[13] and one junior officer, Assistant-Surgeon Flower, were interviewed. Four naval officers were questioned but no naval medical officer gave evidence. Six merchant navy officers who had captained hospital transports, and one medical officer, James Vaux, who had served in a transport, were also called.

Belatedly, certain past or present members of the Cabinet were interviewed, as were certain senior civil servants such as the Controller of Victualling and Sea Transport. The Members of Parliament who gave evidence included Dundas, Stafford and Percy, all of whom had visited Scutari, as well as Layard, the Committee member, who had been with the army when it landed in Eupatoria and had remained in close contact with Raglan, as a political adviser, for about three months. Finally, but significantly, the Committee interviewed, as independent witnesses, the Reverend Sidney Osborne, Macdonald of **'The Times** Fund', Maxwell, who had served in the First Commission, and an Army chaplain, the Reverend George Parker. More medical witnesses might have been called with advantage, as for example Dr. Pyemont Smith, the civilian doctor who had returned to England. In fact Osborne, during his examination, mentioned Smith and expressed the hope that the Committee would call him.

There was more than a hint that the members of the Committee were looking for scapegoats. This comes out particularly in the intensive questioning of Smith, the Medical Director-General. During his prolonged interview he was often baited by some members, personal innuendos were frequent, and attempts were made to trap him into admissions detrimental to his reputation.

The enquiry covered a wide range of subjects but it is sufficient to refer to evidence and comments relating to the medical services.[14] The high ranking officers who had served in the Crimea were questioned mainly on matters of strategy and general policy rather than on medical subjects. The Duke of Cambridge[15], who had been in command of the First Division from June 1854, had paid a brief visit to the Scutari hospitals - he was one of the few high-ranking officers to visit Scutari in the winter of 1854/1855 - and was taken round by Miss Nightingale. He recorded in his diary - "I am very well satisfied with all that I saw there, and think they really have done as much as they possibly could to make it comfortable".[16] In his evidence the Duke suggested that the high mortality rate of the Guards in Bulgaria was due to the fact that they had not been given their accustomed ration of porter! He described the medical men as very efficient. He did not seem to know much about the conditions in which the sick were treated. "The men in the hospital tents were not very comfortable but as comfortable as they could be under the circumstances." Lord Cardigan, who had commanded the Light Brigade[17], reported that his men had received fresh meat regularly. He recognised that conditions in the hospital tents were bad, but otherwise made little comment regarding the medical services. Lord Lucan, former Commanding

Officer of the Cavalry, Division, appeared more concerned about his horses than his men. It was reported that "his evidence had reference chiefly to the inefficient manner in which the horses were provided with food and necessaries, and to the damage they received in carrying baggage".[18] Major-General Bentinck, who had served under the Duke of Cambridge, when asked about the choice of camping grounds indicated that it was not customary to take the advice of a medical man in selecting a camp site.[19] Lieutenant-General Lacey-Evans, who had been in command of the Second Division, said of the regimental hospitals - "With regard to the hospital tents they were pretty well calculated for the reception of the sick and wounded. There were 18 to 20 persons in them; but still a deal of fresh air was admitted .... there was an advantage in the fresh air.".[20] His ideas on sanitation in the camps were revealing,

> The sanitary condition of the army is the business of the general commanding and staff officers. He did not think it necessary to have subordinate sanitary officers. If the officer in command saw anything wrong or if he had any doubt with regard to sanitary measures he might consult the staff medical officers.

Lieutenant-General Burgoyne, chief Engineer adviser to Raglan[21], was questioned about the failure to make a good road up to the camps from Balaclava, a failure which had had such serious repercussions on the transport of medical supplies and the evacuation of the sick and wounded.

The junior army officers were likely to be better informed about the conditions in the regimental camps than were the generals, but they were often cautious of appearing to criticise their senior officers, for fear of adverse effects on their chances of promotion. In most cases they gave confirmation of the inadequate clothing of the soldiers, of the poor diet and primitive cooking arrangements, of the discomforts in the regimental hospitals, and of the difficulty of getting medical supplies. In some respects they seemed to understate the hardships. Captain Blakeley, an officer on half-pay who "went out to the army at the start to offer his services" and had no official attachment, was more frank than some - "the troops were wretchedly clothed and looked half-starved".[22] The single N.C.O. interviewed, Sergeant

Thomas Dawson of the Grenadier Guards, described how the men were grossly overcrowded, and when on duty in the trenches seldom had a full night's sleep.[23] Apart from the green coffee beans he had no complaint about the diet. He confirmed the ragged and dirty state of the clothing and stated that many men had no soles to their shoes. He was full of praise for the doctors, both in the Crimea and at Scutari.

Smith, the Director-General, was faced with an exhausting interrogation which lasted for more than three days.[24] He stood up to this with great credit and was seldom at a loss to answer the loaded questions which were relentlessly directed at him. He reminded the Committee that he had taken over his present post in 1851 at a salary much lower than that of his predecessor McGrigor.

> His duties had become very onerous occupying him in war time fourteen hours a day. From 1851 he had one assistant, Dr. Spence, and two clerks ... In regard to the purveyors of stores, or of medicines ... he was subject to the directions of the Commander-in-Chief, of the Master-General of Ordnance, of the civil authority of the Board of Ordnance, of the Secretary of War, and he hardly knew how much more ... the Department had no power of acting by itself ... he had often to consider for some time what authority to address: and he had often been told when he had addressed the Commander-in-Chief that he ought not to have addressed him. If he had been placed under the direction of the Minister of War and had only one authority to consult and advise with, and whose orders he was to follow, he would have been able to execute his duties with more satisfaction to himself, and much more efficiency to the public service, and half the labour ... If there had been one single power, the public would have known upon whose shoulders to place the failure of any arrangement with respect to the medical wants of the army.

These statements on the divided and confused control of the Medical Department were utterly convincing. Smith was questioned in great detail on the control of army hospitals. He accepted responsibility for the hospitals in the United Kingdom.

> Of hospitals abroad he could not have the same superintendence and direction, because he did not know their exact local conditions. He said that he could not interfere with the proceedings and the arrangements of the hospital medical officers except by giving advice.

This statement had relevance to his answers later in view of his apparent lack of knowledge of the state of the Scutari hospitals. He was also asked about the role of the Purveyor's department in hospitals. He could not exactly describe his position in reference to the Purveyor but considered the War Office, which was responsible for spending, held ten times more authority over this department than he did.

The Director-General was further questioned at length on his preparations for the campaign. He complained of the very short notice he had been given and the uncertainty of the future movements of the army of observation. He described in detail his arrangements for the transmission of lavish medical stores, his deployment of the medical staff, and his immediate recognition that he would require to make provision for an army much larger than the original 10,000 strong. He enlarged on his precaution of sending three senior medical officers in advance to investigate the climate and medical conditions in the countries likely to be occupied. Questioned in detail about the original establishment of the Scutari hospitals Smith indicated he had little to do with this, that the authorities at home knew nothing of the local circumstances, and that arrangements were left to the senior medical officers and the Commander in Turkey, with the help of Calvert the British Consul. He was aware of the poor state of the Barrack Hospital in the summer of 1854 by letters from Menzies and others, but firmly believed that Lord Stratford had been given authority to finance and otherwise help to improve conditions. When he learnt from press reports and other sources that there were grave shortages in the hospitals he was unable to understand this in view of the lavish supplies he had sent out to the East. In retrospect the only way he could account for the alleged shortages was that it had not been possible to transfer from Varna the large residue of medical stores which had accumulated there.

There were long sessions on the lack of satisfactory ambulances and of an efficient ambulance corps. Smith was able to prove that he had done his best to organise these necessities, having sent numerous suggestions and plans to the War Office, as early as April 1854. Equally he defended himself from the charge that he had made no adequate arrangements for sea transport of the sick and wounded, quoting the letter he had written in May 1854 anticipating the need for well-equipped hospital ships.

Smith was able to produce evidence that he had anticipated most problems. For example the need for winter clothing had been clear to him. He had not only made strong pleas to the War Office to provide this but on his own initiative, in the summer of 1854, had organised its manufacture and delivery.

Smith was strongly criticised for failing to check that the supplies he had sent out had arrived at the right destination. He argued that this was scarcely his responsibility once he was assured that they had been taken on board the ships in England. He had, however, made such enquiries as he could through private channels. The Committee also seemed determined to show that Smith had failed in his duty over the hospitals in Scutari. To the question, "You do not consider yourself the chief authority in this country on such arrangements as the Commander-in-Chief might think necessary for the establishment of hospitals at Constantinople?", he replied, "Not at all. I felt I had nothing to do with them, they ought to be entrusted to local authorities and I should have caused confusion if I had interfered". This was a realistic outlook, taking into account the slowness of communications between Scutari and London.

Throughout the whole proceedings Smith was always loyal to his medical officers, never missing an opportunity of praising them for their courage and devotion to duty. He cast no aspersions on those in charge in the East such as Hall and Menzies, although he might have been tempted to criticise them for failing to keep him well informed of the situation in the Scutari hospitals.

Other Army medical officers were questioned. Like Smith, Menzies also had to endure a prolonged examination. Some of his evidence has been quoted in Chapter VI.[25] He was questioned closely about the statements he had made indicating that there were no shortages of essential medical stores or equipment. He blamed the Purveyor for the bad distribution of stores, but rather condemned himself when he added - "whether the supplies are made or not, and in various points, I have no information". He tried to show that he had done his best to have the defects in the hospitals corrected, and complained that little notice had been taken of his suggestions. He pleaded overwork. "His duties were so onerous, and so much of his time taken up in routine business, and in corresponding with the head of departments in the Crimea and at home, that he was unable to visit the hospitals daily." To some questions Menzies made halting replies and he did not create a good impression on the Committee. Forrest was questioned on his brief tenure as P.M.O. at Scutari.[26] He said that "he had found an abundance of medical stores, medical comforts, and medicines, with the exception of opium ... when he came away the hospital was going on very satisfactorily". Some of Dumbreck's evidence has already been recorded (Chapter VI).[27] He was questioned about the hospital at Varna. He had not chosen the site and he agreed that the building was unsuitable for its purpose. When asked about conditions in the Crimea in October he said that "he saw no wants that were not supplied". Surprisingly, "he never had had any direct evidence that green coffee was used", a subject about which the Committee felt very strongly.

Staff-Surgeon Mapleton had served as private physician to Lord Raglan from April 1854.[28] Although most likely stationed at the Commander-in-Chief's headquarters, he must have had opportunities of visiting the regimental camps in the Crimea and of communicating his observations to Raglan. When he was questioned on various subjects by the Committee he came out with some rather strange opinions. He was alone among all the medical officers in suggesting that the uncomfortable stock should be retained by the soldier. He recommended the somewhat unpractical idea that all sick and wounded should be sent home to England from the Crimea as soon as possible, without being admitted to hospital in Balaclava or Scutari. (He regarded all hospitals on foreign soil as dangerous to life!). With such ideas Mapleton was perhaps not the best person to have had the ear of Raglan on medical matters. Assistant-Surgeon Flower does not seem to have had much opportunity to express his views.[29] He was questioned mainly about his own experiences when sent to Scutari because of the effects of frost-bite. He took passage in the 'Victoria' and described how the sick were laid on the bare decks and how they were on board for eleven days.

The six merchant navy captains gave evidence of the use of their ships as hospital transports. Captain Morriş of the 'Andes' described how he was sent to pick up the wounded after the Alma with the ship quite unprepared for this purpose. James Vaux had served as surgeon to the transport 'Harbinger', which was used as a hospital transport.[30] Vaux considered that the ship was grossly overcrowded and reported that the sick had had to use the damp and dirty bedding left over from its use as a troop ship. He stated that after arriving off Scutari it was nine days before all the sick were taken ashore, and that meanwhile repeated requisitions for fresh provisions were ignored.

The past and present Cabinet ministers were not interviewed until April. When the Duke of Newcastle, the former Minister of War, was asked if he had communicated with the Medical Director-General as soon as the expedition to the East was planned he answered - "No, not immediately ... but later through the Secretary-at-War". This corroborated Smith's complaint of the excessive delay before he was in a position to plan for the expedition. The Duke was asked if he had heard from any source other than the public press or private channels of the miseries suffered by the troops in hospital and on passage from Balaclava to Scutari. He answered - "I did not". Equally he denied having received early reports from any medical officers that there was an insufficiency of stores, medical comforts, and medical staff. He said that Smith had assured him that there could be no such deficiencies. The Duke was questioned about the First Commission. He admitted that, having taken the responsibility out of Smith's hand, he had been in error in failing originally to give the Commissioners power to initiate immediate reforms, but later he had directed the Commissioners to advise Lord Paulet (who had succeeded the ineffective Sillery) to take action locally.

The results of the examination of Herbert were more interesting. Officially he had had only financial control over the Medical Department but, as has already been made clear, he had become deeply involved in the affairs of the Scutari hospitals. It was he who had planned the mission of Miss Nightingale and her nurses, and he had made early enquiries into the state of the hospitals. He denied however that he had any responsibility in their control. He stressed Sillery's incompetence, and expressed a poor opinion of Menzies as P.M.O., suggesting that he had escaped censure (or even dismissal) only because he had been invalided. He admitted that all he knew of the hospitals was derived from private reports from Miss Nightingale and the Reverend Sydney Osborne. Asked why he had advocated the employment of civilian surgeons and the establishment of the civil hospital at Smyrna, he replied that this was because the army surgeons were exhausted.

Of the four Members of Parliament who gave evidence that from Layard was perhaps the most persuasive. The evidence of Dundas and Stafford has already been quoted fully (Chapter VI). Percy had been in Scutari for such a short time that he had little to offer, although the Committee seemed to regard him as an important witness. Layard gave evidence about the disastrous conditions in the 'Kangaroo' and other transports involved in the evacuation of the wounded after the Alma. He strongly condemned the chaotic and insanitary conditions of the harbour at Balaclava. Asked about the soldiers' diet, he pointed out that this varied greatly in different regiments, that the wastage of foods was excessive, and that the faults were in distribution rather than in the lack of supplies at Balaclava. He stated that many regimental doctors had complained of shortages of essential medicines.[31]

Finally, the three 'independent' witnesses gave useful evidence. The Reverend George Parker, who had served in the Crimea as a chaplain to the First Division from November 1854 to January 1855, proved a balanced witness.[32] He described the condition of the sick -

> most wretched, lying on the ground with a single blanket ... the medical attendance was very good, so far as the medical attendance went. There was a great want of medicines ... the medical men themselves were most indefatigable, as long as they had health: but in the case of the Scots Fusilier Guards, at one time all the medical men were sick.

Of the regimental hospitals he commented -

> the state of the hospitals was such that had he not been many years in South America and had been accustomed to attend yellow fever patients, he should not have been able to bear the effluvia. A brother clergyman fainted in one of the marquees from the effluvia. This arose from want of means to evacuate: in many cases, perhaps from the actual weakness of the patient, he could not retain anything, and everything went on the ground ... Dr. Hall was at the head of the Department. The witness did not know him by sight: but to his knowledge he never heard of his being in the hospital tents: he might have been there.

The Reverend Sydney Osborne, some of whose observations have already been reported (Chapter VI), arrived at Scutari on 5 November, 1854.[33] His examination went on for two days and his evidence related almost entirely to Scutari. He reinforced his evidence with long quotations from his correspondence with Lord Stratford, the Secretary of War, and other persons of influence. The impression is given that Osborne, who had so many friends in high places, was given much more latitude to express his own opinions than was any other witness. He had been accepted as an authority on hospitals, he had been well briefed by Miss Nightingale, and he had already pressed his opinions on the Duke of Newcastle and other members of the government in private letters and in numerous effusions to the press. Macdonald, as the representative of **The Times** Fund in Scutari, was regarded as a very important witness.[34] His detailed descriptions of Scutari have already been given (Chapter VI). He had much to say about the lack of care of patients disembarked at Scutari from the transports, and the delay in their transfer ashore. The interrogation of Maxwell, the legal member of the First Commission, brought out one significant fact. Questioned on the alleged inefficiency of the Apothecary and the Purveyors, he revealed that he had asked for their records but that these were not forthcoming. In consequence he had searched through their papers himself and found that no adequate records had been kept.

What were the conclusions of the Roebuck Committee? The Committee gave its first report to Parliament on 18 June.[35] This is not the place to discuss the political implications of the report, it is sufficient to note that there was much evidence to prove beyond doubt that too little governmental attention had been paid to the Medical Department for many years and that it had suffered from inadequate financial support. In July the **Association Medical Journal** analysed the report in so far as it referred to the medical service. First of all, Smith, the Director-General, was almost completely exonerated from blame for the errors which had been made. It was admitted that, working as he did under five different authorities he lacked information concerning the campaign and despite his strenuous efforts was greatly hampered in his preparations. Reference was made to the report of the First Commission, which had already confirmed many of the adverse reports of the newspaper correspondents and others. The mismanagement of the Scutari hospitals was not attributed to Smith, whose claim that he had no direct responsibility for these was noted and, perhaps reluctantly, accepted. By implication Hall was censured for his optimistic report after his brief visit to Scutari in October 1854. Menzies was more positively condemned for his ineffective control but there was some admission that the task was beyond him. The Committee appreciated very clearly that the Purveyors were responsible for many of the difficulties which had arisen, acting with an independent authority which was not corrected until late November by new instructions as to their powers. The Apothecary also came in for major criticism. It was agreed that Smith had provided for most contingencies by sending out lavish stores, equipment, and staff. It was suspected that "some dishonesty had been practised in regard to these stores". The Committee noted that it could not investigate this matter but recommended that Parliament should take further action. Major Sillery was criticised harshly for his lack of initiative and his failure to spend money for emergency measures, even although he had been authorised to do so. Lord Raglan was blamed for appointing a junior officer as commandant to the hospitals. Perhaps most strikingly and certainly unfairly, little credit was given to the medical officers, whether in the Crimea or at Scutari, for their tireless devotion to their work in almost impossible conditions, although nearly every witness had paid tribute to the doctors.

The last paragraph of the report must be quoted in full, for in it there is a degree of exaggeration. "Your Committee in conclusion, cannot but remark that the first real improvements in the lamentable condition of the hospitals at Scutari are to be attributed to private suggestions, private exertions, and private benevolence."

> Miss Nightingale with admirable devotion organised a band of nurses, and undertook the care of the sick and wounded ... The Hon. Jocelyne Percy, the Hon. and Rev. Sidney Godolphin Osborne and Mr. Augustus Stafford, after a personal inspection of the hospitals, furnished valuable reports and suggestions to the Government. By these means much suffering was alleviated, the spirits of the men were raised, and many lives were saved.

There was much debate in Parliament over the findings of the Committee. Stafford was one of the most eloquent. On 28 June he paid a belated tribute to the doctors. "Statements have been made before the Commission less generally known than those made before the Sebastopol Committee, which, although they caused the hearts of those who heard them to chill with horror, were highly honourable to the regimental surgeons, who, notwithstanding the risk to their own professional advancement, brought under the notice of the country the sufferings of those committed to their charge. It was not possible to exaggerate the eulogies due to these men."[36] But a vendetta against Smith and Hall had developed. On 10 July Stafford asked whether Dr. Smith had retired and whether Dr. Hall still continued as Medical Inspector of the Army in the East. The reply was given that Smith would continue to act as the head of the army medical department until his successor was appointed. As for Dr. Hall, he had not been removed from his post since during Lord Panmure's term of office he had received no complaints as to the way Hall had performed his duty.

The reaction in the medical press to the findings of the Committee was variable. The **Association Medical Journal** attacked Smith in its leaders until June. "In the name of all that is lucrative and disastrous in the system of medical routine, favouritism, and seniority, let the Director-General of the Army Medical Department take his pension and title while yet the empire of red-tape holds the power to bestow such rewards for such services - and retire."[37] This was written after the Journal had recorded in detail Smith's convincing defence of his actions. Meanwhile the **Lancet** and the **Medical Times and Gazette** had continued to support Smith. But the editor of the **Association Medical Journal** commented -

> no one but an occasional versatile contemporary ... still strives to defend the army Medical Director ... we can only account for this extraordinary and not very creditable advocacy by recollecting that previous occupants of one editorial chair have found favour in the eyes of the Army Medical Department.[38]

The reference was most likely to the former editor of a rival journal, **Medical Times and Gazette,** Spencer Wells, now appointed senior surgeon to the civil hospital in Smyrna. Having published its summary of the Committee's findings, the **Association Medical Journal** then went silent. There were no more leaders condemning the medical service, in fact in the second half of 1855 the journal reported little of the campaign, not even recording the capture of Sebastopol. One reason for this silence may have been the dismissal of the editor, Dr. John McCormack, who had written the vituperative leaders. In addition there was now a new Medical Reform Bill to discuss. The **Lancet** and the **Medical Times and Gazette** took little notice of the findings of the Roebuck Committee except that both expressed pleasure that Smith had been exonerated. Not surprisingly, there was criticism that so much weight was placed on the evidence of unqualified "visitors" to the hospitals.

The Times temporarily ceased reviling Smith and the medical service but was to return to the attack a few months later. **Punch,** which had printed a scurrilous cartoon of Smith, made some amends in an article in which he was given credit for warning the authorities at the beginning of the campaign of the medical risks that would be encountered. The medical profession in general, realising that Smith had received undeserved obloquy, hastened to offer votes of confidence. In August 1855, the Faculty of Physicians and Surgeons of Glasgow elected Smith an Honorary Member. Many other such bodies followed suit. Sir James McGrigor wrote to Hall on 27 June, as follows. "We have had another victory which comes more home to us - to wit the exculpation of the Department in almost every case of the blame intended to be cast on it. Dr. Smith has obtained a victory over his foes, and it is declared that he did everything a man in his situation could have done."[39] It certainly could be said that on balance the Medical Department came out better than most other Departments. As Cantlie suggests, "the 'evils' at Scutari were attributed to the want of an efficient governing authority with a staff to maintain inspection and discipline. This decision meant the ultimate blame lay not on the Medical Department but on the military administration."[40] At the same time it was all too clear that there were no grounds for complacency among those responsible for the medical care of the Army.

In retrospect the findings of the Sebastopol Committee had some important repercussions for the medical services. If there had been any doubts concerning the near break-down of the medical organisation, of the excessive hardships endured by the sick and wounded, and of the deplorable state of the Commissariat those had been at last confirmed officially. As far as medical reforms were concerned, Roebuck's Committee did not have a great impact because before the report appeared the Government had sent out new Commissioners with powers to act locally.

THE SANITARY COMMISSION

The Government had moved quickly in selecting the Roebuck Committee and about the same time it appointed two Commissions to go to the East to investigate conditions on the spot. The first of these was the Sanitary Commission. Whereas the Roebuck Committee was appointed to find fault rather than to secure reforms, this delegation was of a different character. The Sanitary Commission consisted of Dr. John Sutherland[41], Dr. Hector Gavin[42], and Mr. Robert Rawlinson[43], accompanied by three sanitary inspectors from Liverpool (Mr. Newlands, Mr. Wilson and one other). While in practice in Liverpool Sutherland had been associated with the pioneer of urban sanitary reform, Dr. William Duncan, the first Medical Officer of Health to be appointed in Great Britain; and in 1848 Sutherland had become an Inspector under the Board of Health. Gavin, a leading sanitary reformer and the author of several works on public health, had held important government appointments during the outbreaks of cholera in 1849 and 1854, and at the time of his appointment to the Commission was Physician to the Post Office. Rawlinson was a civil engineer under the General Board of Health.

The instructions to the Commissioners, issued by Lord Panmure on 19 February, were couched in terms of considerable urgency.[44] They were ordered to proceed to Constantinople at once to inspect the hospitals. They were to transmit to the appropriate local authorities, Lord Paulet, Admiral Grey and Lord Raglan, a statement of all that needed correction, "whether in the way of arrangement, of reduction of numbers in the wards, cleansing, disinfecting, or of actual construction, in order to secure the great ends of safety and health ... It is important that you will be duly impressed with not resting content with an order, but that you see instantly by yourselves or by your agents to the commencement of the work, and to its superintendence, day by day, until it be finished." In addition the Commissioners were directed to inspect the methods of transport of the sick and wounded to Scutari, the state of the harbour at Balaclava, and the conditions of the camps in the Crimea.

With the First Commission there had been no such sense of urgency, the terms of reference having been indeterminate and the powers granted minimal. Two of the three members of the First Commission had been serving army medical officers, hence, when their advice was turned down by executive officers they could do nothing. In contrast the Sanitary Commission consisted of civilians who could ignore any indifference from local military authorities, and who were empowered to initiate reforms independent of the government. It has been suggested that the brief given to the Sanitary Commission (under the signature of Lord Panmure) was prepared by Herbert (who, in February was still a member of the Cabinet). Kinglake goes further and hints that the author "had received impulsion from a woman's mind", that is, Miss Nightingale had prepared the terms of reference.[45] Her immediate acceptance of the Commissioners and the rapid development of a close and lasting friendship with Sutherland certainly suggest that she approved this new initiative of the Government, while it is clear that she had no faith in the First Commission.

Arriving in Scutari on 4 March, 1855, the Commissioners set to work with great energy. In four days they had inspected three of the main hospitals and sent their recommendations to Paulet.[46] In the Barrack Hospital they found the ventilation of wards and corridors deficient and the privies in a deplorable condition. They admitted however that the hospital "bears marks of much having been done to improve it". They described the General Hospital as scrupulously clean, except for the privies, and the kitchens as excessively damp. They commented on the unhygienic state of the area around both these hospitals, and observed that the close proximity of ill-cared burial grounds was a health hazard. The Palace Hospital (Hydar Pasha) was considered to be very unhealthy in all respects. Firm orders were at once issued to improve ventilation and drainage in all three hospitals. All privies and water tanks were to be cleaned up and further burials were not to be permitted in the vicinity of the hospitals. A strong recommendation was made to reduce the number of patients in each hospital and to stop using the corridors for the accommodation of patients. In addition, an Inspector of Nuisances was appointed to each hospital to supervise the daily cleansing or all areas of the vicinity in which refuse and rubbish had been allowed to accumulate.[47] The hospital at Koulali was visited during the next four days and found to be grossly overcrowded, ill-ventilated, offensive and fever-stricken. Orders were given to correct these evils, although this involved, as with the other hospitals, extensive engineering and much rebuilding.[48] Paulet acknowledged these recommendations on 16 March and indicated that the work would be carried out to the best of his ability.

By 17 March the Commissioners had inspected the two "convalescent hulks" moored off Scutari. They found that both were fever-stricken, ill-ventilated, overcrowded, and dirty, and that the bilge water was grossly offensive. They reported that many patients on board were in conditions of advanced disease and insisted that only convalescents should be accommodated. It was recommended that the numbers of patients should be greatly reduced and that as soon as possible more salubrious convalescent quarters should be found.[49] Admiral Grey, who held responsibility for the hulks, replied the next day in a letter indicating that he was well aware of the defective state of the ships and that he had already lodged the same criticisms. He thought it impossible to improve the Turkish hulk because of its age and rotten condition, but believed that the second ship, the 'Bombay', could be improved. He hoped that the Commissioners would see to it that the use of hulks would soon be abandoned.[50]

In a remarkably short time the Commissioners had acted positively. What mattered was that most of their recommendations were acted upon quickly, the necessary labour force was at last forthcoming, and the work was now directed by skilled engineers and sanitary inspectors. Having initiated such major reforms at Scutari, attention was now turned to the Crimea. With the same energy, measures were taken to correct the sanitary condition of Balaclava and to improve conditions in the hospital transports. Numerous camps were inspected and recommendations made, particularly as to improving the drainage, water supply, and ventilation of huts. The clearance of refuse from the vicinity of the camps, not least the rotting carcases of horses and other animals, was ordered.

Rawlinson stayed on in Scutari to supervise the engineering work, while Sutherland went to Smyrna to inspect the newly established Civil Hospital. Gavin remained in the Crimea, lodging with his brother, a veterinary surgeon.[51] A regrettable accident occurred on 20 April, when Gavin was accidentally shot by his brother and died within a few hours. The loss to the Commission by Gavin's death was considerable. He was replaced in July by Dr. Gavin Milroy.[52] Meanwhile Sutherland remained in the East for more than a year continuing his supervision of all the projects that had been undertaken, and working closely with Miss Nightingale. Rawlinson was injured by a stray round-shot while visiting the front line in June 1855, and he then returned to England, while Milroy stayed on to assist Sutherland in his work.

The Commissioners had sent copies of their preliminary recommendations to Lord Panmure. In April they sent a report to Lord Raglan drawing his attention to the defects of the army camps. Full reports on the work of the Sanitary Commission were published in 1855 and in 1856, but it is not necessary to analyse these in detail. It is, however, relevant to quote from a letter which Sutherland wrote to Lord Shaftesbury and which appeared in **The Times** of 22 August, 1855.[53] In this private communication, Sutherland began by giving a damning account of the harbour at Balaclava - "Nothing could be worse than its condition". But further on in the letter he modifies this opinion, presumably to demonstrate the effectiveness of the activities of the Commission.

> Balaclava is much sweeter than the Thames [incidentally, not a great commendation at the time], and the town is cleaner than nine-tenths of the lower districts of London, Manchester, or Liverpool. Liverpool dock basins smell worse every day than Balaclava did at its worst, when the town itself was held up to the reprobation of the civilised world, from its unburied carcases or filth ... the same may be said of the sanitary condition of the camp ... the camp is in a much better state than the towns and villages at home, out of which the men had come.

Sutherland concluded - "It is also very satisfactory to state that almost every practicable improvement we have advised for the camp we have found already in operation in some part of it ... We have also found the medical authorities thoroughly alive to the nature of the changes required but without the power to carry them out." This statement should have gratified the Medical Department.

The Sanitary Commission was of great significance. Miss Nightingale believed that "the arrival of this Commission saved the British Army".[54] She told the Royal Commission in 1857 -

> The Sanitary conditions of the hospitals in Scutari were inferior in point of crowding, ventilation, drainage and cleanliness up the middle of March 1855, to any civil hospital, or to the poorest houses of the worst parts of the civil population of any large town I have ever seen. After the sanitary works undertaken at that date were executed I know of no buildings in the world which I could compare with them in these points, the original construction of course excepted.[55]

Referring to the Scutari hospitals, Kinglake wrote -

> In the second week of March they [the Commissioners] had already made much
> progress and on the 17th had advanced their works so far as to be in a
> state for producing at once some part of the intended effects. Then came
> on a change which had it been preceded by mummery instead of ventilation
> and drainage, and pure water supply, would have passed for a miracle. Down
> went the mortality.[56]

His suggestion that the mortality rates fell at the end of March because of the work of the Commission is scarcely tenable. It is inconceivable that the work involved in relaying drains and other major improvements was completed in two weeks. More likely the mortality rate fell because the admission rate came down at this time, thus reducing the lethal effect of overcrowding, because the severity of the medical cases admitted from the Crimea lessened at this time, and because the climatic conditions improved.

Hall was to spend much of his retirement refuting the belief that the fall in mortality was because of the actions of the Commission, both at Scutari and in the Crimea, but he did not help his case by sometimes overstating it. It was perhaps excessive of him to write of the Commission as he did. "All dispassionate people will see and admit that the benefits of their labours were more assumed than real, and the results of their mission not commensurate with the expense it cost the British public: for in my opinion neither the health nor mortality of the British Army was in any appreciable manner affected by any reasons adopted at their recommendation; but had they never set foot in the Crimea the result would have been the same."[57] In a later publication Hall produced much evidence that he and his senior officers had made strong representations concerning most of the defects which the Sanitary Commission had claimed to correct, and blamed the executive officers for failing to listen to medical advice. He did not seem to realise that the situation would have gone on indefinitely if the Commission had not intervened and had ensured that reform was quickly effected. There was admittedly some justification for Hall's complaints. It was in the longer term that the work of the Sanitary Commissioners became so important. Ultimately the major improvements which they effected by the exercise of their superior powers created much better conditions in which to deal with the crises which were still to come, and hence prevented a recurrence of the disasters of the first winter of the war in the succeeding winter. The long continued supervision by Sutherland ensured that the improvements made in the spring of 1855 were maintained for the rest of the war, much to the comfort of the sick and wounded.

The findings of the Sanitary Commission were to lead to much argument for some years after the war. It is apparent that its actions were ultimately of great significance, not only in improving the health of the Army during the rest of the war but also of relevance to the reform of the Army Medical Service in the post-war years. The influence of Sutherland as an individual, particularly because of his co-operation with Miss Nightingale, was of great importance. Through her he became involved in Army affairs for the rest of his career. He was to serve on the Royal Commission and was called as a witness on many important aspects of this enquiry. Rawlinson was not subsequently involved in Army affairs but he also appeared as a witness to the Royal Commission.

THE SUPPLIES COMMISSION

On 12 February, 1855 the Government established a Commission, "to inquire into the whole arrangement and management of the Commissariat Department". By this time the public outcry at the apparent mismanagement of the war had reached a peak. It was felt that to placate the critics an impartial investigation should be undertaken. This Commission was of considerable importance, with implications both political and in relation to the whole structure of army organisation. The commissioners were briefed to inquire, in particular, into the delay in the distribution of stores shipped to the East. Their investigations had to deal with provisions, forage, clothing and the means of transport. They were given wide powers to summon and examine witnesses and to call for the production of all records.

Two Commissioners were appointed, Sir John McNeill[58] and Colonel Alexander Tulloch[59]. The mission was a delicate one as it entailed the close examination of regular army officers, many of high rank. The choice of a civilian doctor and a regular army officer of comparatively low rank might have seemed a mistake but the two men were to fulfil their task with great efficiency. McNeill after qualifying as a doctor in 1816 had entered the service of the East India Company as an assistant-surgeon. Following four years in India he became a surgeon in Persia, his competence and his diplomacy leading to his appointment as Assistant Chargé d'Affaires in Teheran. After 24 years of distinguished service in Persia he returned home and became Chairman of the Board of Supervision administering the new Poor Law in Scotland. His wide administrative experience and his special knowledge of the Middle East made him a suitable choice for the leadership of the Commission. Tulloch was a regular army officer and had developed, in contact with Henry Marshall, a considerable skill in statistical analysis. Before the outbreak of war he had been employed mainly in the War Office, where regrettably he had been responsible for the idea of selecting pensioners to form an ambulance corps, in opposition to Smith.[60] He worked well with McNeill, who exerted a tactful control over his younger colleague's outspoken manner. The Commissioners arrived at Scutari on 6 March and went on to Balaclava a week later. They questioned 200 witnesses of all ranks and from all departments.

In their report the Commissioners were highly critical of the Headquarters staff and of the Commissariat Department. They were not concerned with individuals but merely stated the facts, which offered very clear evidence of failure of the administration in dealing with the supplies of rations, clothing, and equipment for the soldiers, forage for the horses, and transport. It was made quite clear that the shortages of fresh meat and vegetables and of winter clothing could have been avoided if the transport system by sea and by land had been managed with more imagination and initiative. They were aware of the problems caused by the failure to construct a good road from Balaclava up to the front. The lack of forage for horses and other beasts of burden was seen as an important factor in the breakdown of the transport system. McNeill, as a medical man, went into the issue of shortages of drugs in the Crimea in some detail, and was particularly critical of the lack of opium, quinine, and lime juice, which he considered was largely the fault of Hall. From the start of the survey, the Commissioners were in close touch with Miss Nightingale, who was well aware of the importance of their investigations in relation to the hospitals and to the care of the soldiers in the Crimea. Miss Nightingale soon had a great admiration for McNeill, which he reciprocated. He was to remain her close friend, advisor, and ally in all her labours during the war and in the subsequent years. It is difficult to assess how quickly the work of this Commission brought changes in the organisation of the Commissariat but one direct effect was the introduction of a more balanced diet for the soldiers.[61] Another change doubtless stemmed from the report, for in June 1855 the Commissariat Department was removed from control by the Treasury and placed under the War Office, an improvement which was highly advantageous.[62]

The Commission made its first full report in June 1855 and issued a more complete version in the following year.[63] The revelations of the gross incompetence of the High Command and of the Commissariat created a sensation among the public. The report gave great offence to senior army officers, at home and abroad, whose administration had been so strongly criticised. Specific references had been made to a few individuals, and these particular officers were the most vociferous. These army officers complained that they had had no opportunity before the report was published of contradicting the adverse opinions which had been expressed, and they at once demanded an enquiry. The Queen herself intervened,[64] and in accordance with the Queen's wish, a Board of General Officers was appointed to investigate the "charges which were thought to have been made against certain officers". Up to this time no resolution of thanks had been accorded to the Commissioners for the ability with which they had carried out their task, and the appointment of a Board seemed to put them on trial for the accuracy of their findings. The Board, commonly referred to as the Chelsea Board, consisted of seven generals, who, after long deliberations, exonerated all the senior officers named in the report.[65] The Commissariat Department escaped censure. Even the incompetent and aged Filder, the Commissary-General, was exonerated, although the Commission had singled him out for harsh criticism. The Government was blamed for administrative errors, particularly the Treasury for its failure to purchase sufficient forage for the horses. As a result of this enquiry the findings of the Commissioners were nullified, causing great and widespread indignation.[66]

Belatedly Palmerston decided to acknowledge the services of the Commissioners by the award of a thousand pounds to each, but both refused the offer indignantly. Miss Nightingale rose to their defence, for to her mind the exposure of the mismanagement by the Commissariat and by many senior officers was well deserved. It was largely due to her later intervention that McNeill was made a Member of the Privy Council and Tulloch was knighted. Controversy over the findings of the Chelsea Board lasted for many years. **The Times**, during the sitting of the Chelsea Board, lost no opportunity to attack the senior army officers. In Kinglake's words, "the great journal assailed with keen, studied invectives the officers defending their conduct ... with the vehement support of the Times and the Public applauding his efforts, Colonel Tulloch was for the moment the hero, conspicuous in the country at large".[67]

Although this one-sided Board whitewashed the senior officers and put all the blame on the government, the findings of McNeill and Tulloch remain a just condemnation of the defects of the army command and of the Commissariat. The report of the Sanitary Commission brought more immediate improvements but that of the Supplies Commission must be seen as complementary. To the medical services the subsequent reorganisation of the Commissariat was of great importance. McNeill's interest in army affairs continued after the war because of his close connection with Miss Nightingale. Both he and Tulloch appeared as witnesses before the Royal Commission of 1857 but curiously were asked no questions about their work in the Crimea, or about the Chelsea Board. Tulloch comes to notice after the war by reason of his published version of the proceedings of the Chelsea Board, which he wrote "out of a sense of injury".[68]

THE PATHOLOGY COMMISSION

Late in March 1855 a Commission was appointed, "to investigate the pathology of diseases in the East". Cantlie suggests that Smith initiated this action.[69] But it seems that Miss Nightingale must be given some of the credit for the scheme. On 22 February, 1855, enlarging on the idea that a medical school should be established at Scutari, she wrote to Herbert,

> there is no operating room, no dissecting room: post-mortem examinations are seldom made ... no statistics are held as to between what ages most deaths occur, as to the modes of treatment, appearances of the body after death etc., and all the innumerable and most important points which contribute to making therapeutics a means of saving life, and not, as it is here, a formal duty. Our registration is so lamentably defective that often the only record kept is - <u>a man died</u> on such a day.[70]

Herbert may well have shown this letter to his successor, Panmure. The instructions given to Dr. Lyons, who was put in charge of the Commission, were therefore precise.[71] He was given the entire responsibility of conducting post-mortem examinations. He was required "to demonstrate the morbid appearances discovered to such medical officers as may feel disposed to attend". With two assistants he was to be given every facility to examine patients in the wards (but not to interfere with their treatment). He was expected to submit diseased tissues to microscopic examination and to preserve illustrative specimens. It was recommended that he observe diseases in Russian prisoners and visit the French hospitals. The instructions concluded: "As the office to which you are now appointed is new in the medical department it is possible, although not probable, that some difficulty may arise in your researches. If by your own prudence or conciliatory conduct, you fail to overcome any such difficulties ... you will report the circumstances to the Secretary of State for the War Department." Panmure anticipated that the investigation would take about four months. Lyons was authorised, if he thought fit, to recommend that one or both of his assistants should remain in the East after completion of the work of the Commission.

Robert Lyons[72], after qualifying in Dublin in 1848, had become an authority in the study of normal and pathological histology. His main assistant, William

Aitken[73], after qualifying in Edinburgh in 1848, had become Demonstrator in Anatomy to Professor Allen Thomson, an influential figure in the Glasgow Medical School. It may be assumed that his experience had been more academic than practical, but he must have had the opportunity of developing an interest in pathology as well as anatomy. It may be observed that there was no Chair of Pathology in Glasgow until 1876, pathology being taught, as in most other schools, by the Professors of Medicine or Surgery. In Edinburgh a Chair of Pathology had been established in 1831, but as late as 1853 Professor Syme and some of his colleagues were still doing their best to abolish the Chair of Pathology, partly because the incumbent was a homoeopathist, but mainly because they did not think pathology merited a separate Chair. This low regard for pathology in many of the British medical schools no doubt accounts for the lukewarm reception given to the Commission on its arrival at Scutari. Hall's biographer comments -

> A pathologist with two assistants was sent to the East, to investigate the nature and cause of the diseases prevailing in the Army. These gentlemen were liberally paid in comparison with Army stipends. What they discovered, or what it was expected they could discover that was hidden from the Medical Officers of the Army, Dr. Hall was at a loss to know.[74]

Lyon's second assistant was a Dr. Doyle of whom little is known, except that like Aitken he was said to be "accustomed to and versed in the operations of the dead-house".

Lyons arrived in Scutari at the beginning of April, and his assistants about four weeks later. It is from the private letters of Aitken that we learn of the somewhat ineffective start made by Lyons.[75] Aitken wrote to Professor Thomson on 28 May.

> I reported myself to the Commandant Lord Wm. Paulet and to the Medical Inspector Cumming. I attempted to find Dr. Lyons but nobody seemed to know anything about him ... There are somewhere between 8 to 10 civil medical officers attached to the hospitals besides we three pathologists, and the Military are dead set against us, I mean the Military Medical men and some of the officials such as the Commandant and old stagers. Many of them look upon our Commission as adding insult to injury and I feel that Lyons is not likely to correct matters. He seems to forget 'more flies are caught with honey than with vinegar', and is already in bad odour - from his taking notice of things he has nothing to do with. When I arrived I found him busy fighting Lord Paulet to obtain the rank of major he somehow thought himself entitled to. He was told we all rank as captains merely for the purpose of drawing rations and nothing else ... I have not formed a pleasant opinion of Lyons, [since] from the way in which he has set about

things we will all do nothing for six weeks to come. He has insisted on their building a large dead house with inspection room and office and will do nothing until that is accomplished ... I have advised him to go up to Head Quarters at the Camp whence all the disease are coming - he is to go on Tuesday (tomorrow) and leave me in charge here in the mean time. It looks as though he wished to prolong the thing unnecessarily.

Aitken was thus left to his own devices and employed his time studying the cases in the hospital. He was glad when some of his friends from Glasgow and Edinburgh arrived on their way to serve in the Civil Hospitals. "I had much pleasure from their being here for really the specimens of the Medicals here are not prepossessing to me."

With this inauspicious start it seemed that the Commission was doomed to failure. Clearly Lyons had not been a particularly good choice to take charge, and Aitken had the more forceful personality. It is likely that Aitken soon made contact with Miss Nightingale and had her encouragement. There is no record that Lyons had any close collaboration with her. Aitken wrote to Thomson early in July -

Dr. Lyons has been in the Crimea during the last three weeks but what he is doing I have no idea as he does not write to us. He left us both here to look after everything that might turn up while the Engineers prepare our Dead House and Inspection Room. I have made a few post-mortems but it is exceedingly disagreeable as the place we have to work in is so small, a little wooden shed and with a temperature varying from 70 to 76 degrees in the shade.

There was a second report in July.

Dr. Lyons is still in the Crimea. He left here about the 12th of June and I was to look after the buildings he set agoing and do what I could in the way of pathology ... the 3rd. Pathologist (Mr. Doyle, an extraordinary hot-headed Irishman) taking charge of the cases at the General Hospital while my duty lay at the Barrack ... I confess that as far as our Commission has gone (although I have seen a good deal to interest me) I do not feel satisfied about it. Now at the time when three months out of our tour have expired we are only about to enter the place provided for us at enormous expense, according to Dr. Lyon's plans. He made himself very disagreeable to Dr. Cumming here and also to Lord Paulet so that we are both looked on with dislike. His plans also if carried out are so to deprive the medical men at the Barrack Hospital from witnessing the inspection of their cases and they are set against him ... Lyons tells me he must go home as he has been appointed to a professorship of physiology in Dublin ... Lyons means to recommend that I shall be appointed to continue as Pathologist. The office is certainly a want in the Army, but the whole system of naming their diseases and their sick statistics would require to be remodelled. It is in a most useless and disgraceful state. The returns sent home are not the least true as to the diseases ... Dr. Lyons is apparently determined to have all the credit, or discredit, of the Commission. He writes the report, we are not to share in it ... I do not know in the least what is the result of our Commission.

In Scutari Aitken did his share of collecting material for the report and he sent this on to Lyons in the Crimea. He now reported - "Dr. Lyons has sent home a first report of a copy of which in scroll he sent me by yesterday's mail that I might read it after he sent it away". We can find no comment of what Aitken thought of this preliminary report but when the final edition was published in 1856 Aitken was given equal credit with Lyons for its preparation.[76]

The report of this Commission does not seem to have made much impact. It is not mentioned in the evidence given to the Royal Commission after the war. There are no quotations from it in the **Medical and Surgical History of the War** published in 1858. A study of the contents of the report does not suggest that many original observations were made. Lyons made the excuse that if he had arrived two months earlier, when the winter diseases were at their peak, his observations would have been more useful. The groups of diseases considered were typhoid, typhus, cholera, and dysentery. Pathological observations were given in particular for dysentery, from 50 post-mortems. Also described were 50 cases of fatal typhoid but it is not clear how many were examined post-mortem. A resume of the pathological anatomy in these diseases was given but detailed statistical information was lacking. The published reviews were critical, one of them as follows.

> With all its undoubted merits we must frankly state that the Report has in some degree disappointed us. The absolute number of post-mortem examinations is not very great - and they are communicated very briefly and in many cases imperfectly ... The chemistry of the fluids has been left untouched, and the microscopic notes are short and unsatisfactory. We have looked in vain for even a microscopical examination of the blood and the absence of these inquiries is not compensated by any researches carried on at the bedside of the patients, for the histories of the diseases are even more meagre than the accounts of the post-mortem examinations.

Such adverse criticism scarcely justified the final sentence of the review - "Their Report is a gain to science, and will always be a document of interest and authority for those who study the medical history of the Crimean campaign".[77]

If the report was not of great value there were at least some good effects following the visit of the Commission and the continued presence of Aitken throughout the war. By the establishment of better facilities for post-mortem examinations and by impressing on some of the medical officers the importance of pathological studies a contribution was made towards an improvement in the standards of clinical practice. It was probably due to Aitken's influence that by the end of the war the medical registers in all the Army hospitals were being much more meticulously kept, and therefore the published statistics were becoming more reliable.

Lyons went home in August to take up the Chair of Medicine and Pathology in the School of Medicine of the Catholic University at Dublin. In addition to collecting pathological information he had treated the sick and wounded while in the Crimea.[78] Aitken stayed on in the East as Consultant Pathologist to the Army until early in 1856 and continued to send to Lyons information for the completion of the report of the Commission. He worked closely with Miss Nightingale in the preparation of statistics. He returned to England with a considerable reputation, and when the Army Medical School was founded in 1860 at Fort Pitt, it was on Miss Nightingale's insistence that a Chair of Pathology was established and that Aitken was made the first incumbent. He remained in this post until his death in 1892.

NOTES

1. E. Cook, **The life of Florence Nightingale** (2 vols., London, 1913), 1:175.
2. P.R. Kirby, **Sir Andrew Smith** (Cape Town, 1965), 305-306.
3. Patrick Laing (1821-1892); L.R.C.S.Ed. 1840; joined as assistant-surgeon 1842; surgeon January 1854; served in the East November 1854-June 1855; retired 1866 as D.I.G. (**Drew**).
4. **Report upon the state of the Hospitals of the British Army in the Crimea and Scutari,** (London, 1855). The title scarcely covers the subjects investigated.
5. Charles White (1832-1878); joined as assistant-surgeon March 1854; served in the East November 1854-November 1855; retired 1862 as S.M. (**Drew**).
6. Robert Cooper (1818-1864); M.R.C.S.; Cooper joined as assistant-surgeon 1843; surgeon 1853; served in the East April 1854-June 1856; retired 1862. (**Drew**).
7. **Kinglake**, 7:281. For Roebuck, see **DNB**; A. Briggs, **Victorian people** (London, 1965), chapter III.

8. Kinglake, 7:313.
9. **Ass.Med.J.** (1855), 400.
10. In fact there were three medically qualified M.P.s: Dr. William Mitchell, Dr. Joseph Hume and Dr. John Brady (C.R. Dod, **The Parliamentary Companion**, London, 1854). None however had anything like the fire and ability of Dr. Thomas Wakley who had relinquished his seat in 1852.
11. **Kinglake**, 7:316-317.
12. Ibid., 308-309.
13. Henry Mapleton (1815-1879); M.R.C.S. 1837; M.D. Edinburgh 1838; joined in 1839 as assistant-surgeon; surgeon 1847; staff surgeon May 1854; served in the East April - September 1854; F.R.C.S. 1859; F.R.C.P. 1860; Head of Medical Board at War Office 1859-1864; retired 1864 as I.G. (**Plarr; Munk; Drew**).
14. The detailed evidence given to the Roebuck Committee can be read in the published report but it is convenient to refer to the very adequate summary of the medical evidence in the **Ass.Med.J.** of April to July, 1855.
15. **Ass.Med.J.** (1855), 422-424.
16. G. St. Aubyn, **The Royal George** (London, 1963), 85. For comment on the service of the Duke of Cambridge in the Crimea, see Chapter III.
17. **Ass.Med.J.** (1855), 424-425.
18. Ibid., 453.
19. Ibid., 403-404.
20. Ibid., 401-402.
21. Ibid., 424.
22. Ibid.
23. Ibid.
24. Ibid., 471-476, 494-503, 575.
25. Ibid., 575-577. 595-596.
26. Ibid., 644.
27. Ibid., 643-644.
28. Mapleton's evidence does not appear in the **Ass.Med.J.** but is in the final report (see note 35 below).
29. **Ass.Med.J.** (1855), 596-598, 643.
30. Ibid., 404.
31. Ibid., 400-403.
32. Ibid., 405-406.
33. Ibid., 544-551,575.
34. Ibid., 425-429.
35. The full report was published in three parts, **First, Second and Third Report from the Select Committee on the Army before Sebastopol: with the proceedings of the Committee. Ordered by the House of Commons to be printed March 1855.**
36. **The Times**, 19.6.1855.
37. **Ass.Med.J.** (1855), 525-526.
38. Ibid.
39. 'Hall/McGrigor Letters', 27.6.1855.
40. **Cantlie**, 2:167-168.
41. John Sutherland (1808-1891); L.R.C.S.Ed. 1827; M.D. Edinburgh 1831 (obituary **B.M.J.** (1891), 2:400; Z. Cope, **Florence Nightingale and the doctors** (London, 1958), 27-41; **DNB**).
42. Hector Gavin (1816-1855); L.R.C.S.Ed. 1835; M.D. Edinburgh 1836; F.R.C.S.Ed. 1838; M.R.C.S. 1843 (obituaries **Ass.Med.J.** (1855), 481; **M.T.G.** (1855), 1:479; E.A. Spriggs, 'Hector Gavin, M.D., F.R.C.S.E (1815-1855) - his life, his work for the Sanitary Movement, and his accidental death in the Crimea.' **Med.Hist.**, 28 (1984), 283-292; **DNB**).
43. **DNB**
44. **Kinglake**, 7:485-487.
45. Ibid., 485-486

46. The preliminary recommendations were printed "for the use of the Cabinet" on 16 April 1855, forming a document of only ten pages. The final report was entitled, **Report to the Right Hon. Lord Panmure G.C.B. etc., Minister at War, of the proceedings of the Sanitary Commission despatched to the Seat of War in the East, 1855-56, March, 1857.**
47. Document of 16 April 1855, 1-4.
48. Ibid., 5-7.
49. Ibid., 9.
50. Ibid., 10.
51. For an account of this incident, see **Lancet** (1855), 1:302; **M.T.G.** (1855), 1:507-508.
52. Gavin Milroy (1805-1886); M.D. Edinburgh 1828; F.R.C.P. 1853 (obituary **B.M.J.** (1886), 1:425-426; DNB; **Munk**).
53. **The Times**, 22.8.1855.
54. Cook, **Nightingale**, 1:220-221.
55. **Royal Commission**, 380.
56. **Kinglake**, 7:391.
57. J. Hall, **Observations on the report of the Sanitary Commissioners in the Crimea** (London, 1857), 51.
58. Sir John McNeill (1795-1883); M.D. Edinburgh 1814; assistant-surgeon I.M.S. 1816; (obituary **Lancet** (1883), 1:932; **Crawford**; DNB).
59. DNB.
60. Kirby, **Smith**, 294.
61. **Cantlie**, 2:163-164.
62. Ibid., 148.
63. **Report of the Commission of Enquiry into the Supplies of the British Army in the Crimea, with the evidence annexed**, 1856. The first version was forwarded from Constantinople in 1856. A second edition was published in England in 1857 and included additional material on the sickness and mortality rates of the army in the Crimea.
64. A. Benson, ed., **The letters of Queen Victoria 1837-1861**, (London, 1908), 3:174-175.
65. **Report of the Chelsea Board** London, 1856.
66. The whitewashing of the High Command by the Chelsea Board greatly angered Miss Nightingale (Cope, **Nightingale**, 69-72).
67. **Kinglake**, 7:326-327.
68. A. Tulloch, **The Crimean Commission and the Chelsea Board** (London, 1857).
69. **Cantlie**, 2:156.
70. Cook, **Nightingale**, 1:229-230.
71. **Brit.For.Med.Chir.Rev.**, 18 (1855), 279-282.
72. Robert Lyons (1826-1886); M.B. Dublin 1848; L.R.C.S.I. 1849; F.K.Q.C.P.I. 1861 (obituary **B.M.J.** (1886) 2:1295; C.A. Cameron, **History of the Royal College of Surgeons in Ireland**, Dublin, 1916, 770-771; DNB).
73. William Aitken (1823-1892); L.R.C.S.Ed., M.D. Edinburgh 1848 (obituary **B.M.J.** (1892), 2:54-55; Cope, **Nightingale**, 85-89; DNB).
74. S.M. Mitra, **The life and letters of Sir John Hall** (London, 1911), 376.
75. 'Aitken Letters.' A large number of the letters sent by Aitken to various people at home have survived, and they give a clearer picture of the Pathology Commission in action than is found elsewhere.
76. A preliminary report, **Report on the pathology of the diseases of the East**, was published in 1856 (reviewed in **Brit.For.Med.Chir.Rev.**, 18 (1856), 279-282). The final report, with the same title, was published in 1856 (reviewed in **Brit.For.Med.Chir.Rev.**, 20 (1857), 30-42).
77. **Brit.For.Med.Chir.Rev.**, 20 (1857), 42.
78. Cameron, **Surgeons in Ireland**, 770. Lyons was awarded the Crimean medal, with a clasp for Sebastopol, and was thanked by the French for rendering assistance to their wounded after the battle of the Tchernaya in August 1855.

CHAPTER XII

THE CIVIL SURGEONS AND THE CIVIL HOSPITALS (1855-1856)

In 1854 there was no organisation by which civilian doctors could be called up in an emergency. Although civilian practitioners were attached to the Militia reserves (which had been formed before 1800), these doctors were available for home service only. In contrast, in France a regulation had been passed to enrol a reserve of civilian doctors to be called up in any emergency, and many were already attached in peace-time to army hospitals. Had the battle of the Alma not taken place at such a long distance from Britain, no doubt volunteers would have flocked to the scene, as after Waterloo. In 1854 there were many doctors fired with the patriotic fervour which had seized the country, and after hostilities broke out some travelled to the East without having acquired commissions in the Army. Richard Mackenzie, for instance, arrived with a letter of introduction from Lord Aberdeen to Raglan, and was at once attached to the 79th Regiment, then in Bulgaria. He was allowed to wear the uniform but had no official rank. There were other such volunteers who had recommendations from persons of influence, and there were those who had introductions directly to certain regimental commanders who felt at liberty to employ them personally and, in some cases, to negotiate for them an acting rank of assistant-surgeon.

A few doctors went out merely as visitors, either from curiosity or in the hope of gaining experience of military surgery as a means of advancing their reputations at home. Thus, the young Glasgow graduate, George Macleod[1], was keen to visit the seat of war. He had an introduction from Sir James McGrigor to Hall. "I now trouble you with a letter in favour of Dr. Macleod, a gentleman of high literary as well as professional attainments: he does not want an appointment but that he may have your sanction to visit in the British Hospitals occasionally and to see what is doing there. Dr. Macleod is the son of the Rev. Dr. Macleod, Dean of the Chapel

Royal, Edinburgh."[2] Macleod took passage early in March 1854 in a private yacht going to the Mediterranean. At Malta he joined a troopship for Constantinople (in which Mackenzie travelled also). For a few weeks he saw something of the work in the Scutari hospitals. Then, as he records in his journal, "made a run to Varna to see if I could get employment ... fever and cholera rampant, (no job)".[3] Somewhat disappointed, he returned home leisurely, visiting various European capitals en route. Shortly after his return he met the mother of Captain George Campbell of the 1st Dragoons, who had been severely wounded at the Alma. Mrs. Campbell asked Macleod to go out and look after her son and to accompany him home when convalescent. Macleod travelled in November by the quickest route and found his patient in the Crimea (presumably in hospital at Balaclava) "in some straits". He eventually had him transferred to Scutari. In this visit of about six weeks Macleod had the opportunity of observing what was happening in the Crimea and at Scutari. On his return with his patient to London, in January 1855, he was interviewed by Herbert, who was always ready to get direct evidence of the state of the medical services from those who could speak from personal experience. Macleod must have made a good impression for very soon he was offered a post of surgeon to the Civil Hospital now being established at Smyrna. He accepted and at once returned to the East. His further activities, originating from these chance experiences, are recorded later.

Herbert and Smith, the Director-General, had from the autumn of 1854 many offers of help from the doctors at home. The shortage of medical officers that was publicised in the press placed considerable pressure on the authorities to bring in the civilian element. Prior to February 1855 there was no firm policy to employ civilians. After the Alma there had been an increasing flow of young recruits to the medical service, but these had only been taken on in the rank of assistant-surgeon, either with a full commission or with a temporary acting rank. Older and experienced doctors were not disposed to accept such low rank and low pay. On 12 February, 1855, **The Times** commented on -

> the want of medical officers qualified by their experience to take

> positions of responsibility in the various hospitals of the Bosphorous, as in the Archipelago ... All medical officers are more or less affected in health by the difficulties with which they had to contend and the individual efforts required of them to compensate for the defects of their departments ... A step in advance has, however, within the last few days been made. We are likely at length to enjoy the admixture of the civil element in the medical administration of the Army.[4]

The latter comment followed an announcement by the Duke of Newcastle, in the House of Lords, on 29 January. "In the present state of the Army and of the hospitals, it will be absolutely necessary, in spite of all opposition and all profound feelings to the contrary, to introduce into the Army Hospitals the civilian element."[5]

Before describing the action taken by the Government to establish hospitals staffed by civilians it is appropriate to record the attachment of civilian doctors to the base hospitals at Scutari which had already taken place. It will be seen that this was a haphazard scheme, neither well planned nor very successful.

From October 1854 onwards a small number of civilian doctors were attached to Scutari and some were seconded to the Crimea for duty. A list is available of "Civil Surgeons" who served at Scutari.[6] The list is incomplete. For instance, Dr. Pyemont Smith spent three months at Scutari (see Chapter VI) but is omitted. The total of recorded doctors is 30. It is not clear how these civilian doctors were appointed and with few exceptions their status in the hospitals is uncertain. Pyemont Smith was possibly sponsored by a charity in Leeds, the Director-General having approved his appointment. One can only assume that most of the others were approved by Smith, that a few were in practice in Turkey, and that some arrived on their own initiative and offered their services directly to Menzies. Their remuneration is not known accurately but we know that as far as allowances and rations were concerned they were rated as army captains, and probably received little more than an assistant-surgeon. According to the official list, 22 of them served entirely in the Scutari Hospitals, six served all their time in the Crimea, and four served both at Scutari and in the Crimea.

Only 18 of these civilian doctors have been so far traced.

In alphabetical order, they are Hugh Birt[7], Anthony Brabazon[8], Charles Bryce[9], William Cullen[10], Patrick Fraser[11], Frederick Gant[12], Henry Holl[13], Edward Howard[14], James Hughes[15], Robert Lyons[16], William McEgan[17], George Macleod[18], Robert Mason[19], Peter Pincoffs[20], Henry Rooke[21], Henry Rowdon[22], Robert Woolaston[23], and John Wordsworth[24]. The average age of those who have been traced was 35 (in 1855), and therefore probably most had been reluctant to join up as assistant-surgeons. All but one (Macleod) had qualified before 1850. About half of this group had hospital appointments or were in teaching posts before the war and half were general practitioners. Three of these men published memoirs: Bryce, Gant, and Pincoff.

Bryce had been sent out to conduct a special investigation. In his memoirs he records how, by the time of his arrival in February 1855, the efficiency of the hospital establishments had greatly improved from the "Fort Pitt routine" of 1854. He worked at Koulali and gave much more favourable reports of its hygienic state than did the Commissioners. Bryce visited all the Scutari hospitals, the field hospitals in the Crimea, and the French hospitals in Constantinople. Of six of the latter he reported that only one was satisfactory, all the others comparing very unfavourably with the British hospitals, being dirty, foul-smelling, and ill-ventilated. He was at great pains to correct the general misconception that the French medical service was superior to the British and was in a good position to judge, since he had worked in a French hospital for a month. He describes how late in 1855 conditions were so bad in the French establishments that the British offered them a hospital of 100 beds, complete with medical staff and stores. At that time the French were suffering much more severely than the British from epidemics of scurvy and typhus. The offer was refused but Linton loaned ten doctors (including Bryce) to give assistance. Bryce emphasises the near breakdown of the French Medical Service in the second winter of the war, categorically declaring that "peace was obligatory on France in the Spring of 1856 because of the sanitary state of her Army".

Bryce paid a generous tribute to the army doctors.

> There is no doubt of the fact that the Medical Department shared in the unpreparedness and miscalculations that depended on hurried actions ... But to the failure to make this department the scapegoat for all the sins of all the chiefs and councils at home and abroad, has succeeded the conviction that no branch of the service, military or civil, displayed higher intelligence and heroism, or answered calls of duty more satisfactorily, than did the medical staff of the British Army, from the Director-General to the acting assistant-surgeon.

Bryce supported his contentions by noting that "a larger proportion of medical officers lost their lives during the war than of any other officers throughout the army". He also paid a tribute to Hall, "for initiating the clearing of camps etc. ... steps seconded and prompted by the Sanitary Commissioners".[25]

Gant wrote an autobiography in his old age and the references to his war service are brief. Of his appointment to Scutari, he wrote "the Crimean campaign had I confess yet other attractions. My love of adventure would alone have led me to seize any opportunity of visiting a land of ancient history". Gant was glad to leave the hardships of the Crimea for Scutari.

> In exchange for the wooden hut without window or chimney to carry away the fumes of a charcoal fire, I was now located in a room having a funnel stove, and windows, a table, chair, and washstand with zinc basin completing my luxuries. In the Crimea meat twice a week was supplied, whether goat or sheep flesh I could not tell ... and this provision, together with rice, yellow Turkish bread and rum in liberal quantity, formed my rations ... In my Turkish domicile I enjoyed an ample supply of all that was needful for the production of energy."

Just before he returned home he had a serious breakdown in health. "Arriving in England May 6, 1856, I was then an emaciated, tottering, back-bowed old man, unknowable to my relations and most intimate friends."[26] However he recovered to live to a ripe old age, when "he wore the thick whiskers and short-cut moustache of the old Crimean officers, and his manners were of the agreeable old-world order".[27]

Like Bryce and unlike Gant, Pincoffs published his experiences immediately after the end of the war, in 1857.[28] When he first arrived at Scutari, in April 1855, he found the total numbers in the hospitals down to 2,000, the Barrack Hospital half empty, and the hospitals "cleaned up" except for the persistence of vermin. The beneficial influences of Miss Nightingale and her nurses "were perceptible". He complained, however, of some lack of cleanliness and that the "English habit of spitting does not improve floors." Although up to this time there had been a general impression that the French hospitals were much cleaner and much better organised than the British hospitals Pincoffs considered that the reverse was the case. Giving his views on the employment of civil practitioners by the Army, Pincoffs considered that they had a better chance of attaining "high professional acquirements" than the military doctors. He thought that the civil doctors should each have been given charge of more beds and the regulars so released for service at the front. He resented the fact that the civil doctors were under the orders of divisional staff-surgeons and deplored the difficulty the civil doctors had in requisitioning medicines and stores directly. Pincoffs believed that the deployment of civil doctors was largely a failure, partly because an original intention that they should not be fettered by army regulations was ignored. He quoted a directive sent by Smith to the Inspector-General of the Scutari Hospitals, in March 1855.

> Her Majesty's Government has decided to resort to the services of a certain number of civil medical practitioners, - to be employed temporarily at the military hospitals with the standing of Surgeons and Physicians: they are to be engaged with the understanding that they are not to be interfered with in the discharge of their professional duties, or in other words they are to be left to the exercise of their own judgement in the treatment of the sick and wounded ... You will take care to place a sufficient number of Assistant Surgeons under their direction to enable them to discharge the duties which will be entrusted to them.

Pincoffs was very critical of the organisation of the Army Medical Department, such as the procedure whereby Army Boards were required to sit and report before approval could be given for the most minor activities. He poured scorn on one army custom. "I have wondered what could be the use of the edifying performance of patients (even cripples) as well as orderlies flying into a tetanic posture, when on the entrance of a medical officer the order 'attention' is bawled out." He deplored the lack of teaching facilities at Scutari for the younger doctors. From the start Pincoffs developed a great admiration for Miss Nightingale, and she regarded him as an exceptional doctor. In fact, much of Pincoffs' book was devoted to suggestions for reform of the Army Medical Service. He was very critical of the way in which the senior medical officers in the hospitals were overwhelmed with administrative duties, at the expense of their clinical responsibilities. In contrast, he admired some aspects of the 'Intendance Militaire' in the French medical service, by which a separate group of staff dealt entirely with the administration. He had strong views on the education of army doctors, particularly in hygiene, feigned diseases, and the different manifestations of diseases encountered abroad. He considered that England was far behind the Continent, throughout which Army Medical Schools had long been established, in Paris, in Vienna, in Copenhagen, in St. Petersburg, and in Berlin, all before 1800.

Of these civilian doctors, Rowdon was the only one to be asked to give evidence to the Royal Commission after the war.[29] He was questioned on his duties and responsibilities at the Barrack Hospital. He indicated that he was subject to no other supervision than that of the Inspector-General and had the entire clinical responsibility for 100 beds. While Rowdon had power to requisition medicines and stores he deplored the fact that junior doctors could not do so. He was critical of the care given by the regular army doctors to their patients. While he approved of the employment of civil surgeons he was against the creation of civil hospitals. In his evidence he made much of the fact that he had been relieved of his post unjustifiably and that on his return to England had received no acknowledgement of his services, which (he averred) had been exemplary. He had sought an interview with Smith in London, who had indicated that Rowdon had "given a lot of trouble" During his interrogation it emerged that Rowdon had had numerous arguments with MacGrigor and other senior officers. Regrettably Rowdon appears to have been a tactless witness and a trouble-maker. His advocacy of the integration of civil doctors in an emergency, provided that their position was clarified, did not carry much weight in view of his personal attitudes and grievances.

The contribution made by this group of civilian doctors may not have been of great significance. However, most had a genuine desire to help, they had given up their practices with no guarantee that they would be reinstated on their return home, and they had exposed themselves to all the hazards of the hospitals, and, in some cases, of the front line. There were no deaths reported amongst them but some contracted serious illnesses. They were given little thanks for their efforts and, unlike those appointed to the Civil Hospitals, no financial bonus to compensate them for loss of income from their practices. It cannot be said that the regular medical officers accepted them at all generously. Aitken's comments on their unpopularity have already been quoted (in Chapter XI). It must be concluded that individual voluntary service was too unsystematic to be of much use, not least because the status in the hospitals of individual volunteers was seldom clearly defined.

Another group of volunteers worked as hospital dressers. A list of 46 Hospital Dressers attached to the medical service shows that all but one were appointed between December 1854 and March 1855.[30] These were medical students who had already entered their clinical years (some medical schools did not favour the release of their senior students). Most were attached initially to the hospitals at Scutari and 24 did all their period of service there. Five were in the Crimea during the whole period of service. Eleven spent part in Scutari and part in the Crimea. Three were temporarily transferred to hospital transports, one of them doing five voyages. Little is known about their duties. At Scutari it seems that in certain wards they did all the dressings. Some of the nurses commented that this was much to their annoyance, since in other wards the nurses were so employed and regarded this duty as theirs by right. It may be presumed that some medical officers took the trouble to teach the students, but nothing appears to have been done in the way of organised instruction for them, such as lectures or demonstrations. For those who were keen to learn, the experience may have been useful in their training. In the Crimea they were probably attached to the general or regimental hospitals, but information on this is lacking. Some stayed on for over a year but most left after three to six months of service.

It has been possible to trace 23 dressers who subsequently went back to their medical schools and qualified. None achieved any prominence in their subsequent careers. Most of those traced became general practitioners with the exception of six who joined the Army after qualification. Those who enlisted were John Atkinson, Robert Elliott, Charles Gray, John Stewart, Joseph Taylor, and Samuel Woodfull.[31] Four of these six were Irish. We can only speculate on what happened to those who cannot be traced. Some may have been put off medicine as a career by the horrors of the winter in Scutari. Some who had volunteered may have been restless characters who sought adventure, and had no real impetus to qualify. Three are said to have died on service (Fell, Harrison, Flewitt). No doubt there were some whose health was greatly damaged. Regrettably no dresser seems to have written of his experiences. In general the employment of medical students was ill-advised, but this question was not discussed by the Royal Commission after the war.

Brief mention may be again made of the small convalescent hospital at Abydos, which has some civilian doctors on its staff. Little is known of these, or indeed of the army doctors attached to Abydos. The hospital admitted 662 patients and was most probably used in the main as a staging post for invalided patients awaiting transport home.[32]

In addition to those civilian doctors who were appointed from Britain through official channels, or at least via official recommendations, there were a number of doctors who were working in the East and who lent their services more or less unofficially. Dr. J. Bowen-Thomson, after working in England, went out in 1843 to the British Hospital in Damascus, and then became an Inspector of Health to the Turkish Government, in which post he brought reforms to the Turkish hospitals. At the outbreak of the war he volunteered to assist the army medical department. It was written that there had been "nothing finer than the conduct of this noble member of the medical profession to the wounded after the battle of the Alma". Nothing more is known of his war service, where he worked, or with whom, until he was taken ill in the Crimea early in August 1855. He was transferred to Scutari but on his arrival, as he was a civilian and his name was not on the official landing list, there was considerable delay before he was taken ashore. He died in Koulali Hospital of "malignant typhoid".[33]

Finally, some civilian practitioners served with the Turkish Army in what was known as the Turkish Contingent. An account of this group of doctors is given in Chapter XVI.

SMYRNA CIVIL HOSPITAL: DOCTORS AND NURSES

The proposal to establish Civil Hospitals staffed entirely by civilian doctors, with a minimum of army administration, greatly offended the army medical officers. The Director-General should have been glad of any means of taking the pressure off his hard-worked staff but Hall resented the scheme. He complained to Smith of the shoal of new arrivals sponsored, officially or sometimes casually, by the War Office, all of whom he considered were drawing excessive salaries. "Certainly the Government has fostered these high pretensions by sending out pathologists, Sanitary Commissioners, and I don't know what 'issioners, with high salaries and no occupation. Then we have female inspectors and Directors of Nurses and I don't know what beside."[34] He was to complain later that "Myers [sic] who has charge of one hospital ... receives £2000 a year, has furnished quarters provided for him, and a free table at the expense of 4s 2d a day". [35] Hall's own pay was only £1,788 a year and his responsibilities were very much heavier. His attitude reflected the feelings of most of the regular officers. To many of them the greatest insult was that the plan suggested that the army doctors were poorly trained, of limited experience, and incapable of dealing with the sick and wounded by themselves. The medical journals published numerous complaints from anonymous individuals. "I object to the civil element as interfering with our promotion ... we who do the work and lie exposed to the dangers of battle while disgracefully remunerated."[36] Again - "The public now labour under the delusion that the soldier ... will come at once under the care of those well-paid civilians and will be indebted to them for that care which it has been falsely alleged was not given by the Army Surgeon".[37] It has to be admitted that the scheme did give rise to misunderstanding. In the estimation of the public the plan seemed to aim at sending out experienced and competent operating surgeons, and there was no understanding that the greatest problems concerned the sick rather than the wounded.

There were fears that the selection of doctors would be made by influence rather than by the recognition of talent, and that the appointments would be in the hands of cliques in the prestigious London Teaching Hospitals. On 22 January, 1855, the War Office sent out a circular to the "Governors of the Principal Hospitals and Dispensaries". "I am directed by Lord Panmure to request your aid and concurrence in his organisation of a special civil medical staff to assist the military staff at the seat of war."[38] It was indicated that civil posts would be safeguarded and that compensation would be made for the loss of private practice. In general the medical press approved the project, but there were some reservations. The **Medical Times and Gazette** considered that senior physicians and surgeons, anxious to volunteer, but unwilling to join up as assistant-surgeons, would offer their services.[39] In a leader, perhaps written by Spencer Wells, the journal gave its opinion.

> The establishment of a Civil Hospital appears to be the most effectual, because the most practical, method of answering those who defend the present system. We, then, are among those who thus rejoice that at Smyrna there is to be opened, for the reception of the sick, an establishment unrestrained by the rules of the service ... the question is to be fairly tried: and if on trial it is found that the Civil Hospitals work better than the military hospitals i.e. than hospitals the surgeons to which are trammelled by the traditions of the service and fettered by codes of Army Regulations, then without doubt a thorough reform of the present system will be allowed to be made. We regret that attempts should have been made to prejudice Military Surgeons against the Civil Hospital. It has been said that its establishment is an insult to the Army Medical Department. We believe the reasons we have used in its favour fully answer this personal argument. Again it is said how well these civil servants are to be paid ... for our part we think the sums in question are too small.[40]

There were further comments a few weeks later in a leader entitled "Civil and Military Surgeons".

> The introduction of the civil element by breaking down the system of routine, by consigning medical duties to be performed by medical men, by giving to the medical authorities the supreme control over the hospitals, and by promoting and encouraging talent and industry without reference to favouritism and seniority - could tend we hope in no small degree to

consolidate the union of the civil and military services.[41] The opinions in the **Lancet** and the **Association Medical Journal** were similar, but were more critical of the chosen site of the hospital and more vociferous in their condemnation of the methods of selection of the civil physicians and surgeons.

In December 1854, as the Scutari hospitals became increasingly over-crowded the need for additional beds, particularly for convalescents, became clear. The selection of the site of an additional hospital rested with Hall. On 3 January, 1855, he received a report from Staff-Surgeon Thomas Moorhead[42], who had been sent to Smyrna to inspect a barracks "proposed as a convalescent station for the British Troops".[43] Smyrna (now known as Izmir) lies on the Mediterranean coast of Turkey. It was nearly four days by steamship from the Crimea and about a day and a half from Scutari. The accommodation offered was a neglected army barracks, with the usual deficiencies of drainage and ventilation. The building was sited near the shore, below the slopes of a crowded and insanitary town, from which open sewers ran in such close proximity that the ground floor was rendered noisome and unhealthy. Moorhead described the building as in good repair, with three floors arranged in a large central block and two small side wings. He estimated that 648 patients could be accommodated in the larger rooms, and 1,112 if the corridors were used. (The lessons of the disastrous overcrowding in the corridors of the Scutari hospitals had not been learned). The water tanks were reported in good order and "the Pasha of Smyrna, himself a medical man, says the supply can be increased". There was nothing in the report about the insalubrity of the environment or of the climate, subjects which were to be argued interminably for the next few months. Moorhead's account was not very detailed and he had glossed over many deficiencies. Hall, however, accepted the report, and, in January he organised the staffing of the hospital, apparently unaware then of the government proposal to send out civilian doctors. He sent Deputy-Inspector William Humfrey[44], assisted by a staff-surgeon, to commission the hospital. These two officers were joined later by Staff-Surgeon Thomas Hunter[45], and five assistant-surgeons. This small staff was to cope with about 600 patients, admittedly convalescents. "Military nurses and orderlies" were also drafted to Smyrna, but there is no record of female nurses arriving until later. Although Smyrna was in Turkey and hence within the official sphere of influence of Miss Nightingale, she does not appear to have been consulted about the planning of the nursing organisation at Smyrna. Patients began to be admitted in large numbers in February, so that when the civilian staff took over there were about 800, in conditions of gross overcrowding. It was reported that in the period between February and March 993 patients were admitted, and that of these 127 died (13 per cent), a high rate for a convalescent hospital.[46] Clearly much had to be done to improve its sanitary condition.

The staff at Smyrna was to consist of a Medical Superintendent, three Physicians, five Surgeons, six Assistant Physicians, ten Assistant Surgeons, and a Resident Medical Officer. In addition a secretary, nine dispensers, and a civil engineer, were appointed. The only military officer was Colonel Henry Storks.[47] The Medical Superintendent was to be paid £2,000 a year, the Surgeons and Physicians £800-£1,000, and the assistants £200-£600. Contracts were to run for one year and on discharge the doctors were to be awarded a bonus of half their annual salary. There was considerable excitement as the names of likely candidates appeared. Competition for the posts was keen, and more than a hundred candidates appeared in the first two weeks. "Are you going to Smyrna?" was the constant question heard in the corridors of the London hospitals. When the final list appeared there was considerable criticism in the medical journals. The first choice for the post of Superintendent withdrew his application within two weeks. At this point the **Lancet** stated -

> We wish we could announce some other resignations in regard to this Smyrna offer, but it would be far better if the project had been abandoned altogether. We cannot but augur much mischief from such a scheme ... of the other appointments made we can only say that most of them are exceedingly objectionable ... God help our country when such men are sent as special messengers of professional amelioration.[48]

In a later leader in the **Lancet**, the question was asked why the successful candidates were mostly from the London hospitals. "We even censure the mode in which the selection of civil practitioners has been made".[49]

There were accusations of "nepotism and jobbing" and the complaint that the majority of the 300 applicants had not even received any acknowledgment of their letters. In both the lay and the medical press there were many comments insisting that the primary need was for experienced surgeons. One was to the effect that surgeons from the mining areas should be selected as they were accustomed to the management of severe trauma.[50] Many of the surgeons who did apply were indeed hopeful of acquiring experience in war surgery, but it was soon all too clear that such opportunities were lacking at Smyrna.

The choice of a Superintendent was obviously of great importance. In January it was announced that Sir John Forbes would take up this post.[51] He was a distinguished physician, editor of the **British and Foreign Medical Review,** and a man of great influence in the medical profession.[52] At 68 he was rather old for a position which was certain to be arduous and difficult, but there was a general approval of his selection and considerable regret when he withdrew. He continued, however, to exert considerable influence in the choice of medical staff. But thereafter trouble began.

It was announced that Dr. John Meyer would replace Forbes, the same Dr. Meyer who had come out with Miss Stanley's party of nurses (as mentioned in Chapter VIII). No-one had heard of him. The **Association Medical Journal** asked - "Who is Dr. Meyer? ... he [has] had no London connection, he might have been to Eton, and he had the M.D. only of a low German university".[53] Worse still, there were suggestions that his appointment was because of his social connections - "married a Shuttleworth, friend of Lord Derby, and it was mainly by Lord Derby's influence he was chosen".[54] Of his clinical and administrative experience in the past little was then known, but he was alleged to have been in the colonial service in Tasmania, in charge of a lunatic asylum.

The criticism of Meyer, often insulting, was to continue for some months. At least one applicant withdrew when he heard of Meyer's appointment. This was Andrew Barclay, a physician in St. George's Hospital. He wrote to the medical press on 24 March criticising various aspects of the plans for Smyrna and attacking Meyer, in particular because of his foreign qualification.[55] However, on 14 April almost all the medical staff at Smyrna signed a letter in reply to Barclay, in which they expressed their complete confidence in Meyer.[56] There is evidence that Meyer returned to England from Scutari late in January to be briefed for his task, and most likely he was consulted regarding the selection of other staff. But Richard Grainger, a senior surgeon of considerable influence in the Royal College of Surgeons, together with Forbes, appear to have had the most say in choosing the candidates.

The following doctors were appointed, in addition to John Meyer[57]. The Physicians were John Barclay[58], Septimus Gibbon[59], and Arthur Leared[60]. The Surgeons were Holmes Coote[61], Carsten Holthouse[62], George Macleod, Thomas Spencer Wells[63], and John Wordsworth. The Assistant Physicians were Charles Coote[64], William Cullen[65], Robert Martin[66], George Rolleston[67], Richard Wilkinson[68], and Barnes Wood[69]. The Assistant Surgeons were Edward Atkinson[70], Edward Complin[71], John Eddowes[72], John Falconer[73], John Hulke[74], Thomas Hornidge[75], John Jardine[76], James Lakin[77], Robert McDonnel[78], and John Streatfeild[79]. In addition, Dr. Ranke, a German, was designated Resident Medical Officer but nothing is known about him. Macleod and Wordsworth had previously worked as civilian volunteers at Scutari, as noted earlier. Complin was the only Smyrna doctor who died while in the East. The average age of the Surgeons and Physicians on appointment was 32: Gibbon and Macleod were both under 30. The average age of the Assistant-Physicians was 31 and of the Assistant-Surgeons 26. At least 12 of the medical staff (including two of the seniors) had been qualified less than five years. About a dozen of those selected had associations with London hospitals - despite the criticism, not an excessive proportion. Of the talent and character of many of these medical officers there can be no doubt when their subsequent careers are examined. Among them we find two Presidents of the Royal College of Surgeons of England and a President of the Royal College in Ireland, five Professors in British medical schools, and numerous distinguished surgeons and physicians who became senior consultants in the teaching hospitals or the larger provincial hospitals of Great Britain. Add to all this the remarkable number of four Fellows of the Royal Society and it is readily seen that the Smyrna group was to make some impact on British medicine and science in the second half of the century.

The first of the medical staff to arrive was Spencer Wells, on 1 March.[80] All the others reached Smyrna by the end of the month, when Meyer took charge. Meanwhile Wells was made responsible for the surgical division. He and his civilian colleagues worked amicably with the military doctors in coping with a large influx of patients. The civil staff gave a farewell dinner to Humfrey and Beatson, since "it was felt that these gentlemen had contended successfully with very great difficulties and had smoothed the way for their successors in a manner which called for public acknowledgment".[81].

Between February and November 1855, 1,887 patients were admitted to Smyrna, of whom 154 died (8 per cent).[82] According to the hospital transport records, 1,685 patients were brought direct to Smyrna from the Crimea. Most of the admissions were between February and May (1,311 cases), but there was an influx in October (419 cases). The average rate of admissions per month was 188, with the highest figure in February (737) and the lowest in September (17). These figures support the doctors' complaints that there was often too little work for them. Most patients were convalescent and the diagnosis was often uncertain. Fevers accounted for 416 admissions, with 38 deaths (9 per cent); bowel diseases for 345 admissions, with 67 deaths (20 per cent); frostbite for 162 admissions, with 18 deaths (9 per cent); scurvy for 137 admissions, with 14 deaths (10 per cent); and rheumatic diseases for 107 admissions, with 4 deaths (4 per cent). Only 32 wounded were admitted, with no deaths.

When the civil staff arrived Smyrna was overcrowded. A report of 17 March stated that "a low form of contagious typhus was very prevalent and fatal, between 90 and 100 patients landed a month before having died".[83] Clearly there was a fever epidemic. There was much argument as to the nature of this fever and as to whether it was brought in by the patients or arose in the hospital. About the same time it was reported -

> The principle cases were either chronic dysentery or diarrhoea, mostly of a scorbutic character - some cases of remittent fever - a few pulmonary affections - and a great number of frost-bites ... In one case hospital gangrene of a very severe type, had appeared.[84]

On 24 March there were

> over 60 cases of frost-bite in hospital. At first the cases of fever had proved so infectious and so many orderlies died ... that a separate portion of the building had been devoted to fever cases, the patients in this division being less crowded. The plan had been in operation a week on the 24th and, as far as could be ascertained, appeared to have been very successful.[85]

After March there was concern about the failure to use the hospital fully and this produced endless discussion about its salubrity. For further details of the medical problems encountered we must turn to the proceedings of the 'Smyrna Medico-Chirurgical Society'. It is likely that this Society, a reflection of the great proliferation of medical societies of all types which was a feature of the profession in Victorian England, was organised by the dynamic Spencer Wells. Meyer was elected President and Wells Vice-President. There were frequent meetings from April until July, and all of these were reported in the medical press.

On 11 April Wells delivered the Introductory Address. He contrasted the organisation of military and civil systems, with the separation in the latter of administrative and clinical duties. He favoured the appointment in Civil Hospitals of a staff of trained female nurses, civilian orderlies and civilian cooks. Of the arrival of the Lady Nurses he had this to say. "I entertained very considerable misgivings as to the propriety or probable success of this experiment. But a very few days served to dispel all forebodings of evil, and to raise my most sanguine hopes of good." He believed the system by which "ladies of education" were put in charge of the female trained nurses was most successful, and "our example being followed at home may be given to a charitable and wider field opened for the labours of the women of England". Wells then went on to discuss a question of great importance: "Should we or should we not segregate cases of this fever which still prevails here?" When he had arrived he had found that the fever cases were scattered throughout all the wards. He had at once proposed that fever cases should be placed in special wards, but Humfrey thought that this would increase infection among the staff. The fever continued to spread and it was soon agreed to treat these cases in a separate ward in the upper storey of the hospital, in uncrowded conditions. Wells had argued that this would expose only one third of the staff to infection, and he was convinced that the policy was successful. In the discussion which followed his paper not everyone supported his contention.[86] Finally, Wells urged his colleagues to undertake clinical research. "We have large opportunities for observation in a new field ... with regard to fevers, for example, we have had but too many opportunities of tracing the progress and termination of this mysterious class of diseases ... let the records of this Society contain the results of our observations whether negative or positive".[87]

On 30 April Leared read a short general paper on fever and on 18 May Gibbon gave a detailed account of "continued fever" seen in an epidemic at Smyrna. On 9 June Complin read a paper on frost-bite, advising conservative treatment. On 30 July Barclay discussed in great detail the much vexed question of the suitability of Smyrna as a site for an Army Hospital. A lively discussion followed and despite some strong criticisms of the unhealthy condition of the hospital it was resolved - "there is no objection to Smyrna as a site for an Hospital for the Army except that its distance from the seat of war renders it unsuitable for surgical cases". These and other meetings reported in the contemporary numbers of the **Medical Times and Gazette** are evidence of the initial enthusiasm of the medical staff. From the frequent references to pathological investigations, and from the careful assessment of the treatment given in different diseases, it would appear that the standards of practice were high.

No more meetings of the Society were held after July. There was now not very much left to discuss, and some of the doctors had already departed. With the new hospital at Renkioi quite advanced it was clear that Smyrna would soon be closed. There were some who believed that the army doctors had purposely cut down admissions, in order to enforce an early closure of Smyrna. However, the **Medical Times and Gazette** of 4 August commented -

> We cannot believe that any such motives as those imputed by more than one writer have been allowed to operate, and think it more likely that the unhealthy character attributed to Smyrna has had its weight, than [that] any medical Chief would have dared detain men in the Crimea who were not likely to recover for some weeks or months, when a large well-appointed hospital was open to them[88].

The doctors at Smyrna spent some of their spare time exploring the surrounding country. This activity came to an end in July, when Dr. McCraith,[89] a local practitioner, was abducted by robbers. "A vigorous pursuit was commenced by Colonel Storks and the medical officers of the civil hospital, with a body of Turkish Guards." Soon Dr. McCraith was released, on payment of a ransom reported variously as from £50 to £500![90] This incident led to many rumours, including a report that some of the Smyrna staff had been kidnapped and that the rest were anxious to leave, "to escape the horrors and dangers of brigandage".[91]

Many of the medical officers were becoming restless, the surgeons in particular because of their lack of opportunities to operate. As early as June, Wells took two weeks' leave and visited the Crimea, Scutari and Renkioi. All this he described in a long letter to the medical press. He reported that there were 2,500 vacant beds at Scutari. Of Renkioi he wrote -"I feel convinced that these buildings, when completed, will form an Hospital, not only superior to any of our own now in existence in the East, but very far superior to any of the French Hospitals".[92] Macleod was the first to be employed officially in the Crimea. He was followed later by Complin, Wordsworth, Eddowes, Hulke, Jardine, McDonnel, Roberts, and Ranke. Holmes Coote and Spencer Wells went to Renkioi in August, but Meyer stayed at Smyrna until the hospital closed in December. By then only Rolleston and three other junior doctors remained, hence it must be presumed that the rest left for home before December. Most of the female nurses also went home, apart from a few who transferred to Renkioi or Scutari. Miss Nightingale was not very enthusiastic about taking on any of them. Storks, the Military Commandant, took over from Paulet at Scutari in September 1855, and Brunton the Engineer, had gone to Renkioi in June, to supervise the erection of the hutted hospital.

It was reported early in March, 1855, that "a great proportion of the military nurses and orderlies, as they are termed, have been replaced by civil orderlies and female nurses from England, and by eighteen lady nurses, under Mrs. Holmes Coote, the lady Superintendent".[93] Nothing has been discovered concerning the selection of "civil orderlies", but most of the "female nurses" and the "lady nurses" were chosen by the committee which had sent out Miss Stanley's party. By this time it appears that Lady Canning had taken charge of the Committee. She was in constant correspondence with Lady Stratford at Constantinople, offering to send out more nurses, at first to Scutari and later to Smyrna. Miss Nightingale did not want more nurses of any kind. Lady Canning wrote -

> Miss Nightingale and Dr. Cumming both say that they have too many ... Miss Nightingale has evidently a great objection to all nurses not immediately under her and as her rights, and of these I think she likes the fewer the better, she is always trying to prevent any more from being sent out. Now if Civil Hospitals are to be, nurses must be employed, otherwise the doctors will not go to them.[94]

As already noted, Miss Nightingale had no interest in the selection of the nursing staff for Smyrna. Indeed she never visited Smyrna, although there is evidence that Mrs. Bracebridge went there about April, presumably at Miss Nightingale's request.

From the start Lady Canning was in contact with Meyer over the despatch of medical comforts to the new hospital. She was soon selecting nurses, and it is possible that some of the newly appointed medical officers, including Meyer himself, were consulted. The committee did not appoint the superintendent of nurses. Lady Canning wrote - "they have got a Mrs. Holmes Coote, wife of one of the surgeons for Smyrna, so that is sure to do well".[95] There was criticism of the appointment of Mrs.

CHAPTER XII

Coote as Superintendent, on account both of her reported salary of £500 and of her alleged lack of previous nursing experience.

On their arrival at Smyrna the first impression made by the lady nurses was favourable.

> The few days these ladies had done their duty had been quite sufficient to convince those who had previously entertained doubts as to the utility of such an order of nurses, of the very great assistance they can and will render. Their extreme kindness and patient attention to the sick - the ready comprehension of directions - the perfect manner in which they were enabled to keep these directions in mind by the use of notebooks - the confidence with which they could be entrusted with wines and spirits ... their excellent cookery of sago, arrowroot, light puddings, and various drinks, have established beyond all question, that if they only continue as they have begun, this experiment in the establishment of hospital sisterhoods must prove a successful one.[96]

This generous appraisal of the lady nurses, much more generous than that accorded to the lady nurses at Scutari, was to be borne out by their further service. Clearly the doctors appreciated their worth and many were to take home a new attitude towards nursing reforms in their own hospitals. Meyer was to report to the Royal Commission after the war that the professional nurses "worked uncommonly well". Of the lady nurses he said - "A good many were found unfit, from one reason or another, and several were sent home, and after that those that remained did very well indeed ... few are experienced but they are intelligent and will carry out the orders given". But of Mrs. Holmes Coote he reported - "Our matron was not particularly good".[97]

One of the lady nurses published her recollections anonymously but the domestic details she gives are not very informative. She noted the death of one nurse from fever, Miss Drusilla Smythe, and stated that many suffered severe illness. Mrs. Holmes Coote resigned about June, transferring to Renkioi with her husband, where she gave birth to a daughter. She was replaced by Mrs. Le Mesurier, whose husband was a medical officer in the Turkish Contingent, but she died at Smyrna later in the year.

How should the Smyrna experiment be assessed? When the Smyrna doctors returned home some said that they had wasted their time, while others believed that the hospital had worked well and set a useful precedent. Meyer was said to have made some critical comments on his staff.

> Many of the young assistants were first rate men, and conspicuous amongst them was Mr. Rolleston. The Seniors made endeavour to treat the Juniors as subordinates in a professional sense, to work as clinical clerks under them. This the young men would not submit to, and the good sense of Dr. Meyer put a veto upon it. He gave them individual care of cases, and looked to the Seniors for general assistance only. He found the junior surgeons, he told me, pretty good physicians, and the junior physicians pretty fair surgeons. The division into physicians and surgeons, but with no rigid demarcation, was found to work well.[98]

As far as can be judged, the medical staff had maintained good relations with each other, turning their hands to anything required of them. In the medical press adverse criticism had been frequent, but in July comments became more favourable - "It very soon became evident that the experiment was in many respects a success".[99] Yet to some observers the hospital had been thought doomed to failure from the start. In retrospect, blame was placed for its limited success on Hall, in particular for choosing a site so far from the Crimea. However when he did this he understood that Smyrna was to be a convalescent rather than a general establishment. It was the authorities at home who made a major error in sending out a staff which included more surgeons than physicians, thus failing to realise that medical cases were certain to out-number the surgical cases.

The experiment at Smyrna did at least show that soldiers could be treated satisfactorily in a hospital with civil staff. The civil administration very quickly corrected defects bequeathed by the original military staff. Sutherland, of the Sanitary Commission, inspected Smyrna and spoke highly of its organisation. It is true that a select Committee on the Medical Department of the Army (appointed in 1856) totally condemned the creation of Civil Hospitals, but this Committee largely consisted of regular medical officers who were biassed in their views.

The Royal Commission after the war made no real attempt to evaluate the work of the Civil Hospitals (or of the Civil Surgeons). Only one member of the Smyrna staff gave evidence, Dr. Meyer.[100] He was questioned in some detail about the differences between military and civil administrations. He stated that the civil administration had many advantages. But his opinions were not given much consideration and no firm views were expressed by the Commission as to the advantages or otherwise of the establishment of Civil Hospitals. Hall's evidence was very different. He stated categorically of the Civil Hospitals - "I think they were of no use and very expensive". When asked why he thought they were of no use he replied - "Because they were built when we had upwards of 3,000 beds vacant in our hospitals ... besides both of them were out of the way for us. I advised that a hospital should be built at Sinope". He agreed however that if the sickness had increased in the army, "they would have been better than nothing". With reluctance he admitted that a few of the civilian doctors had been of use to him in the Crimea. To the suggestion that the Army had benefited from the presence of experienced civilian doctors he replied sharply. "Some who went there had not that experience that their pay would entitle them to have ... some came out for practice ... some of these gentlemen were not men of standing and experience."[101] Hall never got over the fact that in comparison with the regulars the civilian doctors were better paid. The evidence given by Rowdon has already been quoted. Beatson, who had been at Smyrna in February and March, was called by the Commission but was asked no questions about the hospital.

From its conception the Smyrna Hospital was bedevilled by political machinations and by jealousies. Smith had never favoured the scheme but he had to bow to the wishes of his superiors in the Government. When it was clear that the admission rate to Smyrna had begun to fall rapidly, an order was sent to Smith to fill both the Smyrna and Renkioi hospitals with patients. As Hall remarked - "fearful, I suppose, that questions might be asked in Parliament on the subject". Hall had already reported to Smith - "I send you the correspondence about forwarding patients to the civil establishment at Smyrna. Mr. Hawes' reason would amuse you, I think. It was not that they were requiring accommodation but that the expensive civil hospital employed by the Government might have occupation."[102] Hall had never envisaged that the wounded should be sent to Smyrna. On 23

March he had written to the Quarter-Master General - "I am most unwilling to send wounded men there if I can avoid it, the hospital establishments at Smyrna and Abydos are full, and as typhoid fever is reported to have made its appearance in the hospital at Smyrna it would not be desirable to send wounded there during its continuance".[103] Hall's policy was now to hold the wounded in the Crimea until they were fully convalescent. With this in view, he had, by May, increased the hutted accommodation in the Crimea by at least 600 beds. He believed that the wounded should be operated upon urgently near the front and should not be moved in the immediate post-operative period. His reasoning was sound. According to Cantlie, Meyer had complained as early as April that his civilian specialists were idle, and with the lack of acute admissions he could not keep up their interest. The Secretary of State supported Meyer and wrote to the Director-General - "We consider it essential that the civil hospital ... should receive its fair proportion of cases including wounded directly from the Army in the Field".[104] Far from the scene of action, the home authorities had little understanding of the medical and surgical logistics.

THE PRE-FABRICATED HOSPITAL AT RENKIOI

Soon after the plans for Smyrna had been announced there were rumours with respect to the establishment of up to six more Civil Hospitals. In February, 1855, Panmure was reported to have asked Professor Simpson to organise a hospital staffed entirely from Edinburgh.[105] It was even hinted that Simpson himself would go out in charge He had certainly become very interested in the war, but apart from sponsoring some of his young graduates and encouraging the use of chloroform for the wounded he did not become further involved. A deputation to Panmure advocated the formation of a homoeopathic hospital in the East, but this idea was quickly discouraged - "there was no intention to make such a dangerous experiment at the public expense".[106] About the beginning of March, however, a firm decision was taken to organise one other large hospital. The establishment of this hospital involved an extraordinary feat of civil engineering.

On 16 February, Sir Benjamin Hawes, Under-Secretary at the War Office, wrote to his brother-in-law, Isambard Kingdom Brunel, asking him to design a hospital which could be prefabricated in England and shipped out for assembly on a suitable site.[107] To Miss Nightingale Hawes was an arch enemy, opposing by all means possible the introduction of reforms into the Army Medical Service. Of him she was to write - "He was a dictator, an autocrat irresponsible to Parliament, quite unassailable from any questions".[108] Miss Nightingale's subsequent lack of interest in this new hospital may be partly explained by the fact that Hawes initiated the plan - and deserved credit for his untraditional and 'state of the art' proposal.

In 1855 Isambard Brunel was at the peak of his meteoric career as an engineer.[109] Among many other projects, he had completed the Rotherhithe Tunnel under the Thames (begun by his father), and the Great Western Railway. And he had already made a bizarre contribution to medicine. In 1843, while performing a conjuring trick before some children, he inhaled a half-sovereign. Sir Benjamin Brodie was consulted and attempted to remove the obstruction, which he believed was well down the trachea. Brunel himself designed an especially long pair of forceps for Brodie, but there was no success. As his patient was in much discomfort a tracheotomy was done. Meanwhile Brunel sketched out an apparatus consisting of a board on a axle between two uprights, to which he could be strapped and rotated rapidly to the upside-down position, thus using centrifugal force to dislodge the coin. After two attempts the device worked. Brunel wrote to a friend - "At four 1/2, I was safely delivered of my little coin, with hardly an effort it dropped out". The episode of the swallowed coin had much publicity and for several days the British intellectual world waited for Brunel's recovery. Macaulay, on hearing the good news, rushed into the Athenaeum Club shouting "It's out, it's out!" History does not relate whether or not this ingenious technique was ever used again.[110]

Soon after Hawe's request Brunel sent a memorandum to

the Government.[111] He outlined four specifications he thought necessary for a hutted hospital. First, that the units should be easily adaptable to any site, whatever the levels or inclinations. Secondly, that the plan should be capable of expansion to accommodate up to 1,500 patients. Thirdly, that when erected the buildings should provide every possible comfort. Fourthly, that the hospital units should be portable and inexpensive. Brunel proposed that all the wooden ward units should be identical and that they should be connected by covered ways, with detachable sides for use in cold weather. Each unit was to contain two wards, each ward with 26 beds, a nurses' room, surgery, water-closets, and wash places. To each bed 1000 cu.ft. of space was allowed. An elaborate system of ventilation was planned, each hut being fitted with a fan, operated manually, and a rotatory pump which forced fresh air into the hut at floor level. Roof protection was to be provided by a covering of tin sheeting painted white. A separate kitchen unit, constructed of iron, was to be erected, sufficient to serve 1,000 patients. There was also to be an iron building for a laundry. Every detail was considered and planned, including basins, invalid baths, and even supplies of toilet paper (with instructions to the rough soldiery on it use!). An elaborate pumping apparatus, tanks and piping were to be sent out to ensure the ready supply of fresh water. Wooden drainage pipes for the hospital units were proposed. The lighting was to be by candle, as the safest means available.

All these components, it was estimated, could be sent out, for the first phase of providing 500 beds, in five ships. Brunel made a stipulation that all building material and fittings for one unit should be carried in one ship, "so that by no accident, mistake, or confusion, short of the loss of several ships, can there fail to be a certain amount of hospital accommodation provided with every comfort and essential equipment". The specifications were far more elaborate than those of the hospital huts already sent out to the Crimea, which were deficient in ventilation, in comfort, and in many other respects. The cost of Brunel's scheme was estimated at £18 to £22 per bed.

CHAPTER XII

With his usual initiative and industry Brunel completed a contract with the Government in two weeks (much to the chagrin of the War Office Contracts Department). Equally amazing, in another three weeks the first batch of units was ready to leave. Work on the hospital at Renkioi began on 21 May, under the supervision of a Mr. Brunton. He had with him 18 skilled craftsmen from England and there was plenty of local labour. The hospital was ready for use at the beginning of August. It would have been ready earlier if army stores had been sent out as quickly as the building materials.

The first intention had been to site the hospital at or near Scutari, but there was no suitable ground. Sinope, on the Black Sea, was favoured by Hall, because this was nearer the Crimea. Dr. Cowan, a rather young and inexperienced Civil Surgeon waiting at Scutari before going on to Renkioi, was sent (presumably by Dr. Parkes) to inspect Sinope. Dr. Parkes, who was to be Medical Superintendent of the new hospital, stated later that there were transport difficulties and that the climate at Sinope was unfavourable, with frequent damp fog. Renkioi lies on the South-West shore of the Dardanelles, about nine miles from the entrance to the Mediterranean. Parkes described the site: "A healthy soil, abundant and good water, level yet sloping surface, proximity to the sea, good anchorage, tolerably sheltered landing places". Renkioi is 100 miles from Scutari and about the same distance from Smyrna. Parkes estimated that 34 of Brunel's hospital units could be erected comfortably on flat ground, in a long line, or in any other arrangement considered suitable. There was an excellent water supply in the low hills to the South, where a large reservoir was made 70 ft. above the level of the hospital buildings. The position was well-chosen, except that some thought it was too far from the Crimea.[112]

Parkes is said to have discussed with Miss Nightingale where the hospital should be established. She did not apparently have any influence in the planning of both Smyrna and Renkioi, and she did not visit either hospital. She took little interest in the nursing staffs, although both hospitals were within her official sphere of management, as far as nurses were concerned. That she had a poor opinion of Renkioi is shown by a note in Hall's diary in February, 1856. "I have this instant heard that Miss Nightingale has expressed her disapproval of all the sick being sent to Renkioi - as she is all powerful we shall see the result."[113] One cannot but suspect that Miss Nightingale resented the fact that the Government had established the Civil Hospitals without consulting her directly.

Parkes had gone out to prospect in April, 1855. On 6 May he wrote to Panmure to report that a suitable site had been found at Renkioi. He had visited the area with Brunton (the Engineer), Jenner (the Purveyor at Scutari), and Calvert (the British Consul). Some of the details of Brunel's plans were never completed. He originally hoped to have 34 hospital units erected in two parallel lines, providing 1,768 beds. In fact the highest number of beds in occupation at any one time was to be only 642. (Barely 12 huts would have been needed for this number). In a photograph taken from the South side in March 1856 some 15 huts can be distinguished: the huts appear to be quite close together and are connected by short covered ways. A drawing in the **Illustrated Times** about the same date is not very clear, but shows about the same number of units. According to Parkes, accommodation for 300 patients was completed by July, for 500 by August, for 1,500 by January 1856 and, when the hospital closed in March, more than 2,000 patients could have been admitted. In the event, as the accommodation increased the admission rates fell. By March 1856 the hospital had three kitchens and two laundries, as well as separate accommodation for the medical and nursing staff.

A good description of Renkioi was given by **The Times** correspondent on 25 August. He was very impressed,

> Confidence must be placed in the judgement and opinion of Dr. Parkes. He has, after infinite trouble, selected a site which is approved most generally, and no tangible objection of any kind has been raised ... The landing places for the sick are two little bays, one protected from the north wind, the other from south winds ... From the tongue of land which separates them runs a wooden passage, or corridor, which will ultimately be nearly half a mile long. On each side are arranged the 'wooden hospitals'. Each building is formed to receive 50 men ... a longitudinal partition divides each ward into two compartments: at one end are rooms for the wardmaster, orderlies, baths, and necessary stores: at the other end

are lavatories, urinals, and water closets, as complete as at a railway station ... the windows are numerous and supplied with blinds, which do not exclude air: there is an underground apparatus for forcing air into the wards, but if the wind prevails, as at the present moment, there can scarcely be any necessity for artificial ventilation ... Each medical officer has a single boarded compartment, 12 feet by 8 , which serves as a bedroom and sitting room. It is quite innocent of paint or paper and usually contains a camp bed, a wash stand, a deal table and chair; but all the staff appear in good health, cheerful, and contented, and certainly constitute a very efficient and well-informed body of men ... The residence of the Medical Superintendent is but a small wooden hut, divided into four small compartments or rooms, little superior to the rest.[114]

Parkes in his own report described the medical officer's quarters, "10 feet by 8 feet in each unit". He confirmed that each unit was divided into two wards, 80 feet by 40 feet, and that the ridge of the roof was 25 feet from the ground.

Before the site at Renkioi was chosen the selection of medical staff was well advanced. It was planned that there would be a Medical Superintendent, two Physicians, two Surgeons, 15 Assistant Physicians, 11 Assistant Surgeons and one Apothecary.[115] This was a reversal of the proportion of physicians and surgeons appointed to Smyrna, a belated recognition that medical were certain to exceed surgical cases.

Parkes was chosen as Medical Superintendent at an early stage. His appointment was approved by the medical press. He was thought a much better choice than Meyer had been for Smyrna.[116] In addition to Edmund Parkes[117], the following doctors were appointed. The Physicians were William Robertson[118] and Henry Goodeve[119]. The Surgeons were Spencer Wells and Holmes Coote, both transferred from Smyrna. The Assistant Physicians were John Beddoe[120], David Christison[121], John Cowan[122], Thomas Dixon[123], John Francis[124], Robert Hale[125], Thomas Holland[126], John Kirk[127], James MacLaren[128], Alfred Playne[129], Wilfred Reid,[130], William Rooke[131], and George Scott[132]. The Apothecary was John Humphrey[133]. The Assistant Surgeons were Carl Bader[134], George Buchanan[135], John Dix[136], James Fawcas[137], Charles Maunder[138], Bransby Roberts[139], Samuel Stretton[140], and Thomas Veale[141]. In addition to these, there were two Assistant Physicians, Hooper and Parry, and two Assistant Surgeons, Field and Fox, who cannot otherwise be identified. (It is just possible that when in Renkioi they were unqualified and appointed as dressers. However only one dresser, Pagan, is named on the list, and he cannot be traced with certainty as having eventually qualified.) The average age of the five senior doctors was about 40, that of the traced junior doctors 26. Kirk was the youngest, in 1855 being only aged 19. Of the 22 traced junior doctors, 12 had been qualified less than five years, and some had come out immediately after qualification. Of the 13 whose medical schools are known, 12 were from Edinburgh, and 11 from London hospitals.

The careers of Wells and Holmes Coote have already been recorded. Many of the other doctors attained distinction. Three became professors in British medical schools, three became Fellows of the Royal Society, and several became consultants of note in the London and provincial hospitals. Kirk was perhaps the most versatile, achieving a knighthood by his activities in East Africa.

The female nursing staff at Renkioi was not, like that at Smyrna, selected by Lady Canning and her Committee. From her letters to Lady Stratford it is clear that Lady Canning knew about the second Civil Hospital, for she records that Parkes originally asked for 100 nurses, and that the Matron of St. George's Hospital would be in charge. She complained in May - "Miss Nightingale writes so strongly against sending many nurses that Parkes bids fair to go without. I hope he will distinctly write his own orders and they will be obeyed".[142] In the end, only a small staff of nurses was sent, chosen by Sir James Clark and Dr. Parkes. The Matron was Mrs. Newman, and there were four other Lady Nurses, who were given senior positions, and 20 paid nurses. In addition there was a "lady volunteer (unpaid)", who was in fact Parkes' sister. Usually it was possible to attach two nurses to each ward. Like the doctors, the nurses found that for long periods there was not much work to do. Lady Canning wrote concerning alleged hardships experienced by the nurses. "Exceeding discomfort of the Renkioi wooden buildings, very frugal diet, and the fact of so long waiting for any work."[143] As well as nurses, the hospital was well supplied with orderlies, some military and some civilian. Parkes reported that the civilian orderlies recruited in London, although they had had no previous hospital experience, were much more competent than the military orderlies.

Between October 1855 and June 1856 a total of 1,300 patients was admitted to Renkioi, of whom 50 died (4 per cent). Only 50 patients were admitted between March and June 1856.[144] Bowel conditions accounted for 299 admissions with 14 deaths (5 per cent); fevers for 280 admissions with 22 deaths (8 per cent); chest diseases for 203 admissions with 10 deaths (5 per cent); rheumatic diseases for 176 admissions with no deaths; and frostbite for 35 admissions and one death (3 per cent). Wounds accounted for 94 admissions and one death (1 per cent). The mortality ratios compare favourably with those reported for Smyrna, but the cases are not strictly comparable in terms of the severity of disease and of the general condition of the patients.

Parkes in his own report gave the same total of admissions but some additional details about the diseases encountered.[145] He noted that, of 50 deaths, 22 were from "typhus or typhoid", 14 from chronic dysentery, eight from pulmonary tuberculosis and six from miscellaneous conditions. Typhus seems to have been the main concern but isolation was readily achieved (at no time was the hospital overcrowded). Parkes emphasises that a quarter of the military patients came from the Land Transport Corps. "They were thoroughly prostrated, generally scorbutic and had the severest types of the diseases admitted. Hastily enlisted, and comprising many boys or men well past their prime, these soldiers were quite unfitted to withstand the hardships of the Crimea." The camps of this regiment were managed deplorably and understaffed medically. Between May 1855 and March 1856, 1,376 men of the Transport Corps were sent to base hospitals (including Renkioi) and 477 died (35 per cent).[146] Of the medical staff at Renkioi one doctor and one nurse contracted typhus but both recovered. One medical orderly died of typhus.

Because of the low admission rates and the preponderance of chronic cases the doctors had plenty of spare time. The press was rather scathing. "The Civil Surgeon lounges away his time in a comfortable home with a balcony and verandah looking over the Bosphorous or the Dardanelles, smokes his pipe until he is tired, and then with dog and gun, saunters over the hills."[147] A pleasant social life was indeed possible. On 24 September Parkes gave a party for the local Pashas. After inspecting the hospital they were entertained to lunch and in the evening to "dinner followed by games", with 30 ladies present, "young and remarkable for their good looks."[148] Parkes, Wells, Holmes Coote, Goodeve and Hale had their wives with them. Mrs. Wells and Mrs. Holmes Coote each gave birth to a daughter in November. No doubt there were flirtations between the lady nurses and the young doctors. Holmes Coote was later to describe - "The charming and healthy hospital of Renkioi ... The medical men were all paid and being isolated from the outside world could turn their attention to elegant pursuits".[149] Some explored the surrounding country, some went shooting or riding. Bader and Stretton emulated Lord Byron by swimming the Hellespont.[150] Kirk botanised and pursued his hobby of photography. Goodeve (with Calvert the British Consul) did excavations near Chanak. (Calvert had already begun to work on the site, which was taken over by Schliemann in 1872 and was subsequently believed to be that of the ancient city of Troy).

No new patients were admitted to Renkioi after June 1856. The last patient was not discharged until July, when the hospital was finally closed. Many of the doctors had gone home before March. Those who volunteered to serve in the Crimea after being at Renkioi were Buchanan, Cowan, Maunder, Roberts and Rooke. The last to leave Renkioi were Goodeve, Parkes and Wells, who all came home in July.

Two of the Renkioi staff, Beddoe and Buchanan, published memoirs. These contain details of interest, not only about Renkioi but about Scutari and the Crimea. Beddoe supplies the information that Sir James Clark had much to do with the selection of the Renkioi staff. Beddoe arrived at Scutari with Kirk, Christison and Maunder, but although he spent a few weeks there he makes little comment on the hospitals. Next he paid a short unofficial visit to the Crimea, where he met Hulke and Macleod from Smyrna. He records that the civilian surgeons serving in the Crimea were allowed to wear the uniform of a second-class Staff-Surgeon. Macleod, appearing resplendent in his new uniform and cheered by his friends, promptly fell into a puddle. While at Renkioi, Beddoe paid a visit to Smyrna, took part in long expeditions on horseback with Wells, and saw the excavations done by Calvert and Goodeve. He enjoyed life at Renkioi, but gives little account of medical affairs.[151]

Buchanan's account is much more detailed. He arrived in Scutari on 25 June and contacted his friend, Dr. Davidson, a naval surgeon stationed at Therapia. He was taken round the naval hospital and admired its efficiency and cleanliness. At Scutari he sensed an atmosphere of jealousy and disapproval of the civilian doctors on the part of the regulars. On 2 July he paid a short visit to the Crimea where he met many of his Edinburgh friends and Dr. Lyons. He visited the battle-fields and the full horrors of war were brought home to him. He met Cowan who had just returned from his inspection of Sinope, and learnt that Hall, "who at this time had an aversion to civil surgeons", had refused to receive Cowan's report. After a week, Buchanan returned to Scutari. He called on Paulet, "but that nobleman had no good name among the civil staff - acting in a very gruff and unpleasant way to them". Of the hospitals at Scutari he stated - "All the horrors of last winter have given place to the most perfect order and cleanliness". He met Miss Nightingale and noted that "the nursing department was perfect". Cullen told him how he had been nursed by Miss Nightingale during a severe attack of fever, and spoke highly of her assiduous care and kindness. Buchanan himself had an attack of fever and was looked after by Dr. Pincoffs, with whom he had become very friendly.

Buchanan reached Renkioi about the end of July. He says little about the work there but remarks that the population of the neighbouring village of Renkioi "was a capital field of practice for our staff". In particular, there was the opportunity of treating eye diseases, which were very common. His comment on his colleagues is significant.

> I can scarcely say I became acquainted with any of the Renkioi Staff except those I saw elsewhere. I don't remember their names and some I never saw. There being no patients, we never came together professionally.

From this and other evidence it does seem that the Scottish contingent kept very much to themselves and indeed formed rather a clique: the number of patients in the hospital in August was certainly very small. In desperation, "Cowan and I instituted a game of rounders to give us some active employment". Buchanan did not stay on at Renkioi for very long. On 6 September Goodeve and Hale, on their return from a short visit to the Crimea, reported that, as there was now a shortage of surgeons, Hall was more ready to receive assistance. With Cowan and Maunder, Buchanan volunteered to serve in the Crimea, and the three doctors arrived on 15 September. Buchanan was appointed to the General Hospital, consisting of 22 huts, each with 14 beds. His opinion of the regulars now changed, "the utmost cordiality prevailed". Almost immediately he was on duty day and night, attending to the wounded after the final assault on Sebastopol. After a busy four weeks, learning that his father was seriously ill, he sought permission from Hall to return home. Hall was very helpful and waived the condition that Buchanan should have given three months notice, unless sick. He sailed for England on 21 October with his friend Cowan, who meanwhile had gone sick with fever and had been sent to Scutari to recover. While Buchanan was only a short time in Renkioi, his account is eminently readable and gives considerable insight into the attitudes of these young doctors to their service in the East.[152]

CONCLUSIONS

The value of the Civil Surgeons and the Civil Hospitals can now be assessed. There had been much antagonism directed at the hospital at Renkioi. "A certain animus [existed] in attacks upon the only good and perfect thing in the medical way the Government had carried out since the commencement of the war."[153] It was appreciated, however, that the mortality ratio at Renkioi had been less than that of the London hospitals. That the hospital and staff were never used to full capacity can scarcely be advanced as an argument against its establishment. When it was opened in August there was no confidence that hostilities would have ceased before a second winter had passed. Every major war since 1854 has ended with an excess of hospital accommodation, a situation which is far from an indication of bad planning. It is interesting to speculate whether the provision of a comparable hutted hospital before the winter of 1854/1855 might not have prevented the disastrous overcrowding of the Scutari hospitals and saved many lives. Brunel's plan was a nine days wonder in the lay and medical press. There was scant recognition that it could be seen as a major advance in hospital design, and a great improvement on the tented or hutted hospitals provided in the Crimea originally. It is recorded, however, that Brunel's design was adopted by the Federal forces during the American Civil War, and by the Prussians in the Franco-German war of 1870.

In the numerous reports of the Commissions during the war there was little mention of the Civil Surgeons or of the Civil Hospitals. In the official Medical History only an incomplete list of the Civil Surgeons was given and the hospitals received mention only in various tables. No firm conclusions were drawn as to the merits of employing Civil Surgeons or of establishing Civil Hospitals in a future emergency. It was to be many years before a reserve of doctors for service abroad was to be established.

Parkes was the only member of the Renkioi staff asked to give evidence to the Royal Commission.[154] He was questioned closely as to his powers as a Medical Superintendent, compared with those of a P.M.O. in a Military Hospital. He stated that he had been able to get supplies from the Purveyor much more readily than the P.M.O. at Scutari. He had found that he had much more control over the orderlies, whether military or civilian. The general verdict on the Civil Hospitals given by Hall to the Royal Commission has already been noted. As he does not appear to have visited either hospital, even after hostilities ceased in October 1855, he was scarcely in a position to comment fairly. It is curious that, in his long interrogation by the Royal Commission, the Director-

General was not specifically asked to comment on the success, or otherwise, of either the employment of Civil Surgeons or the establishment of Civil Hospitals. The civilians who served during the war received little recognition for their contribution. Hall did make a brief recognition of the work of the group who volunteered to serve in the Crimea and some were awarded the Crimean medal, but neither Hall nor Smith showed any appreciation of those who solely were on the staffs of Scutari, Smyrna or Renkioi. In retrospect, it may be said that, despite all criticisms, the experiments were of value and that many useful lessons emerged.

NOTES

For many of the civilian doctors serving at Scutari, Smyrna, and Renkioi additional biographical notes are to be found in Appendix I.

1. George Macleod (1828-1892); M.D. Glasgow 1853; F.R.C.S.Ed. 1857; F.F.P.S.Glas. 1858 (obituaries **B.M.J.** (1892), 1:637-638: **Glas.Med.J.** 38 (1892), 270-273. For Macleod's surgical writings on the war see Chapter XVIII. He kept a journal of his war experiences, but unfortunately only one volume survives, covering his first visits to the Crimea.
2. S. M. Mitra, **The life and letters of Sir John Hall** (London, 1911), 304.
3. 'Macleod Journal'.
4. **The Times**, 12.2.1855.
5. **M.T.G.** (1855), 1:138-139.
6. **Med. Surg. Hist.**, 1:524-525. The list supplies durations and places of service.
7. Hugh Birt (d. 1875); M.R.C.S., L.S.A. 1836; F.R.C.S. 1844; served in the East March 1855 - April 1856 (**Plarr**).
8. Anthony Brabazon (1821-1896); L.R.C.S.I. 1846; L.S.A., M.D. Aberdeen 1856; served in the East April 1855 - April 1856 (obituary **B.M.J.** (1896), 1:763).
9. Charles Bryce (d.1874); M.D. Glasgow 1835; served in the East April 1855 - May 1856.
10. Cullen transferred to Smyrna - see note 65 below.
11. Patrick Fraser (d.1881); L.R.C.S.Ed. 1828; M.D. St. Andrews 1836; M.R.C.P. 1839; served in the East March 1855 - April 1856.
12. Frederick Gant (1825-1905); M.R.C.S. 1849; F.R.C.S. 1861; served in the East May 1855 - January 1856 (obituary **B.M.J.** (1905), 1:1410-1411; **Plarr**). Gant published **The science and practice of surgery** (London, 1864) and many other texts and papers.
13. Henry Holl (d. 1863); M.R.C.S. 1847; M.D. Aberdeen 1857; served in the East March 1855 - May 1856.
14. Edward Howard (d. 1871); M.R.C.S., M.L.S.A., 1840; served in the East April 1853 - April 1856.
15. James Hughes (d. 1868); M.R.C.S., L.S.A., M.D. St. Andrews 1847; served in the East February 1855 - May 1855.
16. For Lyons, see note 72 to Chapter XI.
17. William McEgan (1817-1857) (**Crawford**). For McEgan's activities, see also

CHAPTER XII

      note 65 to Chapter II and note 55 to Chapter XVI.
18. For Macleod, see note 1 above.
19. Robert Mason (d. 1905); M.R.C.S. 1848; L.S.A. 1856; F.R.C.S. 1865; served in the East March 1855 - April 1856 (**Plarr**).
20. Peter Pincoffs (1815-1872); M.D. Leyden; served in the East April 1855 - April 1856 (G.A. Lindebloom, **Dutch medical biography**, Einthoven, 1984).
21. Henry Rooke (d. 1862); M.R.C.S. 1846; M.D. Edinburgh 1848; served in the East March 1855 - February 1856.
22. Henry Rowdon (1818-1869); M.R.C.S., L.S.A. 1841; F.R.C.S., M.D. St. Andrews 1859; served in the East March 1855 - January 1856 (obituary **Lancet** (1869), 1:131; **Plarr**).
23. Robert Woolaston (1801-1865); M.R.C.S. 1823; F.R.C.S. 1847; M.R.C.P. 1859; served in the East April 1855 - April 1856 (**Plarr**).
24. John Wordsworth (1823-1886); M.R.C.S. 1845; F.R.C.S. 1847; M.R.C.P. 1859; served in the East December 1854 - February 1856 (obituary **Lancet** (1886), 1:525-526); **Plarr**). Wordsworth transferred to Smyrna early in 1855.
25. C. Bryce, **England and France before Sebastopol looked at from a medical point of view** (London, 1857).
26. F. J. Gant, **Autobiography** (London, 1905).
27. **Plarr**.
28. P. Pincoffs, **Experiences of a civilian in Eastern Military Hospitals** (London, 1857).
29. **Royal Commission**, 300-308.
30. **Med. Surg. Hist.**, 1:523-524.
31. John Atkinson (d. 1890), Robert Elliott (1832-1872), Charles Gray (1834-1915), John Stewart (1838-1868), Joseph Taylor (1835-1882), Samuel Woodful (1834-1890). For fuller details, see **Drew**.
32. **Med. Surg. Hist.**, 2: after p.480, "General Hospital Returns. VII. Abydos".
33. J. Bowen-Thomson (1814-1855); M.D. Dublin; practised in Middle East for many years before the war; held a government post in Syria 1852-1854 (obituary **M.T.G.** (1855), 2:249).
34. Mitra, **Hall**, 402.
35. Ibid., 400.
36. **M.T.G.** (1855), 2:41-42.
37. Ibid., 1:420.
38. **Lancet** (1855), 1:225-226.
39. **M.T.G.** (1855), 1:100.
40. Ibid., 186-187.
41. Ibid. 494-495.
42. Thomas Moorhead (1822-1877); M.D. Edinburgh 1842; joined as assistant-surgeon 1845; staff surgeon November 1854; served in the East November 1854 - December 1855, March - June 1856; retired 1876 as D.I.G. (obituary **Lancet** (1877), 1:659; **Drew**).
43. 'Hall/Moorhead Letters', 3.1 1854.
44. William Humfrey (1802-1862); joined as hospital assistant 1826; assistant-surgeon 1827; D.I.G. August 1854; served in the East November 1854 - December 1855; I.G. 1858 (**Drew**).
45. Thomas Hunter (1810-1888); M.D. Edinburgh 1831; joined as assistant-surgeon 1834; staff surgeon August 1854; served in the East August 1854 - July 1856; retired 1859 as D.I.G. (**Drew**).
46. **Lancet** (1855), 2:94.
47. **DNB**.
48. **Lancet** (1855), 1:223.
49. Ibid., 245.
50. **Ass.Med.J.** (1855), 195.
51. Ibid., 167.
52. John Forbes (1787-1861); M.D. Edinburgh 1817; F.R.C.P. 1844 (obituary

B.M.J. (1861), 2:561-562; **Munk; DNB**).
53. **Ass.Med.J.** (1855), 241. In fact Meyer had been to Eton (M.F. Stapylton, **The Eton School List 1791-1877**, Eton, 1884).
54. **Ass.Med.J.** (1855), 376.
55. Ibid., 306.
56. Ibid., 407. The signatories provide a useful list of the Smyrna medical staff in early April, corresponding closely to that published in **M.T.G.** (1855), 1:250.
57. John Meyer (1814-1870); M.D. Heidelberg 1836; L.R.C.P. 1857; F.R.C.P. 1863 (**Munk**). See also B.M.J. (1871), 1:387.
58. John Barclay (1820-1901); M.D. Edinburgh 1842; L.R.C.P. 1846; F.R.C.P. 1859 (E. R. Frizelle and J. D. Martin, **The Leicester Royal Infirmary, 1771-1971**, Leicester, 1971, 111-112; **Munk**).
59. Septimus Gibbon (1825-1909); M.B. Cambridge 1851; M.R.C.P. 1852 (obituary **Lancet** (1909), 1:1360).
60. Arthur Leared (1822-1879); M.B. Dublin 1847; M.R.C.P. 1854; M.D. Oxford, M.D. Dublin 1860; F.R.C.P. 1871 (obituaries **B.M.J.** (1879), 2:653; **Lancet** (1879), 2:633; **Munk; DNB**).
61. Holmes Coote (1815-1872); M.R.C.S. 1838; F.R.C.S. 1844 (obituaries **B.M.J.** (1872), 2:718; **Lancet** (1872), 2:935; **Plarr; DNB**).
62. Carsten Holthouse (1810-1901); M.R.C.S., L.S.A. 1833; F.R.C.S. 1843 (**Plarr**).
63. Thomas Spencer Wells (1818-1897); M.R.C.S. 1841; F.R.C.S. 1844 (obituaries **B.M.J.** (1897), 1:368-369, 434-435: **Lancet** (1897), 1:398-400; **Plarr; DNB**). For Spencer Wells, see note 99 to Chapter I.
64. Charles Coote (1824-1860); M.B. London 1845; M.D. London L.R.C.P. 1853; F.R.C.P. 1858 (obituary **M.T.G.** (1860), 2:517-518; **Munk**).
65. William Cullen; M.R.C.S., L.S.A. 1836; M.D. St. Andrews 1837.
66. Robert Martin (1817-1891); M.D. Cambridge 1851; M.R.C.P. 1854; F.R.C.P. 1859 (**Munk**).
67. George Rolleston (1829-1881); M.B. Oxford 1854; L.R.C.P. 1856; M.D. Oxford 1857; F.R.C.P. 1859 (obituaries **B.M.J.** (1881), 1:1027-1029: **Lancet** (1881), 1:1044-1045; **Scientific papers and addresses by George Rolleston**, Oxford, 1884, XXIII; **DNB**). At the request of the Government, Rolleston prepared **Report on Smyrna** (London, 1887), a detailed account of the topography of Smyrna, with notes on local diseases.
68. Richard Wilkinson; M.R.C.S., L.S.A. 1851: M.B. London 1854.
69. Barnes Wood is untraced.
70. Edward Atkinson (1830-1905); M.R.C.S. 1852; L.S.A. 1853 (obituary **B.M.J.** (1905), 1:631).
71. Edward Complin (1830-1855); M.R.C.S. 1851; L.S.A. 1852 (obituary **M.T.G.** (1855), 2:559-560).
72. John Eddowes (1823-1906); M.R.C.S., L.S.A. 1846; M.D. Glasgow 1850.
73. John Falconer (d. 1895) is otherwise untraced.
74. John Hulke (1830-1895); M.R.C.S. 1852; F.R.C.S. 1857; P.R.C.S. 1893 (obituary **B.M.J.** (1895), 1:451-453; J. Bland-Sutton, **The Story of a surgeon**, London, 1930, 30-34; **Plarr; DNB**).
75. Thomas Hornidge (d. 1895); M.B. London 1852; M.R.C.S. F.R.C.S. 1854, (**Plarr**).
76. John Jardine (? d. 1903); M.R.C.S., L.S.A. 1850.
77. James Lakin (1824-1877); L.S.A. 1848; M.R.C.S. 1849; M.B. London 1851; (obituary **B.M.J.** (1877), 2:424).
78. Robert McDonnel (1828-1889); M.B. Dublin 1850; L.R.C.S.I. 1851; F.R.C.S.I. 1853; M.D. Dublin 1857; P.R.C.S.I. 1877 (C. A. Cameron, **History of Royal College of Surgeons in Ireland**, 2nd ed., Dublin, 1916, 496-499).
79. John Streatfeild (1828-1886); M.R.C.S. 1852; F.R.C.S. 1862 (obituary **B.M.J.** (1886), 1:620; **Plarr**).
80. **M.T.G.** (1855), 1:285.
81. Ibid., 437.

CHAPTER XII

82. **Med. Surg. Hist.** 2: after p.480, "General Hospital Returns VIII. Smyrna".
83. **M.T.G.** (1855), 1:328). But the mortality is here grossly exaggerated.
84. Ibid., 285.
85. Ibid., 347.
86. Ibid., 448-449.
87. Ibid., 430-433.
88. **M.T.G.** (1855), 2:113-114.
89. James McCraith (1810-1901); M.R.C.S. 1833; M.D. Glasgow 1835; F.R.C.S. 1865 (**Plarr**).
90. **M.T.G.** (1855), 2:46,105.
91. **Lancet** (1855), 1:657.
92. **M.T.G.** (1855), 1:648-650.
93. Ibid., 347.
94. 'Canning Letters' 1.3.1855.
95. Ibid., ? June, 1855.
96. **M.T.G.** (1855), 1,347.
97. **Royal Commission**, 34.
98. Meyer made these points to Dr. Tyler, who quoted them in his biographical sketch of Rolleston, in **Scientific Papers and Addresses by George Rolleston** (Oxford, 1884).
99. **M.T.G.** (1855), 2:113-114.
100. **Royal Commission**, 31-32.
101. Ibid., 180.
102. Mitra, **Hall**, 401-402.
103. 'Hall/Airey Letters', 25.3.1855.
104. **Cantlie**, 2:169.
105. **M.T.G.** (1855), 1:317.
106. Ibid., 344.
107. L.T.C. Rolt, **Isambard Kingdom Brunel** (London, 1970), 292-293.
108. Ibid., 292.
109. Rolt, **Brunel**; J. Pudney, **Brunel and his world**, (London, 1974); **DNB**.
110. Rolt, **Brunel**, 137-138.
111. I. Brunel, **Hospital buildings for the East. Memorandum for Government, 1855**: reprinted as appendix to Parkes' Report, see following note.
112. The most useful account of Renkioi is by E. A. Parkes, **Report of the formation and general management of Renkioi Hospital. Addressed to the Secretary of State for War 1 October, 1856**. For a detailed study of the design and construction of the hospital, see D. Toppin, 'The British hospital at Renkioi', **The Royal Engineers Journal** 99 (1986), 225-236; 100 (1986), 39-50.
113. 'Hall Diary', February, 1856.
114. Reprinted in **M.T.G.** (1855), 2:251-252.
115. Lists can to be found in **M.T.G.** (1855), 1:451 and **Ass.Med.J.** (1855), 617. There are slight discrepancies.
116. **Lancet** (1855), 1:351.
117. Edmund Parkes (1819-1876); M.R.C.S. 1840; M.B. London 1841; M.D. London 1846; F.R.C.P. 1854 (obituaries **B.M.J.** (1876), 1:397-398; **Lancet** (1876), 1:480-482; L. C. Parkes, 'Life and Work of Edward Alexander Parkes, M.D., F.R.S. 1818-1876', **J.R.A.M.C.**, 14 (1910), 227-238; Z. Cope, **Florence Nightingale and the doctors** (London, 1958), 80-83; **Munk; Drew; DNB**). For more about Parkes, see Chapter XVIII.
118. William Robertson (1818-1882); M.D. Edinburgh 1839; F.R.C.P.Ed. 1843 (obituary **Ed.Med.J.**, 28 (1882), 382-383).
119. Henry Goodeve (1807-1884); M.R.C.S., M.D. Edinburgh 1829; F.R.C.S. 1844; F.R.C.P. 1850 (obituaries **B.M.J.** (1884), 1:1218; **M.T.G.** (1884), 2:65; **Munk; Plarr; Crawford**).
120. John Beddoe (1826-1911); M.D. Edinburgh 1851; M.R.C.P. 1860; F.R.C.P. 1873 (obituary **B.M.J.** (1911), 2:316; **Munk; DNB**).
121. David Christison (1830-1912); L.R.C.S.Ed., M.D. Edinburgh 1851; F.R.C.P.Ed.

1862.
122. John Cowan (1829-1896); M.D. Glasgow 1851 (obituary **Glasgow Med.J.**, 46 (1896), 192-196.
123. Thomas Dixon (d. 1880); M.D. St. Andrews 1854; L.S.A. 1856; M.R.C.S. 1857.
124. John Francis (d. 1896); L.S.A. 1834; M.R.C.S. 1835.
125. Robert Hale (d. 1860); M.R.C.S. 1839; M.D. St. Andrews 1841; L.R.C.P. 1849.
126. Thomas Holland (1827-1856); M.R.C.S., M.D. Edinburgh 1850 (obituary **M.T.G.** (1856), 1:466).
127. John Kirk (1832-1922); M.D. Edinburgh 1854 (obituary **B.M.J.** (1922), 1:125; M. Gelfand, **Livingstone the doctor: his life and travels** (Oxford, 1957), passim; **DNB**).
128. James MacLaren (d. 1920); L.R.C.S.Ed., M.D. Edinburgh 1854.
129. Alfred Playne (d. 1908); M.R.C.S. 1853; M.B. London 1854; L.S.A. 1856.
130. Wilfred Reid; L.R.C.S.Ed., M.D. Edinburgh 1849; F.R.C.S.Ed. 1855.
131. William Rooke (1833-1888); L.R.C.S.Ed. 1855; L.S.A., M.D. Edinburgh 1856; M.R.C.S. 1858.
132. George Scott (d. 1892); M.D. Edinburgh, M.R.C.S. 1851.
133. John Humphrey (d. 1902); M.R.C.S., L.S.A. 1849.
134. Carl Bader (d. 1891); M.R.C.S., L.S.A. 1855 (E.T. Collins, **The Moorfields Eye Hospital**, London, 1929, 110, 122, 138-139).
135. George Buchanan (1827-1906); L.R.C.S. Ed., M.D. St. Andrews 1849; F.F.P.S. Glasgow 1852 (obituaries **Glasgow Med.J.**, 65 (1906), 354-355; **B.M.J.** (1906), 1:1078.
136. John Dix (d. 1897); M.R.C.S. 1848; L.S.A. 1849.
137. James Fawcas (1835-1871); M.R.C.S., L.S.A. 1835; M.D. London 1858 (**Crawford**).
138. Charles Maunder (1832-1879); M.R.C.S. 1854; F.R.C.S. 1857 (obituary **B.M.J.** (1987), 2:74; **London Hosp.Gaz.**, 22 (1918), 22,97-98; **Plarr**).
139. Bransby Roberts (d. 1919); M.R.C.S., L.S.A. 1853; M.D. St. Andrews 1876 (obituary **Lancet** (1919), 1:688).
140. Samuel Stretton (1831-1920); M.R.C.S. 1853; L.S.A. 1856 (obituary **B.M.J.** (1920), 2:844).
141. Thomas Veale (d. 1860) M.R.C.S., L.S.A. 1854
142. 'Canning Letters', 27.5.1855.
143. Ibid., 28.8.1855.
144. **Med. Surg. Hist.**, 2: after p.480, "General Hospital Returns. IX. Renkioi".
145. Parkes, **Report**.
146. **Med. Surg. Hist.**, 1:460-464.
147. **Illustrated London News**, 17.11.1855.
148. **Lancet** (1855), 2:354-355.
149. **B.M.J.** (1869), 1:565.
150. J. Beddoe, **Memories of Eighty Years** (Bristol, 1910), 79.
151. Beddoe, **Memories**. This work is by far the most detailed account of life at Renkioi, with numerous interesting asides concerning Beddoe's colleagues.
152. A. Buchanan, **Camp life. As seen by a civilian** (Glasgow, 1871).
153. **M.T.G.** (1855), 2:578.
154. **Royal Commission**, 26-29.

CHAPTER XIII

THE FINAL MONTHS OF THE SIEGE OF SEBASTOPOL (APRIL–SEPTEMBER 1855)

THE FALL OF SEBASTOPOL

By April 1855 the investment of Sebastopol was still incomplete and reinforcements of men and supplies continued to be brought in without difficulty, although the failure to defeat the Allies in the field at Inkerman had discouraged the Russians from making any further major attempt to break out of their defence lines. The Allies had become resigned to a long period of siege warfare. As the stranglehold of winter receded they began to be more confident that increasing pressure could be exerted on the enemy. The French now greatly outnumbered the British. In November 1854 each army had held approximately one half of the line of attack: by April 1855 the British were responsible for only a small sector in the centre and the French for two much larger sectors on each flank. However, during the winter the Russian defences had been greatly strengthened. To capture Sebastopol it was not sufficient for the Allies to break through the defence lines at weak areas. Opposite the British sector was the formidable fortress of the Redan, while opposite the French Right attack was the equally strong Malakoff redoubt, in front of which was the Mamelon Hill. Opposite the French Left attack were several small but powerful batteries or forts, such as the Flagstaff and the Garden. Sebastopol could not be taken without first dealing with these key positions. During the late spring and the summer of 1855, trench warfare was waged continuously. Minor sorties to establish advanced positions, or to recapture them, were frequent. Intermittent artillery duels in different parts of the line went on day and night, almost without interruption. From April onwards five intensive bombardments were carried out with the object of reducing the Russian key positions. Not until September was success gained.

The planning of the strategy of the Allies was greatly hampered by differences between the respective commanders. Confusion was also caused by the machinations of Napoleon III. In mid-April, while on a state visit to London, the Emperor produced a plan by which he believed the war would be brought speedily to an end. He proposed that the forces holding the Allied Lines before Sebastopol should be greatly reduced (he considered that repeated bombardments were futile), and that a large army should capture Simpheropol, the important base on the supply line from central Russia. An army of some 45,000, mainly British under Raglan, was to advance on the McKenzie Heights and then to Simpheropol, a distance of thirty miles north. A second force of 70,000 French was meanwhile to be transported by sea from Constantinople to Aloushta on the South-East coast of the Crimea. From there it was to march inland, across quite a formidable range of mountains, to join with Raglan's force. A large Turkish army was already a threat to the Russian supply line from the West. To provide for these two invading armies, a large proportion of the troops before Sebastopol were to be withdrawn and augmented by French reserves via Constantinople. The Emperor anticipated that these manoeuvres would disrupt the Russian supply lines and that Sebastopol, now completely invested, would be forced to surrender.

This grandiose plan was viewed unfavourably by the British Government. Panmure, the Minister of War, considered it a "wild impractical scheme". The Allied commanders saw many objections, considering that any reduction of strength before Sebastopol might encourage the Russians to break out and threaten the Allies' lines of supply. The French commanders were appalled at the expressed intention of the Emperor to come out and lead the seaborne expedition to Simpheropol personally. But on his return to Paris from London, Napoleon abandoned this idea, to the relief of all. He did not, however, abandon his strategy.

Meanwhile, largely on the initiative of the British, a less reckless diversion had already been planned, to capture the Russian port of Kertch, on the Sea of Azov, and thus cut an important sea route of supplies to Sebastopol. A combined naval and military operation was mounted. Some 10,000 troops, of which three quarters were French and one quarter British, were embarked in transports under naval protection. The force set out on 3 May but was recalled shortly before it reached Kertch, the Emperor, still intent on furthering his tactics, having sent a telegraph ordering its return. He was furious at the withdrawal of troops from the Crimea without his permission, and he wanted all the available transports assembled at Constantinople, in preparation for his expedition. Canrobert, the French Commander, saw no option but to obey the Emperor's edict. The British, being the lesser partner in the operation, could not attack Kertch on their own. Exhausted and humiliated by these events, Canrobert resigned his command, and Pelissier took his place. A more resolute man, Pelissier was prepared to ignore the Emperor's telegraphed orders, indeed is said on one occasion to have cut the wires! On 22 May the expedition to Kertch sailed again. The Russian base was captured and destroyed, great quantities of stores destined for Sebastopol were burned, many Russian ships were captured or sunk, and a blockade was established to control all Russian naval movements between the Black Sea and the Sea of Azov. This was a well-planned and successful foray and there were few casualties in the British force.

Pelissier had no intention of supporting the Emperor in his grand strategy. He insisted that the Simpheropol expedition could not be attempted unless some of the key points of the Sebastopol defences were taken, in order that the investment of the town was made more complete and the risk of a Russian counter-attack completely eliminated. With some reluctance, Napoleon ceased to press his plan, and there was a return to a general acceptance that the siege should be continued. It was now hoped that repeated major bombardments would, in time, wear down the defences.

On 9 April the Second Bombardment of Sebastopol had begun. The Allies had 520 guns (of which only 138 were British), and the Russians 938 guns. However, the Allies fired almost twice as many rounds as the Russians, and the casualties in Sebastopol far exceeded those of the

Allies. But since the Russians repaired the damage to their defences each night, no permanent breach was made in their lines. After ten days the bombardment fizzled out, partly because of the reluctance of the French to co-operate in a final assault. The Third Bombardment began on 6 June. Within two days, the French had captured the Mamelon and the British the Quarries, so threatening the Malakoff and the Redan respectively. There followed a pause until 17 June, when the Fourth Bombardment was opened, with an intensity of fire never before witnessed. Under cover of this attack the French attacked the Malakoff and the British the Redan. The advance of the storming parties was not well co-ordinated, and after heavy losses both the British and French had to withdraw. This failure resulted in a profound pessimism among the ranks of the Allies. Two British generals, Brown and Pennefeather, went home; Estcourt, the Adjutant-General, died of cholera; and on 28 June Raglan, his end hastened by a depression following the ignominious failure of the attack on the Redan, died of a fever. He was succeeded by General Simpson, like Raglan a veteran of the Peninsular War, but a man of limited talents compared with his predecessor.

On 16 August the Russians made a final break-out, launching an attack along the Tchernaya Valley and so threatening Balaclava and the lines of communication of the Allies. In an engagement at the Tractir Bridge the Russians were repulsed, with heavy losses, by a combined French and Sardinian force. The British played no significant part in this action, which was a turning point in the campaign, for as a result of their defeat the Russians lost confidence and now saw little hope of holding on to Sebastopol much longer.

On 17 August, the day after the Russian break-out, the Fifth Bombardment was begun, to continue for a week. Following this no assault was attempted. The Sixth (and last) Bombardment opened on 5 September, and the Allied commander planned assaults on the Malakoff and the Redan. After three days and nights of heavy fire, the French, taking the Russians by surprise, succeeded in storming the Malakoff. The British once more attacked the Redan but the Russians were prepared for them.

Exposed to a withering fire from the defenders the British assault parties were forced to retreat in some disorder, sustaining heavy losses. Nevertheless, the joint attack had had its effect on Russian morale. On the night of 8 September explosions were heard from the harbour. The Russians blew up the magazines in the Redan and withdrew. Next morning thousands of Russians were to be seen streaming across a bridge of boats in the harbour, and the whole town was ablaze. The Allies entered Sebastopol, to find it deserted except for the abandoned sick and wounded, dying, or already dead, in the cellars and in the main hospital, now a shambles.

The fighting in the Crimea was over. Not until 29 February, 1856, was an armistice declared, and peace was not established until the Treaty of Paris on 27 April. The Russians still had a huge army poised north of the Crimea, and the Allies had to retain a large force in the Crimea throughout the winter to ensure that there would be no counter attack.

THE MEDICAL CIRCUMSTANCES OF THE SIEGE

The problems which faced the medical services in the Crimea from April to September 1855 differed considerably from those encountered in the winter of 1854-1855. Although conditions had, in many respects, changed for the better much arduous, and often dangerous work lay ahead. In the winter the care of the sick had been the main preoccupation. By the spring the general health of the army had greatly improved. Shortages of medical staff had been corrected. While the regimental medical officers still had a significant load of medical cases to deal with, the monthly totals of admissions for disease were gradually reduced. The fall in mortality rates was dramatic. Now the sick soldier was much less likely to be in an exhausted or debilitated state prior to any attack of illness. The virulence of the camp diseases had lessened, particularly the bowel diseases and fevers (with the exception of cholera). Scurvy and frost-bite no longer presented problems. It was unusual for the regimental hospitals to be overcrowded, and if overcrowding threatened a large reserve of beds in the divisional or general hospitals established in the rear of the camps was available.

The regimental doctors, particularly the assistant-surgeons, served long periods of duty in order to render first-aid to the wounded in the front line, to supervise the evacuation of casualties and, on occasion in times of stress, to operate in emergency in the advanced posts established forward of the regimental hospitals. No longer were the wounded soldiers merely dressed and then hurriedly evacuated, in great discomfort, to Balaclava, and from there conveyed aboard the hospital transports to Scutari, often resulting in a long delay before definitive surgery was performed.

A comparison of the regimental statistics in the three winter months of 1855 (January to March) with those of the six months from April to September is revealing. In the winter period there were 22,554 admissions to the regimental hospitals (with a monthly average of about 7,500). In the following spring and summer (double the number of months) there were 40,627 admissions (with a monthly average of about 6,500). This comparatively small reduction in average admissions does not at first sight suggest a major improvement in the health of the army. However, in the winter months all the regiments were greatly depleted, while from about April the regiments (with the exception of the cavalry) were brought up to a strength approaching the prescribed maximum of 800 to 900 men, and maintained at this level up to the end of the war. Moreover, very few wounded were admitted in the winter while there was a marked increase of such cases in the spring and summer. It follows that comparisons of the mortality rates are much more significant.[1] In the three winter months the ratio of deaths to admissions was 15 per cent, in the succeeding six months the figure was 6 per cent. This steep reduction in the mortality ratio is clear proof of a marked improvement in the health of the army after March 1855.

Between April and September 1855, a total of 7,718 patients was evacuated from the Crimea to the base

CHAPTER XIII

hospitals at Scutari and elsewhere (an average of 1,294 a month). The mortality rates on passage were now negligible, for the hospital transports were more hygienic, more adequately furnished, and better supplied with drugs, food and safe water. Over-crowding did not occur. In addition it was no longer the policy to transfer patients who were still acutely ill. In contrast, 6,405 patients had been sent to the base hospitals in the three winter months (an average of 2,153 a month), producing a considerable mortality on passage.[2] Here, again, was improvement. Reasons for this improvement are not hard to find. Almost all the reports of the regimental doctors contain positive comments. Typical is the report of the surgeon of the 18th Regiment.

> During the months of April and May, the condition of the troops was greatly ameliorated. The increasing mildness of the weather, enabled the men to pay greater attention to personal cleanliness: and improved rations (in which fresh bread and fresh meat held a recognised place), the introduction of a more judicious arrangement of night work, and better clothing contributed to improve the health of the Regiment. The Hospital accommodation, though still limited in extent, was much improved in other respects. An efficient arrangement for washing the underclothing and bedding of the sick was introduced, and overcrowding was prevented by the removal of sick and convalescents to the Hospitals on the Bosphorous... the admission into wards by patients lately suffering from fever was unavoidable; but the free use of lime and other disinfecting agents, with increasing attention to cleanliness, averted all danger; and it is gratifying to be able to state that in no case did the fever, as this time prevalent, prove fatal to men admitted on account of wounds. In the month of April the admissions declined to 187; but seven deaths were returned.

This report refers to most of the favourable changes. No single factor can be isolated as the major reason for improvement: benefits came from a combination of many circumstances.

The last frost of the winter was on 31 March. Thereafter conditions gradually improved, although rain persisted in the first two weeks of April. From May to August the daily temperature rose steadily but the heat was seldom intolerable. In September there was a return to the conditions in April. "That the climate must be said to possess much more of a temperate than a tropical character is evident form the fact that during these months the highest weekly mean temperature was only 79.1°."[3] After March it was seldom that the soldier had to sleep in wet clothing or bedding. By April all the regiments had been lavishly equipped with winter clothing, and indeed there were now complaints from the men that they were too hot! An anonymous officer wrote in April -

> Pray do put a termination to the energies of the Berlin wool interest and try to stop the manufacture of mitts, cuffs, chest-protectors, comforters, socks etc., the very sight of which puts me in a stew this hot weather. Who will send out ice and cool drinks, vegetables, and light summer clothing? Let all warm articles be put in store for the next occasion when they may be required. There is scarcely an officer who is not embarrassed with bales of things which have arrived since the fine weather set in, and which he cannot get rid of at any sacrifice.[4]

The influence of the summer weather on disease was at the time considered at great length, particularly in relation to the second epidemic of cholera (discussed below). An increased incidence of relatively mild bowel disease, usually listed as diarrhoea, was also associated with the warm weather. It might have been expected that the breeding of mosquitoes and the consequent transmission of malarial infections would have increased the number of intermittent fevers representing true malaria, but any increase is difficult to detect because of the indeterminate classifications of fevers. Plagues of flies may well have been associated with some of the bowel infections during the summer months. If the warm weather did favour some diseases, this was balanced by the elimination of the effects of severe cold and damp, so disastrous in the winter months.

From March onwards the hygiene of the camps was progressively improved. This stemmed largely from the fufilment of the recommendations of the Sanitary Commissioners, but also reflected the fact that, as regiments were reinforced, more able-bodied men were available for fatigue duties. The rules concerning the appropriate siting of cooking places and latrines were now much more strictly observed. Increased attention was given to the provision of safe drinking water, and the avoidance of obvious sources of contamination. In the winter months the soldiers had been grossly overworked, and on account of their exhausted and debilitated state they had succumbed all too easily to disease. There was immediate benefit as soon as the regiments were brought up to strength. Shorter periods of duty in the front line and longer rest periods did much to eliminate mental or physical breakdown. Adequate rations were now received regularly in the camps. A more balanced diet was the rule and the cooks were better trained and better equipped. Scurvy had become a rarity, because fresh meat and fresh vegetables were readily available and prophylactic lime or lemon juice was given routinely.

By April some regiments had a proportion of their men in huts, but it was not until the end of the summer that the use of tents was almost completely discontinued. The huts at first were small and often ill-ventilated, but usually floored and weatherproof. At first, most of the available huts were allocated to the regimental hospitals. These had begun to improve before the winter ended. In February, for example, it was reported that the hospital accommodation of the 93rd Highlanders "was extended by the construction of four huts, each capable of sleeping 16 men...". This provided 64 beds, more than sufficient at this time. By April nearly all patients in the regimental hospitals were in huts. In nearly every regimental report comment is made on the great benefits from this change. The accommodation was by no means luxurious. At first few huts were provided with bedsteads, but by the summer either bedsteads or cots were forthcoming. The buildings provided for the 14th Regiment were "28 feet by 16 feet and ventilated by a window at each end, three moveable wooden shutters at each side, and a louvred opening in the roof". Not all the huts were so large or so well ventilated.

Some regimental reports noted that in the hotter weather patients were nursed in tents rather than in huts. During the summer, the Surgeon of the 4th Regiment wrote as follows:

> The most severe cases of wounds and all amputations were placed in circular tents, protected, however, from the heat by a second tent (unserviceable for other purposes) being placed over them... The object was threefold, by lifting the curtain all round full ventilation and a free current of air were obtained - by these means only the swarms of flies, which proved such a curse to the wounded were in some measure kept down - by placing two men only in each tent they received the individual care and attention of one attendant, and suffered no ill effect from the exhalations of other wounds, and imparted none. In most other regiments it was the custom to place the cases of greater severity in wooden huts.

In general the soldier was now nursed in more salubrious and comfortable conditions. The doctors found it much easier to examine and treat their patients in the less crowded conditions.

In retrospect it must be regretted that hutted accommodation for the regimental hospitals had not been available in the winter. The building materials had begun to accumulate at Balaclava early in December 1854, but transport and labour problems prevented delivery to most of the camps. However, in March 1855, the surgeon of the 77th Regiment reported - "All the sick are now accommodated in huts, the materials for which, from the decrease of transport animals, have been carried up on the shoulders of the men."

The failure to provide a well constructed road between Balaclava and the camps before winter set in has already been noted. During the winter months the condition of the existing rough roads or tracks became progressively worse. Wheeled vehicles often had to be abandoned, thousands of horses, mules, and other beasts of burden, sickened and died from the cold, or from shortage of fodder. Stores of all kinds had to be man-handled, work which greatly exhausted the soldiers. The breakdown of the transport system had far-reaching effects on the health of the army. Medical stores, materials for the construction of huts, new tents, winter clothing and bedding, rations, and supplies of fuel were held up at Balaclava after being unloaded in great quantities from the ships, often to rot on the quay-side. Worst of all, the evacuation of sick and wounded to Balaclava became a miserable and often lethal business.

On 2 December, 1854, the Duke of Newcastle wrote to Raglan with plans for the construction of a rail-road to carry supplies of all kinds from Balaclava to the camps. The priority was to ensure the regular delivery of huge quantities of armaments and ammunition by which the attacks on Sebastopol could be maintained and intensified. A contractor had been hired to send out the necessary materials and equipment for a railway and to engage a labour force of navvies accustomed to laying a railway track. The materials and the navvies arrived at the beginning of February. Work was begun within a week and the first section of a single track line, a distance of two and a half miles from Balaclava to Kadikoi, was completed in ten days. By the end of April the more difficult section, advancing up steep gradients to the camps for another four miles, was finished. The rolling stock consisted of simple four-wheeled trucks, which on the flat were drawn by teams of horses, while on the steeper slopes beyond Kadikoi traction was provided by stationery steam engines. According to Hodge, steam locomotives were introduced later, for he wrote home in November that "locomotives are now running on the railway".[5] The navvies worked with great energy. Some thought they were pampered, being allowed extra rations of beef, barrels of stout, and comfortable huts. But the rapid completion of the railway justified these luxuries. The navvies suffered very little sickness, but accidents were not infrequent. On 11 March, Lawson reported that - "the railway is progressing rapidly. The first accident on it occurred last night by the overturning of a wagon when a man was killed, and another was obliged to have his leg amputated".[6]

Some of the army officers thought it would have been better to have built a good road rather than a railway. On 8 February Clifford wrote - "I have little faith in the proposed railway".[7] Few of the medical officers expressed their views, but George Lawson had as a patient a Mr. Upton, who had worked for the Russians and played a part in planning the fortifications of Sebastopol, and on 22 March Lawson noted as follows.

> Mr. Upton says he is quite sure the railway will be the main instrument in the fall of Sebastopol. By its means we shall be able to bring up to the front such quantities of ammunition etc. that we shall regularly blow the place to pieces about them. I hope he may be right in his conjecture, and I believe myself that until this railway is completed, you may not expect to hear anything very decisive.[8]

In retrospect there is general agreement that the railway did prove a decisive factor in the war, particularly by ensuring a constant supply of ammunition to sustain the attacks on Sebastopol. There is less recognition of the importance of the railway, as far as the general well-being of the army was concerned, through its regular delivery of rations and its bringing up of medical stores, material for building huts and countless other necessities. It occurred to some of the medical staff that the sick and wounded requiring stretchers could be transported comfortably on the railway. Cantlie records that after the Second Bombardment, in April - "Some 400 wounded were dealt with, and compared with the cumbersome ambulance wagons the benefit of the new railway was felt in the speed and comfort with which they were evacuated to Balaclava."[9]

Even with the completion of the railway there continued to be much dependence on transport by road. In the summer of 1855 the roads were, in fact, much improved. In November 1854 Hall had sent an urgent plea to Smith for more ambulance wagons, but by May 1855 only a small number had been delivered, scarcely enough to replace those broken down during the winter, and Hall's full requirements were not met until December 1855. He was also kept short of stretchers and litters of the French type for most of the summer, when casualties were at their height. From the start of the war the lack of a well organised 'wagon-train', similar to that organised so effectively by Wellington in the Peninsular Wars, had been severely felt.[10] The belated provision of the railway in the Crimea and the establishment of a Land-Transport Corps in March 1855 transformed the situation.

MEDICAL CONDITIONS (DISEASES)

Of the 40,627 admissions to the regimental hospitals between April to September 1855, 32,887 (81 per cent) suffered from medical conditions caused by disease.[11] In the preceding three months 98 per cent of admissions had been the result of disease. As in the winter, bowel conditions and fevers accounted for a large proportion of cases. While cholera had disappeared it was rampant once more in the summer months. Frost-bite, which had contributed significantly to the admissions in the winter, was no longer a problem, and scurvy was now rarely a primary cause for admission. The cases in this period were distributed as follows: bowel conditions 50 per cent, fevers 35 per cent, cholera 7 per cent, chest conditions 4 per cent, and miscellaneous conditions 4 per cent.

BOWEL CONDITIONS are listed in the regimental tables under the same somewhat indeterminate headings as those used previously.[12] In the six months from April to September 12,595 patients were admitted under these categories. In April there were 515 cases, in May 1,114, in June 2,931, in July 2,650, in August 2,844, and in September 2,541. Out of the 12,595 cases 250 died (2 per cent). In comparison, the mortality ratio (deaths to admissions) from bowel diseases in the three preceding months had been 21 per cent. Although the fall in the mortality ratio must have been influenced by the improved conditions in the camps the major explanation is likely to be that the bowel disorders were now far less virulent than in the winter. Fourteen regiments had no deaths from bowel diseases throughout the spring and summer, although the same regiments admitted 2,333 cases. This supports the view that the vast majority of cases were of a comparatively mild diarrhoea, associated with infection from food or water. Clearly the winter epidemics - severe types of dysentery (or of typhoid fever) with high mortality - had ceased. In the regimental tables the majority of bowel cases were listed under the heading "Diarrhoea." Many of the doctors may have accepted by this time that the differentiation between diarrhoea and dysentery was useless. In the regimental reports we find clinical descriptions which further indicate that these were mild conditions. In the 17th Lancers, during the six months, there were 196 admissions, mostly rated "diarrhoea", with no deaths. The surgeon reported in May - "Diarrhoea extensively prevailed but in a manageable form". He noted in June that of 50 cases of diarrhoea almost all affected young recruits who had recently joined the regiment. He attributed these outbreaks to intermittent exposure to high temperatures in the day and low temperatures at night, and also suspected "unwholesome water".

Additional information on the bowel diseases in this period is to be found in the post-war medical history.[13] In this survey diarrhoea is still discussed separately from dysentery. Comment is made on the great reduction of cases in most regiments from April onwards, and the much lower mortality rate. These improvements are ascribed very largely to "improved hospital accommodation". There is much rather obscure theorisation. A sudden increase in diarrhoea in some regiments is linked with the outbreak of cholera, - "diarrhoea was, during the course of cholera, almost universal in the camp". It is suggested, as in the earlier months of the war, that if a premonitory attack of diarrhoea was recognised and treated cholera might be averted. The statement is made that some forms of diarrhoea could be attributed to the "choleric state of the air". More acceptable is a brief account of -

> diarrhoea dependent on Epidemic Causes ... induced by agencies proper to the season of the year in warm latitudes - exposure to great heat by day, and heavy dews by night, lying on or near damp ground, the use of unwholesome spirits, improper food ....unripe fruit and green succulent vegetables ... This form of disease is so constantly observed that it is unnecessary to refer to it further ... it obtained no great extension either in Bulgaria or the Crimea, and was therefore comparatively unimportant.

This description fits in very well with a modern interpretation of the acute diarrhoea affecting the traveller in hot climates and on unaccustomed diet. With regard to treatment, not much is added to what was said about treatment during the winter. For the "Endemic Diarrhoea" mild laxatives and diaphoretics were commonly prescribed, "but when the symptoms passed into dysentery, leeches, blisters, synapisms, etc. were often resorted to". Although the mortality rate from bowel diseases (other than cholera) was relatively negligible in these six months, the admission rate remained a considerable drain on the strength of the army.

Turning to FEVERS, in the six months from April to September there were 10,817 admissions.[14] In March there had been 2,305 cases recorded, in April the number fell to 1,881, but it rose again to reach in August 2,204, and then to fall in September to 1,373. Of the 10,817 cases 471 died (4.4 per cent). The mortality ratio in the three previous months had been particularly high in a few regiments, suggesting local epidemics of some severity, but in the subsequent six months the cases were evenly spread among all the regiments, yet with a much lower average mortality.

It is difficult to identify the precise nature of the fevers recorded in this period. The majority were labelled 'common continuous fever'. We may turn to the regimental reports in the hope of extracting some information concerning the pattern of these fevers. The 38th regiment had suffered from a severe fever (probably typhus) in the winter, "in some instances petechiae were present and in many cases, the toes had become gangrenous". In March, of 106 men admitted 30 had died (28 per cent). In April the surgeon recorded - "Fever continued not only the most prevalent disease but it still presented, in part, in its grave character ... The cases generally assumed, in April, the continued type which merged after a week or two with the intermittent or remittent types of the disease." In the three months from April to June, 186 cases were admitted with 25 deaths (13 per cent). In the second three months there were 66 admissions and no deaths. In this regiment the pattern of the winter fevers persisted longer than in most other regiments. That a milder form did eventually develop was attributed to - "the mild weather and the facility thence enjoyed by the soldier of washing his clothes and observing personal cleanliness, to the exemption of the severe fatigue duties which developed upon him in the preceding winter, and to the better arrangements and fuller hospital accommodation". The 4th Regiment also had experienced serious epidemics of fever in the winter. In the following six months 298 cases were admitted with 10 deaths (3.4 per cent). The surgeon reported in April - "During the month there was a considerable amelioration in the health of the troops. Fever decreased in number, and assumed in fewer cases a typhoid type, but it is now often accompanied by diarrhoea of an obstinate character ... Relapses of the disease were not less frequent: and over these quinine appears to possess but a slight influence." After May the admission rates for fevers dropped, with milder cases and a low mortality.

In the post-war history the fevers arising in this period were considered in some detail.[15]

> We have seen that fever preserved a low remittent character for some time after the circumstances of the service had been much improved, and the climate had become mild and agreeable, but the rapid decline in the ratio of mortality which occurred in the month of May, indicates in a striking manner, the gradual disappearance of that element of fever, which was derived from the protracted application of the unhappy artificial conditions of life and affords demonstrative proof of the precise period, the exact time, when the system of the reduced soldier was again in a great degree renovated.[16]

In the summing-up there is little new to learn about treatment. The usual medicines were given. Quinine continued to be used hopefully for all fevers, but many of the doctors became sceptical of its value. Mention is made for the first time of tepid sponging for those with high temperatures, an indication of the better nursing and improved facilities in the hospitals. The term 'Crimean Fever' was used to cover most of the fever cases throughout the whole of the war, while recognising that this became a relatively harmless disease from April 1855 onwards. Perhaps this geographical terminology was more realistic than the varieties listed in the regimental tables!

The second epidemic of CHOLERA began in April 1855 with seven cases, of which five died. In May there were 425 cases, in June 1128, in July 297, in August 447, and in September 63, the total of admissions in the six months period being 2,368. Deaths from cholera totalled 1,423 (60 per cent). The mortality was lowest in June (55 per cent) when the admission rate was at its highest, and highest in July (69 per cent) when the admission rate was much lower. (High mortality in April is disregarded as the number of cases was so small.)[17]

There were conflicting opinions about the source of this second epidemic. The surgeon to the 13th Light Dragoons argued that "the appearance of cholera coincided with the drafts of young soldiers from England and it was among them that the disease chiefly showed itself during the three months of June, July and August ... The old soldiers who had been in the country since the landing of the army were rarely attacked and when attacked the disease was much more manageable". (It must be remembered that in 1855 outbreaks of cholera were active in the ports of embarkation in England and Ireland.) Most of the army medical officers had the same view, including Hall, but the surgeon of the 48th Regiment stated that - "he had been unable to decide whether it [cholera] attacked the old or the young soldier, the weak or the strong, the sober or the intemperate ... All seem alike to have suffered, and some of the most rapid and fatal cases have occurred in men of steady habits, and of strong constitution.[18] Although in a minority among the Crimean doctors, this officer, George Shelton[19], had the same view as had many observers of cholera during the civilian outbreaks in Britain, to the effect that no class of individual was likely to escape infection in an epidemic. Some medical officers believed that the fresh drafts of soldiers who brought cholera back to the Crimea had picked it up in Greece, where most transports called on their way to the East. Others saw the town of Balaclava as the main reservoir of infection. The surgeon of the 33rd Regiment noted that the disease "occurred in the persons of lads who had just joined, some of whom fell victims before they had been two or three days in the country, these soldiers had been kept two or three days in the roadsteads of Balaclava and for two days in the filthy harbour itself alongside the vessels in which cholera existed."[20] Linton talked about the new drafts of soldiers exposed to the "emanations of the harbour".[21]

Meteorological influences were blamed by many for the propagation of the disease. Careful temperature records were kept at the Castle Hospital from April onwards.[22] The incidence of the disease in the summer could not, however, be correlated significantly with the hot weather, for in June the admission rate was highest while July and August were much hotter months. The direction of the wind was also believed to be of importance.[23] A North wind prevailed in June, the worst period, and this was thought to have influenced the spread of the disease.

Both in the regimental reports and in the post-war review there is doubt concerning the spread of cholera by contagion. However, the surgeon of the 10th Hussars, Thomas Fraser[24] wrote -

> Hitherto my experience in India ... has accustomed me to regard cholera as non-contagious, my observations in the Crimea however have lead me to form a very different opinion, namely under certain conditions it at least appears capable of being communicated from the sick to the healthy... whether by emanations from the external surface, or from the secretions from the intestinal canal, I have been quite unable to form an opinion.[25]

Clearly there were contagionists and anti-contagionists among the medical officers. At first the anti-contagionists had been in the majority but by the end of the war the contagionists increased greatly in number. The medical officer of the 10th Hussars was almost unique in suggesting (if only vaguely) that "secretions of the intestinal canal" were associated with the transmission of the disease.[26]

In the post-war history there is no discussion at all of the possibility of infection being water-borne. At home, Snow published a paper in April 1855 on the cause of the sickness and mortality in the Crimea.[27] Not only did he draw attention once more to his belief that the "morbid poison" of cholera was often transmitted in an impure water supply, but also he described how other bowel diseases spread in this way. He noted that although the French had suffered more severely than the British from cholera and other bowel diseases while in Bulgaria in 1854, this situation was reversed in the Crimea. "The chief cause of this circumstance probably is that the French, soon after sitting down before Sebastopol, laid down pipes to convey water to the army from the hills above the camp, whilst the British adopted no such measure." Snow quoted much evidence to show that the water supply used in the British camps was grossly contaminated by the corpses of animals, or by human excreta. He stressed also that although tea and coffee were prepared by boiling water (and were therefore safe) the dilution of the routine rum ration with contaminated cold water was a likely source of cholera infection. He concluded - "the chief means of preserving the health of the troops in the camps is to have water conveyed by pipes from some place where it is out of reach of contamination, and until such a measure is taken no water should be drunk that has not been boiled". The failure of the Army Medical Service to take any notice of Snow's work, either during the war or in the post-war survey, is all the more surprising since the Navy had recognised the water hazard as early as August 1854, and there were many individual army doctors who for their own protection against cholera boiled their drinking water.

The treatment of cholera during the second epidemic continued to be ineffective. The post-war history offered a pessimistic summary. "It is quite unnecessary to enumerate the different remedies which were had recourse to ... We shall be scarcely wrong in adopting the words of Surgeon Marlow of the 28th Regiment, who reports that every well marked case of cholera almost always proved fatal, uninfluenced apparently by any mode of treatment whatsoever."[28] The mortality rate in the second epidemic equalled that which had been observed in Bulgaria, even although in 1855 the general condition of the soldier had improved, as had the facilities for the care of the patient. A curious feature was observed - "unlike the disease as it is exhibited in civil communities, the proportion of deaths to the number treated was as large after the pestilence had considerably subsided, as in the earlier period of its outbreak".[29] One suggested explanation was that in the Crimea the disease was not attacking a static community in which some resistance might have developed, but affected in turn and in a virulent manner each wave of men newly arrived in the Crimea. In the camps cholera remained relatively infrequent after September 1855, and it had died out almost completely by the beginning of 1856. But a third epidemic of some magnitude was to break out in November and December 1855, in the hospitals at Scutari.

CHEST DISEASES accounted for almost 1,500 admissions between April and September 1855.[30] In the first three months there were 76 deaths (11 per cent), but in the second three months, despite a large number of admissions, there were only 13 deaths (4 per cent). Most of the deaths were in April and May and were attributed to pneumonia. The incidence of pulmonary tuberculosis apparently did not increase in this period, despite the arrival of many recruits from the crowded industrial cities of Britain where tuberculosis was rife.

The proportion of miscellaneous conditions appearing in the regimental tables was 4 per cent. In the winter months rheumatic conditions had predominated in this group, but the incidence declined greatly in the spring and summer months. No use was made in the statistics of this period of the heading 'unknown'. Once more, we must remind ourselves that this omission does not suggest a greater accuracy of diagnosis, and instead it may well mean that the positive diagnoses categorised were even less accurate than in the previous months.

SURGICAL CONDITIONS AND WAR WOUNDS

According to the regimental reports 5,647 wounded were admitted to regimental hospitals in the Crimea between April and September 1855. Of these 526 died (9 per cent).[31] But the figures are misleading, and a more accurate estimate is to be found in the post-war history.[32] The number of wounded admitted to all hospitals in the period from 1 April, 1855, to the end of the war was 7,746, with 1,083 deaths (14 per cent). After September few wounded were admitted, apart from accidents, so these figures are only a slight overestimate for the period April to September. The discrepancies between the two sources are accounted for largely by the fact that many wounded by-passed the regimental hospitals and went straight to the larger hospitals in the Crimea. In addition, serious cases were frequently transferred from the regimental hospitals to the larger hospitals after three or four days, and this accounts for the higher death rate in the second series of statistics. The number of wounded transferred to Scutari between April and November was about 750. (November is included as many of the September casualties were not transferred until some weeks after injury.)[33] Only one patient died on passage and 25 died subsequently in the base hospitals. These figures confirm that the wounded were mostly convalescent by the time they were sent to Scutari.

As regards the hospital organisation for the reception of the wounded, the situation in the period from April to September, 1855, was very different from that in the first part of the war. The policy regarding the disposal and management of the wounded was later summarised as follows.

> The necessities which compelled the early removal of the wounded had ceased and henceforward the whole of them were treated with their regiments for a considerable time, and ultimately no-one was sent away from the Crimea who was not looked upon as safe and the probable final result of whose case not considered tolerably well ascertained ... To enable us to effect this a large hospital establishment on the heights above Balaclava, capable of holding 600 patients, which was originally planned as a sanatorium, was converted into a hospital for the wounded, and received its first cases on the 13th April ... a general reserve hospital for wounded was also opened on the 11th May in rear of the 4th Division, capable of accommodating 300 patients.[34] [The first hospital referred to was the Castle Hospital.]

The Balaclava General Hospital has already been mentioned. Spencer Wells visited it in June 1855 and described it as "an old stone house with tiled roof and wooden huts near it ... it is very badly situated, near the head of the harbour, some 40 or 50 feet above sea level".[35] In the autumn of 1854 cholera cases had been concentrated there and for the rest of the war it continued to provide medical rather than surgical beds. The total number of beds available is uncertain but was probably about 450. Few wounded were admitted in the period from April to September 1855.[36] The Castle Hospital at Balaclava was opened late in March, 1855. It was a hutted hospital; it eventually accommodated 590 patients in 32 units of different sizes. It was planned as a surgical hospital and few medical cases were treated. Between April and September, 1553 wounded were admitted of which 69 died (4 per cent).[37] The healthy site of the hospital may partly account for this remarkably low mortality. The absence of disease cases cut down the risk of infection from fevers or bowel diseases, so often fatal in the wounded. In addition there is evidence that the cases admitted here were not very severe. A "General Hospital in Camp" was in existence by about April 1855. The site of this cannot be determined, but it was surrounded by camps. It consisted initially of 22 huts, later increased to 26, each hut holding 14 patients, so the total accommodation was 364. One hut was reserved for officers. All the hutted units were well ventilated and floored but the environment was thought unhealthy, owing to the proximity of camp latrines and rubbish heaps. Between April and November the Camp General Hospital admitted 649 wounded, of whom 162 died (25 per cent).[38] This high mortality suggests that many of the most severely wounded were sent to this hospital. The Monastery Hospital was opened later in the summer some distance from Balaclava, but was intended for convalescent cases only. The hospitals for the Land Transport Corps have already been mentioned briefly and were seldom used for the wounded.

It had been Hall's intention to build up a large number of hospital beds in the Crimea and to cut down transfers of both medical and surgical cases to Scutari and other base hospitals as far as possible. He had at his disposal a large number of beds in the regimental hospitals. Few had less than 24 beds in tents, marquees, or huts. The size of a regimental hospital was always flexible, and extra cases could be accommodated in bell tents. Thus, Hall could count on from 2,000 to 2,500 beds in the regimental hospitals alone. With the Castle Hospital and the General Hospital in the Camp he had another 954 beds. In some reports there is mention of Divisional Hospitals but no offical record of these has been found. However, it is possible that regimental hospitals situated near Divisional Headquarters were exceptionally large, and lavishly staffed and equipped, compared with the usual regimental unit. As medical admissions fell rapidly from April onwards Hall could now usually have a good reserve for any sudden influx of casualties.

It can be presumed that during the relatively quiet spells of the siege, when firing was intermittent, casualties were dealt with largely in the regimental hospitals. When a major attack was mounted special arrangements were made for the transport and reception of the wounded. Some major surgery was done in advanced dressing stations and some in regimental hopsitals, but many cases were sent directly to the larger hospitals in the rear for urgent surgery. On 17 June, when a bombardment was expected to be followed by a major assault, Hall sent out this Memorandum.[39]

> 1. As it is probable an assault will take place soon, superintending staff surgeons of brigades will see that everything in the regimental hospitals is in a perfect state of readiness for the reception of the wounded ... 2. A medical officer of each regiment engaged will follow the column and a Staff-Surgeon of Division should be present to give directions ... They will see that prompt aid is afforded to the wounded and get them carried ... to the hospitals in the rear as soon as possible. 3. Superintending officers will make arrangements for forming temporary field hospitals in the ravines, as near to the scene of action as safety will admit. Here those cases that require immediate operation will be attended to, and then sent either to their own Regimental Hospitals or to the General Hospital in the rear of the Third Division.

The organisation and work of a 'Temporary Field Hospital' was described by Assistant-Surgeon James Cowan of the 55th Regiment.[40] He wrote of his experiences on 8 September during the final assault on the Redan.

> General Hospitals, well in the rear of an army on active service, have usually supplied the material for the records of Surgical experience; and,

THE SIEGE ENDED

indeed, it is not to be wondered at, when we consider how much more extended the field of observation is, and the opportunities there afforded of following cases to a conclusion, and of watching them narrowly during their progress. Surgeons in the field have, however, duties of quite a different, and, perhaps, more important character to perform, than their brethren in General Hospitals, and from their practice something interesting may be learned - they have to perform operations on the spot at once - from a coup d'oeil, so to speak, of a case, they must form an opinion, and be prepared to act on that opinion unhesitatingly; they cannot wait, however much it may be desired, for the advice of a colleague or consulting Physician; they must rely on their own knowledge and personal resources; and it is in proportion as these are developed that the practice of one differs from that of another. The Field Hospital of this regiment, situated on the extremity of a slope forming one side of the Woronzoff ravine, where the latter bifurcates and joins the plateau of Inkermann, is about two miles distant from the Redan. The wounded had, therefore, to be brought this distance. Ambulance-wagons and mules carrying litters and chairs, performed the service of transporting those who could not walk, with wonderful rapidity. Before 5 o'clock, p.m., the whole, with the exception of a corporal, who was not found until midnight, were comfortably in bed, and had been nearly all attended to.[41]

Cowan further reported that his temporary hospital admitted 95 wounded, of which ten were at once sent on to the General Hospital in the Camp. Of the remainder 11 were "dangerously or mortally wounded", 52 "severely wounded", and 23 "slightly wounded". Seven major operations were performed under chloroform, including five primary upper limb amputations. A secondary lower limb amputation was done three days after injury. As far as can be judged there were only two medical officers on duty in this hospital, Cowan and acting Assistant-Surgeon George Fair.[42] The hospital was "visited by the P.M.O." on the third day. He gave advice on the necessity of a secondary amputation in one case. He was probably a Divisional P.M.O., but might have been Hall. Cowan had had some experience of battle casualties at the battle of the Alma (having worked with Mackenzie), and at Inkerman. It seems he was in charge of the hospital, while his senior, Surgeon Ethelberg Blake[43], had probably remained on duty at his regimental hospital. It is likely that only a few regiments involved in major assaults on Sebastopol established Field Hospitals of the type described by Cowan. In many cases the additional unit recommended by Hall must have acted only as an advanced dressing station, from which casualties were quickly taken to hospitals in the rear.

Surgical treatment improved throughout the war. From the statistics available it has been shown that there was a reduction in mortality rates, despite the fact that the effects of missiles were undoubtedly more lethal in the second period than previously. Those surgeons who served throughout the whole of the campaign must have become, by their experience, more skilful in diagnosis, operative technique, and general management. A factor favouring improvement in operative technique was the increasing use of general anaesthesia. There is no strong evidence however that the most experienced and most competent surgeons were deployed in such a way that they were always available to deal with the difficult cases. As we have seen, a young assistant surgeon might well do major operations unsupervised in a Field Hospital. Even in the larger hospitals it may not have been the case that the best surgeons were always available. Relatively few names of outstanding operators emerge during this second period, although a handful come to notice by their reports, by official commendations for their work, or by comments from their colleagues. We do not know (with a few exceptions) who were appointed as chief surgeons in the General Hospitals in the Crimea. The idea of specialist or consultant posts had not been developed. There were instances of high-ranking medical officers giving advice in difficult cases, but very often they were merely exerting their seniority rather than demonstrating superior surgical experience.

The improvement in the general health of the army in the spring of 1855 resulted in an increased resistance to the effects of injury and better healing of wounds. The control of scurvy was one important factor. The policy of admitting casualties to hospitals within relatively easy reach of the front line, and of holding them there until convalescent, ensured much better results than previously. In the first period the mortality rates of the wounded had been greatly increased by the hazards of the voyage to Scutari and by the conditions in the hospitals there. The environment in which surgery was performed was also now more favourable, both in the regimental and in the general hospitals. Even in the temporary field hospitals the equipment was better than that available in the first half of the war. There was no more operating on the battle-field, as at the Alma.

The nature of wounds had changed. "At the Alma the musket ball used was chiefly the old-fashioned round ball. At Balaclava the sword and lance played a conspicuous part." At Inkerman, -

> here the bayonet did its work of destruction ... the musket ball used was still the round ball, but a good sprinkling of wounds were due to the conical bullet ... As the siege progressed the conical ball came more into use ... shell of the largest size were employed and the lacerations produced by these were often frightful to look upon ... Round shot of a size never before employed produced wounds not only by actual impact with the individual wounded, but by the displacement of heavy stones from the parapets, and most of the fractures not compound were thus caused. Magazines exploded, producing extensive burns and other injuries. Grape, canister, hand grenades, fougasses, and slugs contributed their quota of injuries.[44]

It was soon realised that the conical bullet inflicted a much more severe injury than the round ball, causing wide-spread damage to soft tissues, viscera, and bone on lodgment in the body. Through-and-through wounds were thought to be less serious if important blood-vessels or viscera were avoided. It was accepted that there was more damage at the exit wound than at the entrance wound. Flying fragments of exploded shells were thought to be less penetrating than round shot. Unexploded shells or large balls were known to carry away limbs, or even the head in the case of a direct hit. (The popular belief that severe contusion "by the wind of the ball" could occur was not refuted.) An analysis of the agents causing wounds in the final assault on the Redan in September reveals, among a group of 1,910 casualties, 1,003 "by musket ball", 654 "by grape, round shot, or shell", and 253 "by sword, bayonet or other means."[45]

Shock was recognised clinically but ill-understood. In some cases where no positive cause of death could be found, an early collapse of a nervous origin (primary shock) was seen as the explanation. There was no conception of the modern idea of wound shock (secondary shock), due to loss of blood or other body fluids. There was uncertainty about the treatment of shock. Stimulants were advocated by some, in the form of brandy or other spirits: depressants were advocated by others, in the form of opium.[46] Chloroform was now seldom withheld in cases requiring operation, but argument still persisted about the desirability of giving a general anaesthetic to the severely shocked patient. The occurrence of one or two allegedly "anaesthetic deaths" during minor operations led to a fairly strong feeling that chloroform should not be used for these cases.[47]

Considerable importance was attached to the diagnostic use of the probe (or, often, the finger) to estimate the direction of the wound track, to assess bone injury, or to locate bullets, fragments of other missiles, pieces of equipment or clothing, or other foreign bodies. Various forceps were available for removing bullets and the like. If necessary the wound of entry was enlarged so that the finger could be inserted as far along the wound track as possible. (Of course, such exploratory procedures may well have increased the risk of sepsis in wounds.) It was, however, of some benefit to remove missiles, separated fragments of bone and foreign bodies as soon as possible.[48]

At this time the significance of gross soft tissue injury (particularly of muscle) was not appreciated, either in relation to secondary shock or to subsequent infections such as gangrene. According to the official history, the accepted mode of dealing with a gunshot wound was as follows.

> When laceration was extensive and the displacement of soft tissues considerable, as was usually the case in shell wounds, the injured parts were replaced as nearly as circumstances would allow, and as soon after the infliction of injury as possible, they were then retained there by artificial means ... a piece of lint, wetted, and just so many turns of bandage loosely applied as would suffice to keep it in position, was usually considered sufficient dressing by most of the army surgeons, even in large lacerated wounds, and over this most of them placed loosely a single fold of wet lint, rewetted from time to time as it dried, or kept wet by 'irrigation', but the original dressing was seldom disturbed, unless for some special reason, for two and sometimes, three days ... If the laceration was very extensive, and there was difficulty in keeping the parts in position we did not hesitate to use sutures, although these wounds are contused and lacerated ... After the first dressing most of the surgeons used the water dressing i.e. moist lint covered with oiled silk or gutta percha tissue. Some covered the wet lint with a second portion spread with spermaceti, or calamine ointment ... at a later period stimulant washes were often requisite. A simple flesh gunshot wound was often healed in from one to two months. In wounds with injuries to bones most of the surgeons relied on the same means, but a few under these circumstances preferred warm lintseed poultices, as soon as suppuration had been set up ... Slinging wounded limbs, both where fracture existed and where it did not was found to add materially to the comfort of the patient.[49]

No doubt in practice there were many different methods of dealing with wounds. The techniques favoured above may represent the views of Thomas Matthew, the editor of the surgical section of the post-war medical history. He had first served at Scutari as a staff-surgeon and then in the Varna hospital; he had later been medical officer of the transport 'Cambria' which carried wounded to Scutari after the Alma and had thereafter worked in the Balaclava General Hospital.

The technique of wound management, without any suggestion of cleansing or disinfecting the affected area, without excision of grossly damaged soft tissues, and without (in most cases) relieving tension by laying open the skin and deeper layers, would appear to have carried a high risk of infection. However the practice of packing wounds tight with 'charpie', or other material which was inevitably septic, had been discarded.[50] If sutures were used care was taken that these were not tied too tightly. Healing of gunshot wounds by 'first intention' was not expected and infection was accepted. "When a musket ball was lodged in the soft tissues, an abscess, in the great majority of cases, formed about it in from 8 to 14 days time."[51] Such localised abscesses were usually easy to deal with, often discharging spontaneously through the wound track. Diffuse inflammations seem to have been surprisingly rare. Sloughing of wounds was not uncommon (attributed by some to a dry 'sirocco' wind from the South-East), but was, however, usually a superficial condition and seldom the cause of secondary bleeding or of fatal complications.[52]

The incidence of GANGRENE of a serious nature was rarely reported except after major injuries of the limb arteries. "Except for this form of sloughing ulceration nothing at all resembling hospital GANGRENE was at any time seen amongst the wounded at the Crimea."[53] In fact, Hall was influenced in retaining the wounded in the Crimea because of reports of hospital gangrene amongst the wounded transferred to Scutari during the winter. There was, however, at least one epidemic of gas gangrene in the Crimea.[54] From the description it seems to have been a fulminating infection with severe toxaemia, collapse, and death often in less than 24 hours from the onset of symptoms. This epidemic broke out in June in the General Hospital in the Camp. It affected mainly patients who had undergone major amputations. The incidence and mortality rates are not stated. The epidemic remained local and did not recur. Some associated the lethal nature of this complication with a coincidental outbreak of cholera. In some of the regimental tables "gangrene" is listed as a separate entity, but it is never clear whether this is a complication of war wounds, of frost-bite (in the winter), or of medical conditions. It can be said that all the conditions which favoured gangrenous infection of wounds were present. In addition the circumstances of trench warfare with the risk of implantation of anaerobic organisms (the cause of gangrene) or fragments of dirty clothing might have been expected to raise the incidence of this serious complication. It does not seem, however, that the soil in the Crimea was as infective as of the highly manured fields of France in the 1914-1918 war. The low incidence of tetanus in the wounded also suggests that anaerobic organisms were not common in the Crimean battle fields.

Only 21 cases of TETANUS were recognised between April and September 1855, of which 11 were in the latter month.[55] The clinical picture was well-known and it is unlikely that many cases were missed. Of the 21 cases only one survived, the interval between wounding and the onset of symptoms being 17 days. Most of the deaths were within an incubation period of five days (still a circumstance of grave prognosis). The true cause was of course unknown, but weather conditions were often suspected, such as a high humidity with low barometric pressure. The association of tetanus with wounds of all kinds was well recognised but injuries to nerves were thought to be particularly prone to this complication, supporting a theory of "direct irritation of nerve endings". Treatment was of little avail. Morphine in heavy dosage or chloroform by inhalation was used to control spasms, with occasional success. The incidence of tetanus being much lower than in previous wars, this was thought to be due to the abandonment of earlier dressing techniques which involved the packing of wounds "with charpie or other irritating substances". A small epidemic occurred in the Second Rifle Brigade. Four soldiers developed the disease and all had been injured on the same day, sustaining flesh wounds only. All developed symptoms four days after injury and all died (two within three days of the onset of the symptoms). A factor may have been that all four were operated upon in the same dressing station or operating room, hence the infection may have been implanted by contaminated ligature material, instruments, dressings, or operating room dust.

Plagues of flies were a great problem in the hot weather.[56] The surgeons went to great length to try to diminish this source of irritation to the wounded by nursing them in separate tents (as already described). All sorts of applications were used to prevent eggs being laid in the wounds, creosote in water being one of the most useful preparations since it also destroyed any larvae which had hatched out. The infestation of wounds with larvae (or maggots) was looked on with horror by doctors and nurses alike, and seen as evidence of gross neglect on the part of those managing the case. It was not realised that maggots could have a beneficial effect at certain stages of healing.[57]

Although blood letting was still used in the management of some medical conditions it was now less popular for the wounded. The illogicality of withdrawing blood from those already exsanguinated was more generally recognised. "Because a man was shot through the chest or other important part, the surgeon did not there and then pull out his lancet and bleed him till he fainted." Traditions died hard, however - "in inflammations following gunshot or other wounds, the army surgeon had ceased as a rule to apply them [venesections]".[58] But there was still support "for the abstraction of 12 ozs.

of blood at the commencement of inflammation", in the belief that in some obscure way this would promote a beneficial 'adhesive' inflammation. From unofficial accounts of treatment of the wounded there are in fact several accounts of the free use of bleeding. For example, Assistant-Surgeon Thomas Birnie[59], in a report of gunshot wounds of the head and chest, describes the management of a patient with a penetrating chest wound. After admission he was bled to the extent of 48 ounces. Next day eighteen leeches were applied to the chest. Three days later he was very ill. "He was now bled again to the extent of twenty ounces in the erect posture till syncope was nearly reached: was again relieved by the depletion." Despite all this the patient did recover, "although 68 ounces of blood may appear a large quantity to take in so short a period".[60]

A detailed account of the types of wounds in this period and their frequency and mortality is now given, with some comparison between the experiences in the earlier and the later parts of the war.

The records of the wounded after April 1st, 1855 were kept much more accurately than previously. In the first period a heading, "Particulars not known, no records of them have been kept, or, the records have been lost" was used, and in this group there were 1,815 cases. No such heading was repeated in the tables of the second period. The classification of wounds for the second period was made largely on a regional anatomical basis: Gunshot Wounds of the Head, of the Face, of the Neck, of the Chest, of the Abdomen, of the Perineum and Genito-urinary Organs, of the Back and Spine, and of the Extremities. Sword, Lance, and Bayonet Wounds were listed separately with no regional differentiation. There was a heading Miscellaneous Wounds and Injuries. "Gunshot" wounds covered those from all varieties of missiles.[61]

The 898 HEAD WOUNDS treated after 1 April represent 12 per cent of the admissions for all wounds in this second period.[62] (In the first period head wounds represented only 5 per cent of the wounded). There were 668 "Simple Flesh Wounds" of which 466 were classified as "slight". These latter require no special comment, and none was fatal. Simple dressings were applied and suture was rarely done. There were 212 "severe" flesh wounds, from which seven men died (3.4 per cent). In these fatal cases there was usually delayed recognition of fractures or brain injury. There were 63 cases labelled "Cranial Fracture without depression of the bone", and from these 23 died (36 per cent). This high mortality was attributed in some cases to a depressed fracture not having been recognised clinically and in others to an apparently simple fracture proving later to be associated with gross brain damage. Such cases were treated initially by "calomel or antimony, with or without purgatives, and venesection should be had recourse to as a prophylactic against inflammation." In a few cases a delayed cranial exploration was done to exclude a more serious condition than that at first diagnosed, but the results of these late interventions were very poor. In a small group of cases there were delayed operations of a minor type to remove fragments of sequestrated or dead bone. In general non-operative treatment was applied in this group.

"Depressed fracture of the skull (with confusion)" might be readily diagnosed if there was an open wound but if in a closed injury could easily be missed. There were 76 cases in this group and 55 died (72 per cent). It was recognised that in a missile wound the inner table of the skull was often more severely damaged than the outer. In 50 cases no attempt was made to decompress the brain by elevation of the depressed fracture and 36 died. In 26 cases the depressed bone was elevated but 19 still died. These operations were sometimes easy and depressed fragments of bone were readily manipulated to relieve compression on the brain, although in some cases the trephine was necessary so that leverage could be effected through the trephine hole. The high mortality was therefore associated with infection acquired at the time of wounding or at operation.

Meningitis, brain abscess and diffuse brain infection were the common and lethal complications of these wounds. In many cases the full extent of brain damage remained uncertain. In some a second serious fracture, remote from the obvious site of injury, ('contre-coup' fracture), might not be recognised. Whether operation was done or not, purgatives were given, such as calomel (in fact an acceptable means of reducing swelling of brain tissue). Bleeding was quite often employed for the unconscious patient. Some surgeons were content to apply leeches locally, rather than to do venesections. Of the few patients who recovered from major surgery many developed 'brain fungus' of the herniated brain substance, paralyses of various types, or permanent mental changes. "Penetrating wounds of the cranium" and "Perforating wounds of the cranium" can be considered together although separated in the tables. Of these there were 93 cases, and all which died. It was reported that these presented "some of the most terrible and hopeless cases which it is the lot of the military surgeon to witness, and many of them, in a scientific point of view, are mere curiosities .... these are of necessity, and, it may be said, happily, mortal wounds, and, beyond mention that such occur, seem to require no notice."

In March 1856 the veteran Guthrie communicated to the **Lancet** a series of 15 detailed reports of head injuries treated in the Crimea.[63] Seven of these reports were written by Rooke, who had been transferred to the Crimea from Renkioi and attached to the Camp General Hospital. One report was furnished by Ranke, another civil surgeon, transferred from Smyrna to the Crimea. Six reports were given by regimental medical officers. Finally Maunder, from Renkioi, reported on a very unusual case which was a complicated facial injury rather than a cranial injury. In this instance Staff-Surgeon Mouat had attempted to control severe bleeding (with temporary success) by ligating the common carotid artery. These cases are mentioned because the descriptions of the operations done (such as trephining) are much more detailed than those in the illustrative cases of the post-war review. It is interesting too that there were seven deaths in the series and six post-mortem examinations were done. Cranial surgery had not advanced greatly by 1855 and the experience of war reflected that in civilian life, in which the results of surgical intervention were no better.

Gunshot WOUNDS OF THE FACE totalled 573, but only 14 men died (2.4 per cent).[64] There were 299 "slight" and 116 "severe" flesh contusions or wounds. In 113 cases bony structures were penetrated, and of these 9 died (8 per cent). Of the 46 cases associated with eye injuries, 3 died. In general the healing of facial wounds was remarkably rapid and without serious infection. If there was severe bone injury then the problems of treatment were considerable. Plastic procedures were limited to the careful suture of eyelids. More elaborate techniques such as rhinoplasty (reconstruction of the nose) were left to the surgeons at home. Gunshot WOUNDS OF THE NECK numbered 147, of which three died (2 per cent).[65] Of flesh wounds 47 were "slight" and 76 "severe" (of which two died). There were two laryngeal injuries, one involving larynx and oesophagus, and one involving the trachea. All these recovered. Wounds involving the great vessels of the neck are not included in this section.

Gunshot WOUNDS OF THE CHEST accounted for 6 per cent of all wounds and totalled 474, of which 117 died (25 per cent).[66] There were 154 "simple" and 126 "severe" flesh contusions or wounds. Two of the latter died, probably of a post-traumatic pneumonia. There were 25 cases of injury to the ribs or cartilages (without pleural or lung injury), of which one died from pneumonia. Lesions of the contents of the thorax without penetration of the chest numbered 17, with ten deaths (59 per cent). Unfortunately details of these cases are sparse, only four being described and these briefly. Three were due to shell explosions causing rib fractures in two cases and no fracture in one case. The fourth case was fatal and the injury was due to a round shot hitting the scapular area but causing no fractures, producing a "total contusion of the lungs". It is possible that in such cases occurring in close proximity to an explosion the condition was similar to that now defined as 'blast lung'. "Wounds opening the chest cavity" numbered 147, and 120 died (82 per cent). It was thought that a 'through-and-through' wound was less likely to be fatal than one in which a missile lodged in the lung. Some of these patients died of haemorrhage within hours. Those who survived the immediate period after injury almost inevitably developed empyema or lung abscess, which was often fatal. "It seems very doubtful if every case in which the ball was fairly lodged within the pleural chest lining did not terminate in death." In the immediate period following injury, internal or external bleeding (or more rarely haemoptysis) were the main hazards. In very few cases could the source of haemorrhage be located, far less controlled, yet such bleeding was known to stop spontaneously. Venesection was sometimes thought of value. The only immediate surgery recommended was the removal of fragments of bone or missiles lying close to the surface and perhaps traumatising the lung. A limited probing with the finger was permitted. Chest wounds were not sutured but merely covered by a light dressing. In the surviving patient inflammation or suppuration was considered inevitable. On occasion a localised abscess might discharge spontaneously through the wound track, while in late cases a circumscribed abscess might be suspected and drained by a well-placed incision. Even if bullets or other missiles were believed to be retained in the chest explorations were not attempted, as the exact location of the foreign body was seldom known. It was often policy to leave the surviving case to recover by natural processes, and in a few instances this did happen.

Gunshot WOUNDS OF THE ABDOMEN were reported in 268 cases (3 per cent of all wounds), leading to 131 deaths (49 per cent).[67] There were 35 "slight" and 66 "severe" flesh wounds of the abdominal wall without penetration of the abdominal cavity. None of those with slight wounds died, but 17 with severe wounds did so (26 per cent). No explanation of the high mortality rate in the latter group is given. It is possible that severe haemorrhage was the cause of death in some instances, and gross infection or gangrene followed extensive muscle damage in others. There were only four cases of "Visceral Rupture without an external abdominal wound" (closed rupture). All these patients died. Autopsies appear to have been done, as two ruptures of the liver, one of the spleen, and one of the intestines are listed. Such injuries were due usually to direct blows from large fragments of stone blown off the parapets.

The classification of wounds penetrating the abdominal cavity is confusing but a simple division can be made into those penetrating the peritoneal cavity without damaging viscera or causing severe bleeding, and those penetrating with visceral damage or severe bleeding. Only five of the former are listed, with three deaths, but there are 101 of the latter with 95 deaths (94 per cent). Many patients with penetrating abdominal wounds died of severe bleeding within a few hours of injury. Shock was thought to cause early death in many instances. Of those patients who survived the first few hours, most died later of infection varying from peritoneal abscess to general peritonitis. Surgical intervention was rarely performed except in cases where viscera protruded through the wound. If intact, the viscera were returned to the peritoneal cavity and the wound closed. Very occasionally if the bowel was perforated and prolapsed through the wound, it would be left exteriorised as an enterostomy or colostomy with some hope of recovery.

In the post-war review the emphasis is very much on non-operative treatment. The illustrative cases include none in which suture of perforated bowel was done. We are left with only vague indications of attempts at reparative surgery. "Few cases, also, came under notice where suture of the gut was required, or had recourse to and where such occurred they were, without exception, fatal." The message seemed to be that exploration should not have been attempted for penetrating wounds of the abdomen, but that "our endeavours were directed to assist in 'procuring the agglutinative process' if possible, or, at all events, not to thwart nature in her efforts for effecting that object". Thus, "bullet wounds were dressed by a wet compress of lint, or a piece of adhesive plaster; while shell lacerations were brought together by sutures inserted through the skin and cellular tissue ... [recovery depended on] quiet, restriction both in the articles of food and drink, occasionally small lumps of ice ... abstinence from aperients or even enemata, for several days, [and] the exhibition of opium, with treatment of the symptoms of peritoneal inflammation as they arose." Venesection in the acute phase was not recommended, thus following the teaching of Guthrie. Of the ten cases of abdominal injury summarised in the post-war review only one had venesection as treatment. While a handful of recoveries were reported after non-operative treatment it had to be confessed that "almost all the cases died ... and in hardly any of the recoveries can the fact of penetration of the abdominal cavity be considered indisputable".

The use of general anaesthesia might have encouraged a bolder approach. In civil life, at this time, there were very few abdominal procedures attempted other than those for the drainage of an abdominal abscess, for strangulated hernia, or, rarely, for removal of a chronic ovarian cyst. Spencer Wells, who was later to put abdominal surgery on a new footing by his work on ovariotomy, seems to have observed in the base hospitals (or on his brief visit to the front) some rare and unexpected recoveries following penetrating wounds of the abdomen.[68] He was thus encouraged in the belief that the peritoneum could deal with severe infection remarkably well and that the risks of abdominal exploration had been exaggerated. No other serving surgeon seems to have returned from the war with any such optimism concerning the future of abdominal surgery.

Gunshot WOUNDS OF THE PERINEUM AND GENITO-URINARY ORGANS totalled 57, with 17 deaths (30 per cent).[69] The fatal cases were mostly associated with bladder or urethral rupture. Gunshot WOUNDS OF THE BACK AND SPINE totalled 355, with 48 deaths (14 per cent)[70] There were 157 "slight" and 116 "severe" flesh contusions or wounds, the latter leading to 20 deaths. Most of these wounds were inflicted by exploding shells, the soldier at the time of injury lying on his face for protection. In such cases muscle damage was often extensive and the risk of sloughing or gangrene high, hence "the patient died of exhaustion and worn out by suppuration". Of ten cases with "fractured spine but no nerve injury", six died. Of 22 "spinal injuries with nerve damage", 21 died. Usually there were gross fractures in these cases, with severe contusion or even severance of the spinal cord. If there was survival from the haemorrhage and shock of the injury, death was almost inevitable from ascending meningeal infection, or from the septic consequences of bladder paralysis, since catheterisation, necessary in such cases, was then always a septic procedure.

Gunshot WOUNDS OF THE EXTREMITIES (i.e. limbs) accounted for 4,754 admissions (62 per cent of all wounded).[71] Of these patients 273 died (6 per cent). Three minor sub-groups are first distinguished: those with direct or primary injury to the larger arteries (but no compound fracture), those with direct injury to major nerves (but no compound fracture) and those with penetration of the larger joints.

Of the first sub-group there were only 13 cases, with nine deaths, major arterial injuries in the limbs being much more common as secondary to compound fractures. In this small group of isolated injury to vessels, the first problem was control of bleeding. It was generally accepted that an immediate amputation should be done for severe injury to the femoral artery, since if ligation alone was done gangrene was almost certain and would demand secondary amputation. Below the knee local ligation was thought worth while. Survival of the upper limb usually followed ligation of the brachial artery. The high death rate in this small group is most likely explained by excessive loss of blood before controlling the bleeding vessel (either by ligation or by primary amputation), and by a significant incidence of secondary haemorrhage or infection in the amputation stump. Of the second sub-group, injuries to nerves, there were 23 cases with 7 deaths. Much was made of the high incidence of tetanus in this group, accounting for five of the seven deaths. The brachial plexus was involved in five cases, the sciatic nerve in five cases, the median in five cases, the ulnar in four cases, and in two cases the nerve is not specified.

Of the third sub-group there were 121 cases, with 23 deaths (19 per cent). These were penetrations of major joints, with bone injury confined to the immediate vicinity of the joint and without excessive soft tissue injury. Unfortunately the specific joints involved are not mentioned in 33 cases, but as 11 of this undocumented group died (33 per cent), it seems likely that a majority of lower limb cases were included. Reported injuries of the upper limb totalled 47, with seven deaths; and of these 17 involved the shoulder joint, with three deaths. Reported injuries of the lower limb totalled 41, with seven deaths. Ten involved the hip joint, and three died "from the severity of the injury" before any operation could be done. The seven who survived were transferred to other hospitals for delayed operation, amputation in one case and "joint resection" in six. The survival of these seven patients after secondary operations is not certain. Reported injuries of the knee joint totalled 23, with three deaths. The opinion about treatment of these cases was expressed as follows. "Gunshot wounds of the knee joint are generally looked upon as demanding either amputation or excision and were those operations attended with less danger it might seem right to have recourse to one or other in almost all cases in which the bone is implicated beyond the most trifling amount ... the risk to life from such a wound treated without operative interference is very considerable." It appears that about half of these cases were treated without operation initially and 15 had to have secondary operations, all but one being an amputation. These secondary amputations were most likely done for sepsis and "proved a very formidable operation, terminating fatally in a large proportion of cases". In the statistics of this group there must be some overlap with cases in which excision of a joint was done. (Joint excision is discussed below).

The three sub-groups of wounds of the extremities just discussed are not altogether satisfactory categories. With joint injury it was not really possible to draw a clear line between a local joint injury and a major compound fracture. Few so-called primary arterial and primary nerve injuries were in fact isolated, since all were certain to have soft tissue injury of varying degree and some had associated fractures. The majority of gunshot wounds of the extremities, having no claim to fall into the above sub-groups, are now discussed as a general category. General gunshot wounds of the extremities numbered 3,785, with 213 deaths (6 per cent). This total is divided into upper limb injuries 1,279, with 47 deaths (4 per cent) and lower limb injuries 2,456, with 176 deaths (7 per cent). Many minor injuries are included in this series, hence the comparatively low mortality ratios.

To begin with upper limb injuries. In the first group of upper limb injuries, "slight flesh contusions and wounds" numbered 689 with no deaths, and "severe" flesh contusions or wounds numbered 500 with 8 deaths. The fatal cases in the latter group must have followed gross muscle injury with severe blood-loss or severe infection. One major amputation was required as a secondary procedure following a severe flesh wound. In the second group, "Simple Fractures of the Long Bones following contusion by round shot, shell, or stones", there were 27 admissions with two deaths: "these injuries occasionally required amputation, the whole substance of the limb having been disorganised." In the third group, "Contusions or Partial Fracture of Long Bones, including Fracture of the Clavicle and Scapula", there were 102 admissions with 12 deaths (12 per cent). There were cases in which localised fractures occurred from the passage of a missile. The bones were either grazed or cracked, but occasionally there was a localised comminuted fracture (strictly speaking, these were compound fractures). Most of the deaths in this group were instances of fractures of the scapula or upper end of the humerus, associated with chest injuries.

In the fourth group, "Compound Fractures", there were 310 admissions, with 22 deaths (7 per cent). These were defined as "complete compound gun-shot fractures of the long bones." The humerus was involved in 167 cases, with 13 deaths (8 per cent); both radius and ulna in 66 cases, with two deaths: the radius alone in 38 cases, with 3 deaths: the ulna alone in 37 cases, with 4 deaths. The mortality rate for all forearm fractures was 6 per cent. These upper limb compound fractures varied greatly in their severity. Included were "limbs torn off by round shot or shell", for which amputation was inevitable. For less destructive lesions the results of conservative management was regarded as encouraging. The indications for primary amputations for injury of the humerus were "extensive longitudinal splintering of bone" and "gross destruction of soft parts." The number of amputations done for compound fractures of the humerus is not clearly indicated. Severe comminuted fractures were not necessarily indications for amputation, since loose fragments of bone or the detached head of the humerus could frequently be removed by a relatively minor operation. For fractures both of the humerus and of the bones of the forearm secondary amputation was more frequently done than primary amputation. The amputation rate (for primary and secondary operations combined) was about 65 per cent for fractures of the humerus, and less than 35 per cent for forearm fractures. The conservative treatment of upper limb compound fractures involved simple methods of splinting. "No complicated or expensive apparatus was thought necessary." Sepsis was almost inevitable. In some cases healing was hastened by drainage of localised abscesses and removal of fragments of dead bone or of missiles; in others amputation had to be done for progressive inflammations. The figures are not clearly stated but secondary amputation for advanced sepsis almost certainly accounted for many of the deaths in this series.

There were 407 admissions for wounds of the carpus, metacarpus and fingers. The rate of invaliding was high in these cases because of residual disabilities.

Turning to lower limb injuries. In the first group, "Simple Flesh Contusions and Wounds", rated "slight", numbered 792, and those rated "severe" 836. There were 49 deaths in the latter group (6 per cent). This significant mortality rate must have been related to haemorrhage or sepsis in the bulky muscle groups of the legs, particularly in the buttocks and thighs. As many as seven amputations were required for severe soft tissue injuries. In the second group, "Simple Fractures of the Long Bones by Contusion of round-shot, shell, or stones", there were 23 cases, with one death. In the third group, "Contusion or Partial Fracture of Long Bones" there were 43 cases, with one death. These consisted of "partial longitudinal fissures, without displacement", occurring in the track of a missile (in fact compound fracures).

In the fourth group, "Compound Fracture", there were 384 cases with 100 deaths (26 per cent). The femur was involved in 174 cases, with 64 deaths (37 per cent), the tibia and fibula in 144 cases, with 27 deaths (19 per cent), the tibia alone in 44 cases, with six deaths (14 per cent), and the fibula alone in 22 cases, with three deaths (14 per cent). Conservative treatment was discouraging for lower limb compound fractures. The percentage of cases in which amputation was avoided and the patient survived was eight for fractures of the femur, 19 for fractures of the tibia and fibula, 36 for the tibia alone and 41 for the fibula alone. From the information available it seems that amputation, primary or secondary, was done in about 80 per cent of compound fractures of the femur, 70 per cent of the tibia and fibula, 50 per cent of the tibia alone, and 60 per cent of the fibula alone. Proportionally more primary amputations were done for lower limb than upper limb compound fractures. Both primary and secondary amputation for compound fractures of the lower limb caused high mortality rates, but the exact figures are unknown. For thigh amputations a figure of between 65 and 75 per cent is likely, for lower leg amputations 35 to 40 per cent. Conservative treatment was selected for lower limb compound fractures where it was thought that soft tissue damage was not excessive. It was much less likely to be used for fractures of the femur than for lower leg injuries.

In the fifth and sixth groups a variety of injuries of the tarsus, metatarsus and toes is listed. In total there were 120 admissions, with eight deaths. Fatalities most likely followed gross destructive lesions of structures of the foot in which amputation was probably the only answer but was perhaps delayed too long.

Conservative treatment for compound fractures consisted of simple dressings applied on the principles already described. Some form of splintage was routinely used. For upper limb fractures, as already noted, the simplest devices were used. For lower limb fractures use was made of simple long splints, MacIntyre's splint, or more rarely, the double inclined plane. Minor surgery to remove fragments of bone was adopted when necessary. Abscess formation was frequent and drainage often occurred spontaneously through the wound. The severe infections with spreading cellulitis, pyaemia or septicaemia were treated by amputation, but this seldom saved life. Healing was always slow even in the more favourable cases, with chronic sinus formation, slow union of the bones, and, occasionally, non-union. Antiseptic solutions (such as Burnett's Zinc preparation) was sometimes applied to the wounds. A generous diet was given, and wine freely prescribed. There was the inevitable faith in quinine for any febrile reactions.

Sword, bayonet and miscellaneous wounds totalled 169, of which 11 died (7 per cent).[72] In the second period of the war there were few of these types of wounds.

AMPUTATION deserves separate discussion. Between April 1855 and the end of the war 470 major amputations were carried out, with 204 deaths (43 per cent).[73] Most of these were done for wounds received in the siege. After September numerous secondary amputations were carried out on those wounded during the six months of fighting before Sebastopol. Unfortunately the tables quoted do not specify the reasons for amputation. However comparison is possible between the different sites of amputation. Major amputations of the upper limb numbered 204, with 43 deaths (21 per cent). Amputations at the shoulder joint numbered 37, with 13 deaths (35 per cent), at the elbow 102, with 27 deaths (26 per cent), at the forearm 59, with 3 deaths (5 per cent); and at the wrist one (who survived). Some comparative statistics of primary and secondary amputations are also available.[74] Primary amputations of the upper limb totalled 182, with 32 deaths (18 per cent), while secondary amputations totalled 19, with 9 deaths (47 per cent). Major amputations of the lower limb totalled 291, with 156 deaths (54 per cent). There were seven amputations "at the hip joint" and all died (100 per cent); 39 "at the upper end of the thigh" of which 34 died (87 per cent); 65 "at the middle third of the thigh" of which 39 died (60 per cent); 60 at the lower third of the thigh of which 34 died (57 per cent); 101 "at the lower leg" of which 36 died (36 per cent); and 12 "at the ankle joint" of which 2 died (17 per cent). Amputations through the knee joint were not listed separately. All told, there were 251 primary amputations of the lower limb of which 127 died (51 per cent) and 40 secondary amputations of which 27 died (68 per cent).[75]

The technique of amputation varied greatly. "As a general rule, flap operations were performed in preference to the circular in primary cases, but in secondary ones, more especially when the patient was much reduced, the circular method had many advocates." Clearly the planning of flaps must have been influenced greatly by local skin loss in the original trauma. The healing of amputation stumps was seldom straightforward. Sepsis almost inevitably supervened to cause abscess formation and a chronic discharging sinus. In many cases the cut end of the bone became infected and it was months before dead bone was discharged and the wound finally healed. A large proportion of amputation cases spent long periods in hospital in England under treatment for stump problems.

A comparison of the mortality rates for amputation between the first and second periods of war might be thought to offer some evidence of improvements in surgical management as the war progressed. Unfortunately the records in the first period are not satisfactory. From one source it appears that 256 amputations and resections were done with only 22 deaths "in the Field Hospital" (the number of resections was probably very small). This represents an exceptionally low mortality of 9 per cent. A fuller story is however told in a subsequent table in which it is shown that of 216 cases of primary amputation "transferred from the Crimea", 14 died "on passage", and 41 died "in secondary hospitals" (i.e. at Scutari). This gives a total of 77 fatal results and a mortality rate of 30 per cent for all primary amputations in the first period. The comparable rate for primary amputations in the second period is 43 per cent. But the apparent increase is misleading, for the statistical returns before April 1855, particularly those after the battle of the Alma, are notoriously incomplete. In the post-war survey a table showing mortality rates for amputations in previous campaigns is given but the figures are not readily comparable. Some comparison is also made with London and Paris hospitals.[76] The London results are better than the Crimean results but the Paris results are worse. For the purpose of comparison, statistics relating to a large contemporary series of amputations in Glasgow Infirmary are of value. A total of 461 amputations produced, 177 deaths (38 per cent), 197 being classed as primary amputations, with 61 deaths (31 per cent), and 264 as secondary amputations, with 116 deaths (44 per cent). It seems likely that surgical management in relation to amputation was at a level of competence in the Crimea little different from that in civilian life, at least in the later period.

A limited number of joint resection operations was carried out throughout the war. These are recorded for the second period in the amputation tables.[77] They totalled 47, with 12 deaths (26 per cent), 36 being primary operations and 11 secondary operations. (Such conservative operations were well established in civil life, particularly to deal with tuberculous joints, as an alternative to amputation). The shoulder joint was operated on 14 times, nine primary operations with two deaths and five secondary operations with no deaths. The elbow joint was operated on 17 times, 13 primary operations with three deaths and four secondary operations with no deaths. In the lower limb the hip joint was operated upon six times, five primary operations with four deaths, and one secondary operation which was fatal. The knee joint was operated on only once and the patient died. The remainder of the operations listed were on minor joints with no deaths. The object of these resections was to remove comminuted fragments of bone from the vicinity of joints. In the shoulder joint it was the head of the humerus which was most often resected, but occasionally the socket on the scapula was also removed. At the elbow complete resection of the joint was sometimes done, removing comminuted areas of bone from the articular surfaces of the humerus and the ulna in most cases. The functional results were usually remarkably good but in two elbow resections secondary amputations had to be done for sepsis and the patients both died. In the hip joint, excision of the head of the femur was the usual resection procedure but the results were very poor. Nevertheless local resection was advocated in suitable cases rather than amputation at the hip joint. The experience of resection at the knee joint was confined to one case and sepsis proved fatal. It was not considered that this operation was advisable for the knee joint. In civilian surgery, joint excisions implied that all the synovial membrane (or lining) of the joint was removed, together with a limited amount of underlying bone. The operation in military surgery was more crude and in some instances several inches of the adjacent shaft of a long bone was excised (with the inevitable production of a flail joint). These operations were seldom attempted in the first period of the war but became more popular and increasingly successful in the second period. That the military surgeons were, even in a limited way, prepared to apply joint resection for the wounded was an indication of their readiness to apply new techniques.

THE DOCTORS IN THE FRONT LINE

The routine duties of the junior medical officers during the quieter periods of the siege were described by Spencer Wells after his short visit to the battle front in June, 1855.

> During the time I spent in the camp the only active operations before the enemy took place in the siege batteries and trenches opposed to the defences of Sebastopol. The men employed in our works are exposed to wounds from rifle-bullets, round shot, shell and their fragments, splinters of stone, and bayonet thrusts in case of a sortie. They are accompanied, not only in the batteries, but in the advanced works, by Medical officers, whose duty it is to suppress haemorrhage, and afford any such assistance as the wounded men may require before removal to a place of greater security. Formerly both men and Medical officers remained twenty-four hours in the works, but of late they have been relieved every twelve hours. The relief party leaves the camp about 3.30 a.m. and half-an-hour before sunset. A walk of something more than half-an-hour, along natural covered ways formed by ravines, brings the party to the batteries in the first parallel, from which trenches are carried to the advanced works. On the relief arriving, the party employed returns to camp. Wounds from shot and shell sometimes occur during the transit to and from the camp, as the enemy have information from deserters the direction taken by the working parties and the hours of relief. The Medical officers are accordingly accompanied by an orderly, who carries such instruments and necessaries as may be immediately required, either in the walk, or during the twelve hours of duty. In each of our batteries in the first parallel, a sort of hut, in a tolerably sheltered spot, is used as a surgery. One Medical officer is always stationed there, and sometimes two or more. Others accompany the men into the advanced works. When a man is wounded the nearest Medical officer is immediately called to him, and often has to run the gauntlet of several embrasures at which the Russians are directing their shot, before he arrives at his patient; so that he not only runs as much risk as a combatant, but very often considerably more. The man having received such attention as he immediately requires, is carried on stretchers, or supported if he can walk, to the hut in the battery of the first parallel, where more assistance is given if necessary, and he is afterwards conveyed to a sheltered spot in the ravine leading to the camp where ambulance

wagons are always in waiting to carry wounded to the Regimental Hospitals - a distance, probably, of a mile. Here the French system differs from ours. Where we put men into ambulance wagons the French have advanced Field-Hospitals and a Medical Staff for the performance of primary operations. Most of the Medical men with whom I conversed seemed to think this plan better than ours, as a mile in an ambulance wagon can be better supported by a man with a dressed stump than with a shattered limb.[78]

There are many other accounts from army medical officers. An anonymous letter was published in **The Times** describing a surgeon's experiences in April.

> In my last letter I told you I was going to the trenches. Well, I went and I had enough of it ... We paraded at a quarter-past six p.m. I had a bandsman attached to me to carry the pack, containing lint etc. As we are not allowed to take down servants with our breakfast now, I had to take everything I wanted myself. I accordingly took in my haversack a tin canteen to boil water in ... some red herrings, biscuits, rum and a plate and knife and fork, a little firewood, a candle and some matches. I also had my wooden barrel with water in it, slung on the other side my telescope, cloak and macintosh: altogether I was in heavy marching order. My orders were to stay in the surgeon's hut and to do the best I could with the wounded. There are four assistant-surgeons in the trenches, one, an artilleryman, who goes wherever he is most wanted: a naval man: and two line-assistant surgeons who stay in the first parallel. The firing stopped for the night shortly after I went down ... I came back to the hut and seeing a nice soft board I took possession and was soon sound asleep. I got up about six o'clock when the firing commenced. About 7 o'clock in walked the artillery surgeon with his face bandaged up. He had gone to the advanced battery at daybreak, where he had a number of men wounded, and got hit himself. He said that someone must go there, as the men were being hit every minute. Well I was rather in a fix ... Now I had been told we were to stay in the hut and not to leave it, and if I sent anyone forward, and he got hit, the authorities would come down on me for doing so, and if any man got hit, and no help at hand, they would equally be down on me: so I thought the best thing I could do was to go myself. I accordingly went forward, and found that during the short time the other surgeon had been away, five new men had been wounded ... every shot fired by the enemy threw up a perfect shower of stones, some of them very large: and as they fired at us all day, everyone was hit more or less, some very severely: fortunately, although this morning I am black and blue, and my back aches from a large stone that fell on it, I was not hurt .... The escapes we had were most wonderful .... A man got his hand blown off, they sent for me at once, at this time there was a perfect storm of shot coming on the unfortunate battery ... and it took me nearly a quarter of an hour to dress the wound, it was such a bad one, and I am sure if one shot came past me, twenty did.[79]

Assistant-Surgeon Edward Wrench[80] of the 34th Regiment wrote a vivid account of his experiences in the siege, many years after the event.

> During the winter months one assistant surgeon (the full surgeon never went on trench duty) accompanied each trench guard, which was relieved every twelve hours, in each attack. When the winter was over the guard and medical officers remained on twenty-four hour duty. Until late in the siege no shelter was provided for the surgeons; they had to brave the elements as well as the shot and shell and to attend the wounded under

> extraordinary difficulties ... on one occasion a round shot killed two stretcher bearers and took off the leg of the patient while the surgeon was dressing him for a previous wound. I was on duty in the right attack at both the assaults on the Malakoff and the Redan ... The first assault on June 18th failed all along the line ... the few survivors had to retreat leaving all their dead and many of their wounded on the ground. Most of these were gradually carried under cover .... I was for eight hours engaged in dressing wounded in a recently captured Russian rifle pit, occasionally running out to attend to such as were too severely injured to be moved. Some, alas, lay so completely in the line of fire ... that neither friend nor foe could render them any assistance, so there they lay untended for fifty-two hours. And yet after this terrible ordeal I found one man of my regiment still alive when I was able to approach him under a flag of truce on the third day.[81]

The medical officers who accompanied their regiments into the final attack on the Redan underwent the most hair-raising experiences, as quotations from a letter written by an acting-assistant-surgeon in the 55th Regiment reveal.

> At parade General Codrington gave a short address, informing us that we were to act as supports to the storming party ... to enter the Redan, and insure the possession of it to the stormers ... so off we marched to the middle ravine. It was sharp work for at twenty minutes past twelve our signal was up ... so we all shook hands and moved down the trench as fast as we could ... I kept up with my regiment as well as I could, for the wounded falling around me kept me back. I bound them up and then made a run after the regiment until arrested by others, and so on until I got to the end of the sap which led to the open. To go further was useless, already there was such a crowd of wounded, so I took up my position there - no enviable one, for grape and shot came bounding among us wounding those beside me, two Riflemen fell dead almost on top of me. I had plenty to do - I was so busy ... Officers and men kept crowding on, mowed down by the grape from flanking fire which rushed over and amongst us, throwing up dust and stones, which dealt us no gentle raps. I was struck twice, once on the back by, I think, a grape shot, but I had no time to look, and once on the foot by a rifle ball ... when I was hard at work among the wounded, the soldiers around cried out, 'Doctor, you must get out of the way, they are retreating!', so I looked up and saw our men rushing helter skelter into and over the open to the trenches in the rear of us. I did not know exactly what do do so I drew my sword (which by the way got very bloody that day, but not with Russian blood) and went on with my dressing until I had finished all about me, and then thought of moving off. I could not leave poor Captain Richards, as we all expected the Russians would be among us: so there was nothing for it but to put him on my back and carry him till I got a stretcher ... then I went down to the trenches again, dressing any wounded I found on the way.[82]

These extracts give a good indication of the difficulties facing the regimental doctors throughout the siege. Although conditions were worst during the major bombardments and assaults, even in the quieter periods the doctors in the front line underwent great discomfort and danger. There were many acts of heroism. Of the three awards of the Victoria Cross to doctors (out of 111 awarded for gallantry during the Crimean War), one was won at the battle of Balaclava and two on 8 September during the final attack on the Redan.[83] The three awards can be seen as a general recognition of the self-sacrifice and courage of all the medical officers who served with devotion and at such risk in the front lines. The three doctors were all men in their early twenties. Thomas Hale[84] was serving as an assistant-surgeon with the 7th Foot, a regiment which suffered heavy losses in the major assaults. His citation for the Victoria Cross reads -

> Date of bravery: 8 September, 1855. One, for remaining with an officer who was dangerously wounded in the fifth parallel on 8 Sept. 1855, when all the men in the immediate neighbourhood retreated excepting Lieut. W. Hope and Dr. Hale: and for endeavouring to rally the men .... Two, for having on 8 Sept. after the regiment had retired into the trenches, cleared the most advanced sap of the wounded, and carried into the sap, under heavy fire, several wounded from the open ground.

Henry Sylvester was serving as an assistant-surgeon with the 23rd regiment (the Royal Welsh Fusiliers). His citation for the Victoria Cross reads:

> "For going out on 8 Sept. 1855 under heavy fire, to a spot near the Redan, where Lieut. and Adjutant Dyneley was lying mortally wounded, and for dressing his wounds in that dangerous and exposed position." This officer was also mentioned in General Sir James Simpson's despatch of 18 Sept. 1855, for his courage in going to the front under a heavy fire to assist the wounded.[85]

From the start of the war the army medical officers resented the lack of recognition of their work, both by the high command and by the government. The medical press constantly drew attention to this neglect. The honours awarded to the doctors during the war were sparse. After the war ended a correspondent to **The Times** wrote - "The regimental surgeon who went through the cholera campaign in Bulgaria, who was at the Alma and Inkerman and at Balaclava, who has had to struggle through the terrible winter of 1854, and contend with typhus, disease, cholera, and wounds ... works on with his 14 s. a day, with no decorations or honours, and no local brevet or advanced rank".[86] However, there were occasional mentions in despatches, local commendations from regimental colonels to Divisional Commanders, and more rarely Raglan made some recognition of the work of individual doctors. After the attack on the Redan on 18

June, Assistant-Surgeon Thomas Brady[87] and Assistant-Surgeon J. Phelps[88], both of the 57th Regiment, were commended for "coolly and zealously attending the wounded under the enemy's fire." Assistant-Surgeon Arthur Greer[89] of the 21st Regiment, and Assistant-Surgeon Wrench of the 34th Regiment, were commended "for treating the wounded under heavy fire." The names of Assistant-Surgeon John Gibbons[90] of the 44th Regiment and Assistant-Surgeon William Jeeves[91] of the 38th Regiment were brought to the notice of Lord Panmure, "for the judicious arrangements of the medical department on the memorable 18th of June, in the attack on the Redan, and their zealous and humane exertions in the field exposed to a most galling fire". Significantly the **Lancet**, publishing this citation, remarked that - "We trust Lord Palmerston and Lord Panmure will see this recommendation is carried out, and becomes not merely an empty compliment on paper".[92] On 14 September a special report was sent to the Commander-in-Chief praising the service throughout the whole siege of Staff-Surgeon John Bent[93], Surgeon Richard Elliot, Surgeon James Fogo[94], and Assistant-Surgeon Arthur Taylor. But such official recognition was relatively rare.

Nevertheless, throughout this exacting period the morale of the medical officers remained high. Almost without exception they took the rough with the smooth and served to the best of their ability. There were periods of relaxation. At times there were opportunities to explore the country and visit the more distant camps (most of the doctors had their own horses). There was great fellowship, particularly among those who had joined up during the war. Nothing gave more pleasure than unexpected reunions with friends in other regiments, or in the navy, who had been fellow-students. The letters and diaries of the younger men convey a great sense of camaraderie. Despite all the horrors of the war there was an almost schoolboy enjoyment of life, even in the conditions under fire. In general the quarters of the doctors were now reasonably comfortable. The supply of luxuries for the table was profuse. Even before the winter ended George Lawson could write home -

> I am in right good health, living on the fat of the land ... shiploads of good things are continually arriving, and from them we are able to buy all

we can desire ... sherry very decent, can be had at about 3 s. a doz. ....
What do you think of my extravagance? I saw a fine fat pig about to be
killed on board one of the transports and in a luxurious mood I purchased
one half of the animal for which I had to pay the small sum of £6.12s.[95]

Although the army doctors carried on with the utmost loyalty they still saw it as right to seek some betterment of their conditions of service. At the end of August a Memorial was sent to Lord Panmure by 49 surgeons serving in the Crimea.[96] Believing that reform of the medical department was now under consideration, they asked that the government should "extend to us a fair share of those honours and rewards which have of late been so liberally bestowed on all other branches of the service." They asked that, for the purposes of promotion and other rewards active employment in the field should be reckoned as equivalent to three times the amount of ordinary service, (as was the custom in other armies in Europe). They expressed a grievance concerning the appointment of civil practitioners to the charge of any patients in hospitals, seeing this as retarding the promotion of the regular officer and as a slight to his clinical and administrative ability. They submitted that a surgeon's relative rank should be that of a field officer. They complained bitterly about their low pay (13s. per day), considering their great responsibilities and hazards. There were complaints also concerning the slowness of promotion, the restrictions on leave, and the poor conditions of pay on retiral. About the same time the assistant-surgeons (there were 106 signatures) forwarded their own Memorial.[97] The complaints were similar, but in particular they complained of their low military rank and pay (as a result of which they had no proper standing in the army) and the long delay before they could have any hope of promotion. They suggested that five years should be the maximum period for promotion to surgeon. Smith was shown this Memorial but at first he refused to forward it to Lord Panmure. Smith regarded as completely false the statement that "promotion appears at the present time to be conducted on no definite plan." Lord Panmure did eventually see the Memorial but merely remarked that assistant-surgeons were too young and inexperienced to decide on these matters! It was to be some time before the complaints of the junior doctors were to be rectified.

In general there were now fewer criticisms of the army medical service, although attacks on Smith and Hall had not ceased in the public press (and in at least one of the medical journals). Yet there was still a strong faction only too ready to seize on any adverse report. The opportunity came when an anonymous letter appeared in **The Times** of 5 July.[98] This happened just when Hall believed that he had at last a really efficient organisation for the reception and treatment of the wounded. As was soon to be revealed, the letter had been sent by Assistant-Surgeon Bakewell, who had already attracted notice by his communications to the press earlier in the year (as mentioned in Chapter X). Bakewell asserted that on 11 June, when a major assault was expected, he had been put in charge of a reception ward in a general hospital (probably the Camp General Hospital). He had found it was ill-equipped to deal with the wounded. He alleged there were serious shortages of drinking vessels, water, medical comforts, suitable diet, adequate bedding, and splints, and that he had had only one inexperienced orderly to assist him. These complaints raised a public outcry, Bakewell's account being at first accepted quite unequivocally. When the letter became known in the Crimea, a Committee of Enquiry was quickly convened, primarily to establish whether or not there were any grounds to suspect gross negligence in the preparations made for the reception of casualties. The verdict of the Committee was categorical - "by the concurrent testimony of the Medical Men ... never was a hospital better provided or patients more humanely treated ... and never a more unfounded representation made to the public". Bakewell was summarily dismissed from the service for making such criticisms publicly, and although his father wrote to Lord Panmure in protest, he got no satisfaction.[99] Bakewell's allegations were refuted by some of his colleagues. Assistant-Surgeon Greig stated that Bakewell had not known how to set about applying for necessities and affirmed - "I have never yet applied in vain for anything". Two civil surgeons now in the Crimea, Macleod and Rooke, firmly contradicted Bakewell's charges.[100]

In retrospect it does seem surprising that a very junior staff assistant-surgeon such as Bakewell was put in solitary charge of a ward in a General Hospital, with no senior officer to whom he could appeal for help or lodge any complaint. Bakewell returned to England and for the next few months continued to fight his case, largely on the grounds that he had not been permitted to furnish evidence at the Enquiry. In December he quoted evidence from two patients admitted under his care, both confirming that his letter was true in every detail. After his discharge from the army Bakewell held various hospital posts in Britain and wrote prolifically in the medical journals. In November 1855 he produced a paper on the diseases he had encountered at Scutari. His opinions were dogmatic and there was veiled criticism of his seniors. From this paper it emerges that shortly after he sent off his ill-fated letter he had been admitted to hospital with cholera. He recovered despite (in his opinion) the wrong treatment by his colleagues!

Surprisingly, no doctor was killed in action or seriously wounded but between April and September 1855, five army doctors died of disease. Those who were transferred sick to Scutari and died there are listed in Chapter XIV.

Surgeon Christopher Macartney[101] died on 11 April of erysipelas "before Sebastopol". He was then serving as surgeon to the 77th Regiment, and had been wounded at the Alma (which may account for one report that he died of wounds). After surviving the winter siege he died after an illness of six days. Surgeon Walter Simpson[102] died on 31 May of intermittent fever "in the camp before Sebastopol". He was then serving as surgeon to the 17th Regiment, which did not land in the Crimea until December 1854. Assistant-Surgeon John White[103] died on 2 July, of fever after cholera, "in the camp before Sebastopol". He was then serving in the 31st Regiment. Assistant-Surgeon Malcolm Ancell[104] died on 10 August in the Crimea. He was then serving with the 11th Hussars. He had served in Scutari until late in September 1854 when he became a medical officer of the hospital transport 'Courier' for one voyage. Assistant-Surgeon John Longmore,[105] died on 22 August of cholera, "before Sebastopol". He was then serving with the 19th Regiment, to which his better known brother, Thomas

Longmore, was surgeon. The accidental death of Dr. Hector Gavin, of the Sanitary Commission, has already been noted (in Chapter XII). Of the civil surgeons from Smyrna and Renkioi transferred to serve in the Crimea none died.

THE NAVAL BRIGADE (APRIL-SEPTEMBER 1855)

The Naval Brigade continued to make an important contribution during the six intensive months of the siege. As well as manning the gun emplacements and the trenches, the Brigade took an active part in all the major assaults. 'Ladder parties' were provided for storming the Russian fortifications. The casualties sustained in this role were exceptionally high.

Exact information concerning the hospital admission and mortality rates for medical conditions between April and September 1855 is not readily found. There is, however, considerable evidence to show that, as in the winter, the naval camp remained remarkably healthy in comparison with the army camps. We know for example that the Naval Brigade Hospital (originally in H.M.S. 'Diamond', but expanded to a hutted hospital of 72 beds in May 1855), admitted until the end of the war 742 cases, of which about one third were for wounds or injuries and two thirds for medical conditions. The medical cases included about 270 with bowel conditions and almost 80 with fever. There was no serious outbreak of cholera in the Naval Brigade. There were 32 deaths in the total of 742 cases (4 per cent), but most deaths followed wounds. This remarkably low death-rate is accounted for by the fact that serious cases, whether medical or surgical, were transferred quickly to Therapia.[106]

It has been calculated that throughout the whole war the sick rate in the Naval Brigade was 10.5 per cent (of which 7 per cent were wounded).[107] This contrasts with the very much higher sick rates in the army, particularly in the infantry regiments engaged on the same tasks as the Naval Brigade. From another source it is learned that only 44 officers and men of the Naval Brigade died of disease throughout the whole period of its service in the Crimea.[108] It can be assumed that less than half that number died between April and September, 1855. Not even the cavalry regiments could boast of such a low death rate from disease (allowing for the fact that the Naval Brigade averaged a complement of 1200 throughout its service, and cavalry regiments were often down to 300).

Statistics of killed and wounded between April and September 1855 can be derived from the report of 1857.[109] Of a total of 66 who died, 26 were killed outright and 40 died after severe wounds, while 265 recovered from wounds. It is not clear how many of these had severe and how many minor wounds. Even in the relatively quiet periods between the major bombardments few days passed without a death or without one or two men being wounded. The greatest losses were sustained during the assaults, in particular on 18 June when 15 men were killed and 46 wounded. Of the 26 men killed outright more than half had severe head injuries (at least four were decapitated). As already noted, the sailors were reckless in the extreme in their reluctance to keep under cover during fire. Of the serious injuries recorded a high proportion involved the limbs, the lower twice as frequently as the upper. Seven upper limb amputations were done, with two deaths, and 12 lower limb amputations, with six deaths. Very few men were admitted to hospital with severe chest or abdominal wounds. Only one penetrating wound of the skull was operated upon.

Some general conclusions concerning the wounded are reached in the 1857 report. "Fractures of the skull, with depression of the bone, were always dangerous, and too often mortal, as were wounds of the chest and abdomen, whether caused by bullets or pieces of shell." A high mortality rate in compound fractures of the thigh was noted.

> When the brigade was first landed an opinion prevailed that cases of compound fracture of the thigh would be met with in which it would be proper to attempt to save the limb .... Two cases were at length brought into the camp respecting which the majority of medical officers were of the opinion that amputation should not be performed ... the injury to the bone and soft parts [being] comparatively slight in both cases; the external wound was small and situated on the outer side of the limb in one, in the

other above the knee. The result in the former was, after great suffering, death: in the latter, although the patient still lives, his ultimate recovery appears to be hopeless. Experience has therefore forced on us the conviction that to attempt to save the limb in any case of compound fracture of the thigh the result of gunshot, is to endanger the patient's life: and the result of secondary amputation has not been such as to trust to that chance of saving life after failure of the first attempt.

The naval surgeons ashore therefore quickly accepted a policy of primary amputation, which was their choice afloat. During the whole period the Brigade was in the Crimea, 16 amputations for compound fracture of the thigh were done and ten died. Of six amputations below the knee all recovered. Of ten amputations of the upper arm one died and of five at the forearm three died.

It is not always clear where these primary amputations were done. There was probably a sick quarters in the naval camp where urgent operations could be performed. Surgeon Duigan records - "An account of the progress of the cases could not be kept, as they were immediately drafted from the Field Hospitals after the first indications were surgically fuflfilled .... In the ravines leading from the camp to the batteries ambulances were stationed for the transmission of the wounded to the Field Hospitals."[110] It is possible that some kind of casualty clearing station, similar to the field hospitals set up in the ravines by some regiments, was used by the naval doctors.

Duigan in his account does not give anything in the way of statistical information. He was more interested in the effects of different missiles. "The weight of metal employed, and the size of the projectiles thrown, by the opposing forces against each other's works, far exceed that of any previous siege .... some of the wounds which resulted were perhaps, for these reasons unusually severe, or, at least, novel in their characters." He describes in grisly detail the gross destructive effects of exploding shells, usually killing outright. Wounds from round shot caused by direct hits were equally lethal, "Most of the men killed by shot had their heads knocked away, either completely or in part." Bullet wounds were frequent, for the advanced trenches manned by the Naval Brigade were constantly under fire from the Russian rifle pits, often at only forty yards range. The destructive effect of the conical bullet was well recognised. The naval medical officer's duties were as testing as those of the army. "The duties of the siege fell heavily on the Medical Officers of the Naval Brigade, five of whom do that duty, and out of the five two go on trench duty ... on the whole this trench duty is very trying and hazardous: and in performing it the Medical Men run the same dangers if not more certainly not less than the executive officers who are generally stationary in the battery, while the Medical Officer, as ubiquitous as possible, is rushing in all directions to succour the wounded."

In a second report Duigan records the final attack on the Redan. "As may be expected, when hostile troops met in the ramparts, wounds of the most terrible and fatal character were received..."[111] There is evidence from Duigan's reports, and from many other sources that there was a close co-operation between the army and the naval medical officers in coping with the wounded in the batteries, in the trenches, and during the assaults. On evacuation from the front line the soldiers invariably went to an army hospital and the sailors to the naval hospital.

As in the earlier months, the morale of the Naval Brigade remained high. In July, Lushington, the commander, was promoted and succeeded by Captain Henry Keppel, an equally able officer who had the same caring attitude for his men. Keppel published his reminiscences and these reflect the irrepressible spirit in the Naval Brigade and the light-hearted attitude towards the high risks of death.[112] He describes how new recruits were introduced to the front line. "The new arrival affords the best sport and is prepared for. The dirtiest stretcher, on which some bleeding body has lately been carried, is at hand. The shell bursts: the new arrival is struck behind the ear by moist clay, is immediately seized, laid on the dirty stretcher, carried off without resistance ... and upset in the ditch, which generally holds water. Of course he is received with cheers".[113] Keppel frequently visited the hospital. "I found one of my poor fellows carving a heart on a ring, part of his own thigh bone ... on asking him what he was going to do with it he replied 'To send it to my girl, Sir!'"[114] He recognised too well the recklessness of his men. "My silly fellows unnecessarily expose themselves in spite of warnings and examples ... an amateur youngster must mount the parapet and borrow a sergeant's musket to take a shot at a Russian ... he had a Minie ball through his thigh in a moment."[115]

No medical officer attached to the Naval Brigade was killed or wounded despite the frequent exposure to enemy fire. As far as can be traced there was only one death from disease. Surgeon Percy Chapman,[116] recorded briefly as of the Naval Brigade, died in camp in August.

A large force of Marines was maintained until the fall of Sebastopol near Balaclava, as described in Chapter IX. Some of the force took part in the expedition to Kertch. There were 225 deaths in the whole period of service in the Crimea, but only 13 were under the heading "killed or died of wounds".[117] The fatalities from medical conditions were high and conformed very much to those in the army regiments. In eleven months there were 78 deaths from dysentery, 42 from cholera, 22 from fever and 70 from other diseases. The low incidence of wounds is readily explained by the fact that the marines sustained a purely defensive role, to protect Balaclava in the event of a Russian attack. The sickness rate was far higher than that of the Naval Brigade. Although the camp was in charge of naval medical officers landed from warships (as with the Naval Brigade) it does not seem that hygiene was supervised very effectively. The unhealthy site of the camp, near Balaclava harbour, probably accounts to some extent for the high rate of cholera and dysentery. Whether or not there was some difference in the way in which the marines adapted to camp life, as compared with the sailors, is unknown. It is possible that sheer boredom caused a general decline in morale and discipline. There are hints too that the commander of the Marines was not of the calibre of Lushington or Keppel.

In July 1855 it was reported that Surgeon James Elliott[118] had been court-martialled, dismissed the service, and sentenced to two years in prison. He had entered the Navy as an assistant-surgeon in 1848. In 1854 he was serving in H.M.S. 'Britannia' and during the cholera epidemic he had been commended for his work. He was promoted to surgeon in November 1854 having just been attached to the marine force at Balaclava.

> Mr. Elliott who served during the whole winter ... on the heights of Balaclava had no ordinary difficulties to encounter in the execution of his duties .... He had the sole charge of 1500 men, 400 of whom were sick at one time, chiefly with dysentery and cholera .... Mr. Elliott himself dwelt in a tent pervious to every shower of rain, after the earthen cave in which he was first located had fallen in, with about a ton of earth upon him, when he himself was suffering from dysentery ... the difficulty was often extreme in visiting his patients, spread over such an extent of ground, particularly on snowy weather, when he often had to crawl on all fours .... It was not to be wondered at, under such trying hardships, that Mr. Elliott's own health should have given way ... he ought at once to have officially represented his own long continued illness and his utter inability to perform such effective duties ... this was the more necessary as he had to deal with a commandant who was increasingly 'taking notes' and never so happy as when he could get the doctor into hot water.[119]

The chief charge brought against Elliott was of having neglected a private who was dangerously ill. There were other accusations of neglect and he was accused of calling the men under his care a 'rotten set'. "The witnesses at his trial were marines and soldiers, some of whom he had punished for neglect of duty, and he himself declined to say a word, or call a witness in his defence."[120] The main charge was subsequently refuted by many observers, since Elliott had at once responded to the call for help but had to walk half a mile from his quarters to those of the sick man. In the meantime the patient had rapidly become worse and died before Elliott arrived. The sentence passed was undoubtedly a harsh one considering the circumstances. No allowance was made for the fact that Elliott was exhausted and sick. The affair caused a considerable outcry in the medical and lay press, more especially when the unfortunate Elliott, now incarcerated in Exeter gaol, died on 1 December, 1855, of a brain disease.[121] His relatives appealed against the injustice which had been committed. The 'brain disease' was attributed to the hardships Elliott had suffered in the Crimea.

There may have been two sides to the question. Elliott was perhaps seen by his senior officers and by his patients as a difficult person with whom to deal. As far as can be ascertained none of his medical colleagues came to his support, but it would have been difficult for them to criticise their own commander, Admiral Lyons, who had approved the verdict. In the medical journals at home, however, many doctors wrote in support of Elliott and expressed the opinion that a gross injustice had been perpetrated. At a time when recruitment to the naval medical service was at a low level the affair was scarcely a good advertisement. Elliott was as much a casualty of the war as any other doctor who died on service, but officially he went into oblivion.

MISS NIGHTINGALE VISITS THE CRIMEA

In April 1855 Miss Nightingale felt that things were at last going relatively well at Scutari and that the pressures on the hospitals had greatly diminished. She now saw it as her duty to visit the Crimea to inspect the hospitals there and to try to introduce the new arrangements for laundries and kitchens which had been so successful in the base hospitals.[122] She may well have wished to establish her position more positively with regard to the nurses who had already gone to the Crimea, but her authority at this time with reference to the Crimea was not absolutely clear, her original appointment having been as Superintendent of Female Nurses in the Military Hospitals in Turkey.[123] The nurses in the Crimea were under their own Superintendents, although in some quarters it was understood that Miss Nightingale did have the ultimate responsibility for their deployment and discipline. Her visit to the Crimea was approved by the War Office, but only in the capacity of 'Almoner of Free Gifts in the British Hospitals in the Crimea', not as Superintendent of Nurses. She did in fact accept that her official duty was to plan the distribution of comforts provided by **The Times** fund and from other sources. Hall considered that she had no authority either to inspect hospitals in the Crimea, or to direct the nurses serving there. Hall was probably informed by Raglan about the projected visit but maintained a passive attitude. As far as can be made out, there was no meeting during this visit, although letters may have been exchanged. There is no mention of Miss Nightingale's visit in Hall's diary. Hall was certainly touchy about any further hospital inspections. The Sanitary Commission had already reported adversely on the Balaclava General Hospital, and he did not want any more criticism.

Well aware of this delicate situation, Miss Nightingale sailed from Scutari on 2 May in a transport, and, as she reported, she was "taking back 450 of her patients, a draft of convalescents returning to their regiments to be shot at again."[124] The party included her main lieutenant, Mr. Bracebridge (Mrs. Bracebridge had been left at Scutari in charge of the nurses and of the distribution of gifts), M. Soyer, who had also decided to give the army at the front the benefit of his advice, and four nurses, including Mrs. Roberts, Miss Nightingale's favourite amongst the professional nurses and her aide-de-camp. There were also two cooks and three faithful personal attendants, one a drummer boy aged only twelve years! On arrival at Balaclava the party established quarters on board ship as there was no suitable accommodation ashore. The members of the Sanitary Commission at once came on board to pay their respects. On the first day Miss Nightingale rode in a small cavalcade to call on Lord Raglan and Dr. Hall at their headquarters, four miles from the harbour. She found both were out. It is not clear when she did eventually succeed in meeting Raglan, and it is almost certain that she never met Hall. She went up to the front line. At a mortar battery, Soyer, with his flair for publicity, requested her to ascend the rampart and seat herself on the central mortar. He then declaimed, "Gentlemen, behold this amiable lady sitting fearlessly upon the terrible instrument of war! Behold the heroic daughter of England, the soldier's friend."[125] This set the pattern of her visit. For the next few days she moved about the camps, and was received with great enthusiasm by the soldiers, to whom she was now a legend. Setting out each day, on foot or on horseback, she exhausted herself visiting the regimental and general hospitals, planning the nurses' duties, distributing gifts and comforts, discussing the building of new huts, and, with Soyer, planning new kitchens. Raglan had given orders that anything she recommended was to be carried

CHAPTER XIII

out. She found that the Sanitary Commission had already achieved considerable improvements.

In the Balaclava General Hospital some of the nurses viewed her visit with suspicion. Mrs Davis, with whom she had already crossed swords, greeted her with some sarcasm, "I should have as soon expected to see the Queen here as you".[126] But these were minor rebuffs and in a short space of time she was able to set in motion some much needed reforms. Soyer was equally successful and even gained the co-operation of Hall in his plans to improve the kitchen at the Castle Hospital. The nursing superintendent there, Miss Shaw Stewart, was glad to see Miss Nightingale, to take her round the wards, and to seek her advice. Miss Nightingale found time to spend with the patients, to issue comforts, and to give encouragement. George Lawson happened to be admitted with typhus at this time. The senior medical officer of the hospital wrote to Lawson's parents - "Miss Nightingale who has come up here has just called to see him [Lawson] and taken a great interest in him".[127] She arranged that an excellent nurse, Miss Elizabeth Woodward, should look after Lawson and, when he was convalescent, travel home with him.

Shortly after her visit to the Castle Hospital Miss Nightingale nearly collapsed. Mrs Roberts tried in vain to make her rest. Soon it was clear that she was ill with a high fever. She was carried on a stretcher to the Castle Hospital and admitted under the care of Staff Surgeon Henry Hadley.[128] Nursed by the faithful Mrs Roberts she lay for nearly two weeks in a critical condition. When she was beginning to recover Raglan came one night to visit her. Mrs Roberts asked who he was, and he (allegedly) replied - "Oh only a soldier but I must see her, I have come a long way, my name is Raglan, she knows me very well."[129] Miss Nightingale heard and recognised his voice, and insisted on seeing him. It seemed likely that she had contracted typhus. Her recovery was very slow. Her progress was followed with alarm and then relief, by everyone in England from the Queen downwards, and by all the soldiers in the Crimea. She refused the advice that she should

THE SIEGE ENDED

convalesce in England or in Switzerland, and insisted on returning to Scutari.

A strange incident is said to have occurred when the invalid was ready to leave the Crimea.[130] One version is that the transport 'Jura' had been chosen for her journey, by Dr. Hall or Dr. Hadley, and that when she was taken on board she learned that the ship was going straight to England. At the last minute she was transferred in a fainting condition to a steam yacht belonging to Lord Ward, and after a rough voyage landed at Scutari. The implication was that Hall had arranged her passage in the 'Jura' for the very reason that it was going straight to England, so making sure that he would be rid of her completely! Bracebridge, who was very antagonistic to the senior army doctors, was quite convinced of this plot. Miss Nightingale's early biographer, Cook, does not even hint at the episode but implies that the arrangement for Miss Nightingale to travel in Lord Ward's yacht was in fact not made at the last minute.[131] A modern biographer, Woodham-Smith, accepts the attempted abduction without question, quoting a letter to Herbert on 15 October in which Miss Nightingale states - "It was quite true that Doctors Hall and Hadley sent for a list of vessels going home and chose one, the 'Jura', which was not going to stop at Scutari, and put me on board for England, and Mr Bracebridge and Lord Ward took me out at the risk of my life to save me from going to England."[132] Another modern biographer, O'Malley, although she does not appear convinced of the story, repeats Bracebridge's belief that an attempt was made to highjack Miss Nightingale. She quotes a letter from Miss Nightingale written to her Aunt Mai (Mrs Smith). "It is quite true that Doctors Hall and Hadley sent for a list of vessels going home and chose one, the 'Jane'[sic] ... because it was not going to stop at Scutari."[133] Biographers such as Woodham-Smith who have been strongly biased against Hall are particularly ready to seize on this story.

Yet for Hall to have acted like this would have been exceedingly rash, knowing of Raglan's strong support for Miss Nightingale, as well as that of Herbert and other ministers at home. That Miss Nightingale was transferred from a transport to a no doubt more comfortable private yacht is factual, and apparently she and her friends came to believe, no doubt sincerely, that the transport was sailing non-stop to England. But it was most unusual for any transports to go through the Bosphorous without stopping to coal and to land or take up passengers. In addition, all ships were stopped at the entrance to the Bosphorous from the Black Sea in order to declare their cargo and movements. Thus, had Miss Nightingale travelled in a transport her friends could still have easily ensured that she disembarked for Scutari. (The 'Jura' is listed as a transport which carried stores to the East in 1854, but does not appear on the 1855 shipping lists).[134]

In her short time in the Crimea Miss Nightingale had been able to give much useful advice and to accelerate improvements in the camps and hospitals. She had found out much about the nurses already in the Crimea, and assessed the merits or otherwise of the superintendents. Most of all, she had seen for herself how the soldier lived and worked in the field and she now knew much more about his discomforts and hazards. She returned from the Crimea more than ever determined to improve his lot.

NURSES AND OTHER WOMEN IN THE CRIMEA

Nurses were first introduced into the hospitals in the Crimea in about February, 1855 when eight of Miss Stanley's party went there. The request for their services came, it is said, from Lord Raglan. Miss Nightingale disapproved of the move. Initially all were attached to the Balaclava General Hospital in charge of Miss Langston, head of the Sellonite nurses who had come out with Miss Stanley. Miss Langston went home in April, a nervous wreck, and was replaced by Miss Weare, aged 70, a "fussy, gentle, old spinster", who was a great admirer of Dr. Hall. The cook at Balaclava was the irrepressible Elizabeth Davis. When the Castle Hospital was opened later in the year Miss Shaw Stewart was put in charge of a small group of nurses. She also had come out with Miss Stanley and was a lady of some social position, with considerable nursing experience in

England. Unlike most of the Stanley nurses she admired Miss Nightingale. Miss Nightingale did think that Miss Stewart had "a streak of queerness" and that she was not easy to deal with, but saw her as one of the most able administrators. Indeed at a later date Miss Nightingale appointed Miss Stewart as her successor in the East, should she die or have to give up the task. Also at the Castle Hospital was Mrs Drake (a professional nurse of the original party which came out in October 1854), who was highly regarded by Miss Nightingale. There is no record of any nurses being attached to the Camp General Hospital. But after September 1855 a number of nurses were sent to the Monastery Hospital and to the Land Transport hospitals.

Mention has already been made of Miss Clough who, much to Miss Nightingale's disapproval, after arriving in the East with Miss Stanley, insisted on going to the Crimea.[135] At first Miss Clough, with seven other nurses, was attached to the General Hospital. They lived, slept, washed, and ate in two small white-washed rooms. "Our rations are biscuits, meat of the coarsest kind, a bottle of wine among four, tea without milk, eggs none, butter, salt, bread, flour none." After a few days Miss Clough was contacted by Sir Colin Campbell (with whom her deceased officer friend had served). He invited her to come and work in the hutted hospital of the Highland Division, near Balaclava. She was accommodated in a hut especially built for her and looked after by a soldier and his wife. She was immediately very busy, for the 'Superintendent' had taken ill and required special nursing care. If the 'Superintendent' was a female she must have been the wife of an officer or a soldier appointed unofficially. Miss Nightingale at once wrote reprimanding Miss Clough for taking up an appointment in a regimental hospital. Miss Clough replied reminding Miss Nightingale that she had no authority over nurses in the Crimea. "I was the first woman to propose to come out here, to brave all the dangers and privations of Balaclava, and it would be strange if Miss Nightingale were to have it in her power to deprive me of my office and occupation." Miss Clough had many influential friends including Lord Raglan, "then I have the chief of all, Sir Colin, so I think the Nightingale will have a tough job to unseat me".

This powerful lady soon established her position. She was the only woman in the hospital. She wrote home - "It is odd to be seeing constantly men and no women, and the deference with which they treat me is a relief ... I have no trouble whatever. I am looked on as a hospital nurse, with this difference that I am a gentlewoman." There was much sickness in the camp and in early April three of the doctors were ill, including the Surgeon, John Furlong of the 42nd Highlanders.[136] Miss Clough by her efficiency and untiring efforts became quite a celebrity. She was visited by the Ambassador, Lord Stratford, and his daughters, who were in the Crimea late in April. When Miss Nightingale came in May she did not go near Miss Clough, and the latter wrote - "she has not returned to my territory, fearing I suppose the cool, or warm, reception I might give her." However, late in June Miss Clough became seriously ill with a relapsing fever. She refused at first to return to England or to convalescence in Constantinople. At the end of August acute symptoms recurred. She was admitted to the Castle Hospital and a passage arranged on a steamer sailing for England. She was taken on board but died soon after the ship left, on 21 September. Miss Nightingale was informed of her death and arranged for the burial at Scutari. She wrote to Miss Stewart - "Poor Miss Clough! I little thought that the first time I should see her face would be in death." A suitably enigmatic remark, for Miss Nightingale had never expressed the slightest approval of Miss Clough's notable service. She sorted out Miss Clough's effects and learned for the first time that the officer whose grave she had longed to visit was the Hon. Lauderdale Maule, brother and heir presumptive of Lord Panmure.

Furlong, the army doctor with whom Miss Clough had worked closely, paid her this tribute - "She was the greatest use in the hospital and made herself liked by all". Hall, too, recognised her contribution, but not least admired her firm stand against Miss Nightingale. Some saw Miss Clough with her strong character, energy and endurance as the equal of Miss Nightingale. "Miss

Nightingale seems to have lost no opportunity to disparage Miss Clough while she lived", writes the latter's biographer, and he adds that the disparagement continued after her death. It may be suspected that by winning the support of Lord Raglan, Lord Stratford, Sir Colin Campbell and other notables, Miss Clough not only increased the antagonism of Miss Nightingale but also caused much jealousy: "Was she a rival too near the throne?"

When Sidney Herbert had asked Miss Nightingale to take out a party of nurses in October 1854 he had never contemplated that a military hospital within the range of the enemy's guns should be staffed by a female superintendent. The experiment, devised by Sir Colin Campbell and approved by Lord Raglan, was an outstanding success. More is known of Miss Clough's work than that of any other of the Balaclava nurses, although it is clear that Miss Stewart contributed greatly to the efficiency of the Castle Hospital. It is uncertain how many nurses were employed officially in the Crimea between February and September 1855, but thereafter the total was considerably increased. In the original group the majority were antagonistic to Miss Nightingale and owed her no allegiance. Miss Weare and Mrs Davis found it more satisfactory to deal directly with "that kind gentleman Dr. Hall". Between April and September, as well as Miss Clough one other Crimean nurse died. This was Mrs Drake, on 9 August, "of a low fever". Miss Nightingale wrote to St. John's House in London, where Mrs Drake had trained, - "I have lost in her the best of my women here".

With the coming of spring, well-to-do relatives, friends and the curious came out in large numbers from England, on tours advertised by the shipping companies, or in private yachts.[137] Some of the officers' wives who had been in Bulgaria had succeeded in joining their husbands in the Crimea. Mrs Duberley was still there, her position as the most prominent lady sharing the hardships of the campaign now somewhat overshadowed by the arrival of Lord and Lady Paget. Paget, who had gone home on leave after the destruction of his cavalry at Balaclava, now returned, but more as a spectator than as the active commander of a cavalry division. His beautiful young wife, Agnes, became the toast of the army. While the carnage continued, she and her fashionable friends picnicked, dined, danced, went on conducted tours of the battle-fields, attended parades and reviews, patronised the race meetings (now an established recreation), and no doubt flirted and intrigued to their hearts' content. At the end of April, Lord Stratford brought a party of ladies and gentlemen from Constantinople to tour the front. While a few officers, such as the austere Colonel Anthony Sterling of the Highland Division, viewed this influx of ladies with considerable distaste, most enjoyed the unexpected bonus of female company. Raglan was not averse to the ladies and Lady Paget became his close companion - and indeed was to be the only female present at his death-bed (a proceeding not approved in military circles). This was of course an army with senior officers largely recruited from the aristocracy. The ordinary regular soldier had an accustomed deference to the upper class and did not appear to resent the privileged position of the visitors. He rather enjoyed the spectacle of the ladies riding through the camps, and also appreciated that certain ladies visited the sick and wounded in hospital, often bringing gifts.

Life was otherwise for the soldiers' wives and the female camp-followers who had contrived to stay with individual regiments. A few were on the strength officially, as cooks or laundry-women, or as workers in the regimental hospitals. When Miss Nightingale visited the Crimea in April, although not enthusiastic about females working in the regimental hospitals, she expressed approval that two of these women were to be given official status as nurses. Certain women even went up to the advanced lines, often under fire, to render first aid or to help to bring in the wounded. In a special category was a West Indian Creole volunteer, Mrs Seacole, who had been brought up in a British garrison in the Caribbean. She had tried to go out to the Crimea as a nurse with Miss Nightingale's first party, but had not been accepted. She then decided to set up a hotel and store as near the battle front as possible. On her way to the Crimea she called on Miss Nightingale in another attempt to be accepted as a nurse, but again was thwarted. Somehow she reached Balaclava with her stores, and by her extraordinary powers of persuasion had the 'British Hotel' built for her, mainly using drift-wood collected from the harbour. It became a social centre for officers and men alike, where provisions and comforts of all varieties could be purchased at a fair price, where a meal or a drink could always be supplied, and where even lavish parties could be arranged. Her establishment, a sort of privatised N.A.A.F.I., was extremely popular and a boost to morale.[138]

Mrs Seacole, like many West Indian women, had been recognised in her own country as a remarkably skilled 'doctoress'. She now ran an out-patients clinic, providing herbal remedies and dressings for men who thought more of her skills than of those provided by the medical service. In the winter, as the sad procession of wounded passed her doorway on its way to the harbour, she gave the men endless cups of hot tea. Because of her constant cheerfulness and kindness everyone came to know her. She usually got wind of forthcoming actions and made her way to the front carrying a large bag full of bandages, lint and medicines. Often under fire she tended the wounded until they could be taken to hospital. Mrs Seacole emerges as a legendary figure. The doctors knew her well and although they thought her rather a quack, they were appreciative of her good works. George Lawson wrote of her-

> She did not spare herself if she could do any good to the suffering soldiers. In rain and snow, in storm and tempest, day after day she was at her self-chosen post, with her stove and kettle ... brewing tea for all who wanted it. Sometimes more than 200 sick would be embarked in one day, but Mrs Seacole was always equal to the occasion.[139]

It was appropriate that at the end of the war the authorities, not usually notable for their imagination, awarded Mrs Seacole the Crimean Medal.

The names of many other women who served in the Crimea with great courage and devotion remain unknown. Those wives who were widowed suffered greatly, for there was no organisation in the Crimea to help them. Some made their way back to Scutari, where they could get assistance from Lady Blackwood who, with her husband, had taken over the task of caring for such unfortunate women. A number of wives died in the Crimea. Some are recorded in the regimental cemeteries but many died who must have been buried in unmarked graves, or graves without a permanent record. A stone near the Tchernaya River bore this inscription. "To the memory of Margrett Starret late wife of James Starret Pt. 95th Regiment who landed in the Crimea on the 14th of September 1854. This woman travelled with the regiment through the campaign until such time as pleased God to call her to Himself ... being in the 23rd year of her age."[140] Below this inscription was written "Woman British". Many infants and young children also died. In the burial ground of the Light Division was a stone, "Sacred to the memory of Charlotte Elizabeth Bayford who departed this life Nov. 9th 1855, aged 16 months." There were other such poignant memorials but it is likely that many infants or children were buried in unknown graves. Yet the sparse records indicate that not only were children born in the camps but that some survived infancy, despite the unfavourable conditions.

Assistant Surgeon John Ogilvy[141] reported his obstetric experience.

> An incident took place in our camp yesterday, which while it may amuse your readers shows what a Crimean practitioner may have to do ... Corporal B. of ours, came about noon yesterday to report to me that his wife was very much griped and wished to see me. This enterprising lady had, in spite of remonstrance and reproof, struggled up to the camp from Balaclava about three weeks ago .... I proceeded to visit her in the hole her mate had prepared for her. This was an excavation six feet long, three broad and two deep. To cover it a small pyramidal tent was placed over the opening ... Brushing away a foot or two of snow that almost buried the interesting habitation I stooped and wriggled my head and shoulders within the door ... She was far advanced in labour: a smiling, although occasionally distorted, countenance evinced that she suffered but little pain. Our parturient females of the expedition appear to be retrograding towards the nomadic immunity from severe and long-continued labour pains.

Ogilvy was able to complete a rapid and successful delivery.

> From the rapidity of the execution I was obliged to tie the funis [cord] with the mother's apron string and sever it with my clasp knife, as no more appropriate instrument could be procured at the moment ... the happy mother, the only female in the camp save her child, at once proceeded with the help of her anxious husband, to wash and dress their little daughter, which looks most lively and blooming today, though thanks to the booming of the Russian guns, it made its appearance two months sooner than it ought. Owing to the individual interest and kindness of our Brigadier (Major-General Codrington) the mother and child want for nothing, and are comparatively comfortable.[142]

Edward Wrench had a similar experience in December, 1854. "I was called to the lines of the 27th Regiment, only a few hundred yards in the rear of the trenches and truly under fire of the Russian guns ... and in a bell tent, with the patient on the ground, I delivered a soldier's wife of a living child".[143] It may well be that many births took place without medical assistance, since there may have been reluctance to reveal to the authorities that a child had been born for fear that the mother would be sent away from her husband. They were a tough breed these soldiers' wives, prepared to follow their regiments to the ends of the earth!

THE DEATH OF LORD RAGLAN

By June 1855 Lord Raglan was a tired and disappointed man. The failure of the allied attack on 17 June and the death of General Estcourt from cholera on 24 June were the final blows. According to Kinglake, Raglan visited the dying Escourt[144], but this is unlikely from the report of Raglan's illness written by his personal physician Joseph Prendergast.[145] Prendergast states that Raglan became unwell on 21 June with a relatively mild diarrhoea. He had improved by 25 June and was able to get up and he "passed the day at his usual avocations (except riding), diarrhoea apparently having ceased". Early next morning he had a "copious fluid evacuation." Prendergast called in Hall for a second opinion and he agreed with the treatment by arrowroot wine and astringents. On 27 June the diarrhoea continued and in the evening the record ran - "the pulse and voice feebler". Alexander was then asked to see Raglan and he "wholly co-incided in the treatment pursued", now lead acetate and opium pills two-hourly. On the morning of the 28th Raglan had again slightly improved, but in the afternoon he became much worse. Prendergast recorded, "from this time the pulse, breathing, temperature of surface, all indicated approaching dissolution". Raglan died at 8.40 p.m., aged 67.[146]

In Mitra's biography of Hall a different picture is given of Hall's intervention. From this account, it is suggested that Hall was in fact alarmed at Raglan's condition and "on expressing his apprehensions to Prendergast, the latter said he thought much of what he saw was nervousness". Hall suggested that a further opinion should be sought. According to this account, Alexander considered "his Lordship had not a single unfavourable symptom".[147] It may be that Prendergast was rather slow in appreciating that his patient was seriously ill. Prendergast wrote to his brother on 27 June describing Raglan as "not very well - partly from atmospheric, partly from moral depressive causes, and recent loss of success, Estcourt's death, General Brown's illness, etc." Both in his official report and in his private letters Prendergast gave no firm diagnosis and cholera was not mentioned as a possibility.[148]

It is widely considered that Raglan died of cholera. Certainly the premonitary diarrhoea with temporary improvement, the relapse with frequent fluid stools, the reported cramps, and the final and rapid circulatory collapse, are very suggestive of cholera. Miss Nightingale, in her confident way, dismissed this diagnosis and attributed Raglan's death entirely to strain and exhaustion.[149]

There are many accounts of the final scenes at which Prendergast, General Airey, Lord Burgesh, Lord George Paget, Lady Paget and several others were present.[150] Mrs Seacole got wind of the event and (so she records) was allowed to peep at the dying Field-Marshall through the door![151] Kinglake was not present but this did not prevent him giving a long and detailed description of Raglan's last hours, affirming that "the expression on Lord Raglan's countenance in the moment of death seemed to tell of - not pain but - care".[152]

Raglan's death came as a shock to the army in the Crimea and to all at home, at a time when morale was low. Many of the soldiers had never seen him but most were aware of him as a figure-head and some believed he had had their interests at heart. Private Gowing was perhaps rather sanctimonious - "We did not know until he was taken from us how dearly we loved him."[153] From among the officers Clifford wrote on 20 June - "I see no one to replace him .... Lord Raglan has passed quietly away without leaving a single enemy. Everyone who knew him loved and respected him and rightly so ... he was gifted with the most sensitive feelings and kind heart."[154] But on 7 July Clifford had this to add: "I have felt the death of poor dear Lord Raglan very much and I cannot understand how many appear not to care the least about it".[155] In a critical account of Raglan's career, Russell summed up thus. "Still there was a simplicity about his manner, something of the old heroic character, which would have compensated for graver defects, if their results had not been, in many instances, so unfortunate to our arms.[156] To Kinglake Raglan remained the hero, the outstanding general and diplomat, of whom there could be no criticism.

Prendergast wrote: "the death of the Field Marshall has proved a personal loss as well as national. No one could live in intimacy with him without good feeling being brought into play."[157] But to most medical officers Raglan was probably seen as a remote commander-in-chief who showed little appreciation of their work, who had at times reprimanded the medical service unfairly, and who had not appeared to exert himself unduly to mitigate the hardships and suffering of his soldiers. However, Miss Nightingale felt the loss of Raglan deeply.[158] He had been her ally and had given her considerable support. Raglan was succeeded by General James Simpson, an ineffective commander-in-chief. He showed little interest in the medical service. Miss Nightingale found that he did not communicate with her as had Raglan, and she thought that he was opposed to her for some unstated reason.

NOTES

For the military background to this chapter, up to the death of Raglan, Volumes VIII-IX of **Kinglake** have been frequently consulted.

1. Comparison of statistics from regimental tables in **Med. Surg. Hist.**, 1.
2. Statistics from "Vessels which arrived at Scutari etc ..." **Med. Surg. Hist.**, 2:471-475.
3. Ibid, 31-32.
4. **Illustrated London News**, 14.4.1855.

CHAPTER XIII

5. Marquess of Anglesey, ed., **Little Hodge: his letters and diaries of the Crimean War 1854-1856** (London, 1971), 138.
6. V. Bonham-Carter, **George Lawson, Surgeon in the Crimea** (London, 1963), 160-161.
7. C. Fitzherbert, ed., **Henry Clifford V.C.: his letters and sketches from the Crimea** (London, 1956), 166.
8. Bonham-Carter, **Surgeon**, 162.
9. **Cantlie,** 2:155 (no source given). The only other reference to this use of the railway I have found is in W. Russell, **The British Expedition to the Crimea** (London, 1858), 315. Dr. Sutherland tried but failed to get "a carriage or truck fitted up on the railway" to convey the sick Mr. Stowe, Almoner of **The Times,** to Balaclava. This episode does not suggest a routine use of the railway to evacuate the sick.
10. **Kinglake,** 7:337-339.
11. Statistics from regimental tables in **Med. Surg. Hist.,** 1.
12. Ibid.
13. **Med. Surg. Hist.,** 2:58-106.
14. Statistics from regimental tables in **Med. Surg. Hist.,** 1.
15. Ibid., 2:159-167.
16. Ibid, 159.
17. Statistics for cholera in this period are from Tables in **Med. Surg. Hist.,** 2:86-87. Note that these indicate only the cases in regimental and general hospitals in the Crimea. The second epidemic is discussed in **Med. Surg. Hist.,** 2:72-85.
18. Ibid, 2:74.
19. George Shelton (1811-1875); M.B., T.C. Dublin 1842; joined as assistant-surgeon 1845; surgeon May 1854; served in the East for the duration of the war; retired 1882 as S.G. (obituary **B.M.J.** (1895), 2: 1067; **Drew**).
20. **Med. Surg. Hist.,** 2:73-74.
21. Ibid, 74.
22. Ibid, 399-464 "Meteorological observations recorded at the Castle Hospital by Dr. Jephson ... and Staff-Surgeon G.P. Matthew ... from April 1, 1855 to June 30, 1856".
23. Ibid, 76-77.
24. Thomas Fraser (1819-1890); L.R.C.S.Ed., M.D. Edinburgh 1845; joined as assistant-surgeon 1845; surgeon March 1855; served in the East for the duration of the war; retired 1875 as D.I.G. (**Drew**).
25. **Med. Surg. Hist.,** 2:78.
26. Ibid.
27. J. Snow, 'On the chief cause of the recent sickness and morbidity in the Crimea', **M.T.G.** (1855) 1:457-458.
28. **Med. Surg. Hist.,** 2:80.
29. Ibid.
30. Statistics from Regimental Tables in **Med. Surg. Hist.,** 1.
31. Ibid.
32. **Med. Surg. Hist.,** 2:258-259 "Return of Wounds and Injuries received in action", Tables 3 and 4, covering from April 1 to the end of the war.
33. Ibid., 2:471-485 "Vessels which arrived at Scutari etc ....".
34. **Med. Surg. Hist.,** 2:254-255.
35. **M.T.G.** (1855), 1:648-650.
36. **Med. Surg. Hist.,** 2, after p. 480, "General Hospital Returns. III. Balaclava".
37. Ibid., after p. 469, "General Hospital Returns. IV. Castle Hospital".
38. Ibid., after p. 480, "General Hospital Returns. II. Camp Hospital."
39. **Lancet** (1855) 2:93.
40. James Cowan (1832-1859); M.D. Edinburgh 1853: joined as assistant-surgeon April 1854, died on service. (obituary **Ed. Med. J.** 5, (1859), 95-97; **Drew**).
41. J.H. M'Cowan [should be Cowan] 'An account of the wounded of H.M.'s 55th Regiment', **M.T.G.** (1856), 1:205-206.

42. "Gair" in Cowan's account was probably George Fair M.D., who served as a staff assistant-surgeon November 1854 to June 1856 and was attached to the 55th Regiment in June 1855.
43. Ethelbert Blake (1818-1857); M.D. Edinburgh 1841; joined as assistant-surgeon 1841; surgeon 1853; served in the East for duration of the war; retired 1867 as D.I.G. (**Drew**).
44. **Med. Surg. Hist.**, 2:262.
45. Ibid., 264.
46. Ibid., 265-266.
47. Ibid., 266-272.
48. Ibid., 272-273.
49. Ibid., 273.
50. 'Charpie' was composed of lint or other rags which were inevitably septic. Condemned by many surgeons long before the war it was still frequently used in 1854, particularly by the French, for packing open wounds and dressings.
51. **Med. Surg. Hist.**, 2:274.
52. Ibid.
53. Ibid., 275.
54. Ibid, 275-276.
55. Ibid., 279-285.
56. Ibid., 274.
57. In 1940, a chapter in Hamilton Bailey's text-book on War Surgery discussed the use of maggots in wounds. But the technique was not revived in the 1939-1945 War.
58. **Med. Surg. Hist.**, 2:261.
59. Thomas Birnie (1827-1889); L.R.C.S.Ed. 1849; joined as assistant-surgeon 1853; served in the East for the duration; retired 1879 as D.I.G. (obituary **B.M.J.** (1890), 1:111; **Drew**).
60. T.R. Birnie 'Cases of gun-shot wound of the head and chest', **Lancet** (1856) 1:681-682.
61. Unfortunately the tables in **Med. Surg. Hist.** are confusing. See, however, "Return of wounds and injuries received in action. Table 3. Cases after April 1 to end of war, non-commissioned officers and men only." (**Med. Surg. Hist.**, 2:258) and "Return of wounds and injuries received in action. Table 4. Cases throughout whole war." (**Med. Surg. Hist.**, 2:259).
62. **Med. Surg. Hist.**, II:286-303.
63. G.J. Guthrie, 'Wounds of the head communicated by G.J. Guthrie', **Lancet** (1856), 1:257-260,310-312.
64. **Med. Surg. Hist.**, 2:304-310.
65. Ibid., 311-312.
66. Ibid., 313-326.
67. Ibid., 327-333.
68. J.A. Shepherd, **Spencer Wells** (Edinburgh, 1965), 32-33.
69. **Med. Surg. Hist.**, 2:334-335.
70. Ibid., 336-338.
71. Ibid., 339-364.
72. Ibid, 365-367.
73. Ibid, 368-379.
74. Ibid., 373.
75. Ibid.
76. Ibid., 370-371.
77. Ibid., 374-379.
78. **M.T.G.** (1855), 1:648-650.
79. **The Times**, 14.5.1855, and reprinted in **Ass.Med.J.** (1858), 476-477.
80. Edward Wrench (1833-1912); L.S.A., M.R.C.S. 1854; joined as assistant-surgeon December 1854; served in the East for the duration; F.R.C.S. 1859, resigned 1862; in practice in Derbyshire (obituary **B.M.J.** (1912), 1:983-984; **Plarr**; **Drew**).
81. E.M. Wrench 'The errors of the Crimean War', **B.M.J.**, (1899), 2:205-208.

CHAPTER XIII

82. **M.T.G.** (1855), 2:382.
83. J. Smyth, **The story of the Victoria Cross** (London, 1963).
84. Thomas Hale (1832-1908); M.R.C.S. from King's College 1854; joined as assistant-surgeon December 1854; staff assistant-surgeon March 1855; served in the East for the duration; served in India during the Mutiny; M.D. St. Andrews 1856; retired 1876 as S.M. (obituary **B.M.J.** (1910), 1:56; **Drew**). A memorial to Hale can be found in Acton Church, Cheshire.
85. For Sylvester, see note 60 to Chapter V. Sylvester's own account of the action which earned him the V.C. is in **B.M.J.** (1879), 2:1045; and the citation is in **M.T.G.** (1857), 2:556.
86. Quoted in **Lancet** (1856), 1:717.
87. Thomas Brady (1827-1871); M.R.C.S. 1850; joined as assistant-surgeon 1852; served in the East May 1854 - November 1855; retired 1869 as staff-surgeon (**Drew**).
88. Thomas Phelps (b. 1830); joined as acting assistant-surgeon August 1854; served in the East for duration of the war.
89. Arthur Greer (1831-1877); L.R.C.S.I. 1852; joined as assistant-surgeon 1852; served in the East for the duration of the war; retired 1877 as D.S.G. (**Drew**).
90. John Gibbons (1826-1882); M.R.C.S. 1849; joined as assistant-surgeon 1850; served in the East for the duration of the war; retired 1882 as S.G. (obituary **B.M.J.** (1882), 2:1234; **Drew**).
91. William Jeeves (1828-1875); M.R.C.S. 1852, L.S.A. 1853; joined as assistant-surgeon April 1854; served in the East for the duration of the war; retired 1873 as S.M. (**Drew**).
92. Lancet (1855), 2:19.
93. John Bent (1817-1874): M.R.C.S. 1839; joined as assistant-surgeon 1838; surgeon 1852; served in the East 1855 - June 1856; S.G. 1874 (obituary **B.M.J.** (1874), 2:725; **Drew**).
94. James Fogo (1928-1899); M.R.C.S. 1844; joined as assistant-surgeon (O.M.D.) 1844; surgeon April 1855; served in the East for duration of the war; F.R.C.S.Ed. 1877; retired 1882 as S.G. (obituary **B.M.J.** (1899), 2:885; **Drew**).
95. Bonham-Carter, **Surgeon**, 165-166.
96. **Lancet** (1855), 2:236.
97. M.T.G. (1855), 2:380-381.
98. The Times, 5.7.1855.
99. **M.T.G.** (1855), 2:226-227.
100. **The Times**, 8.8.1855.
101. Christopher Macartney (1818-1855); M.B. Dublin 1840; joined as assistant-surgeon 1844; surgeon March 1854; served in the East from June 1854 until death; buried in the Light Division Cemetery in the Crimea (**Drew**).
102. Walter Simpson (1820-1855); M.D. Edinburgh 1843; joined as assistant-surgeon 1844; surgeon March 1854; served in the East from December 1854 until death; buried at Cathcart Hill Cemetery in Crimea (**Drew**).
103. It is not known where John White qualified. He joined as acting-assistant surgeon on 23 December, 1854, aged 26; and may have served at Scutari as staff assistant-surgeon before joining the regiment.
104. Malcolm Ancell (1830-1855); joined as assistant-surgeon April 1854; served in the East from September 1854 until death (**Drew**).
105. John Longmore (1835-1855); M.R.C.S. 1852; joined as acting assistant-surgeon during the war but period of service uncertain. That he served with the 19th Regiment is confirmed by his name being on the regimental memorial in York Minster.
106. **Parl. Report., Naval Brigade Hospital,** 71-72.
107. Keevil, 4:150.
108. J. Colborne and F. Brine, **The last of the brave** (London, 1857), 64.
109. **Parl. Report., Naval Brigade,** 28-36.

THE SIEGE ENDED

110. D.J. Duigan, 'Some accounts of the wounded in the recent bombardments of Sebastopol', **M.T.G.** (1855), 2:234-235.
111. D.J. Duigan, 'Some further accounts of the wounded in the last bombardment of Sevastopol', **M.T.G.** (1855), 2:494-495.
112. H. Keppel, **A sailor's life under four sovereigns**, (3 vols., 1899), the Crimean period in Vol. 2, chapters LV-LXI.
113. Ibid., 2:286.
114. Ibid., 288-289.
115. Ibid., 297-298.
116. Richard Percy Chapman; surgeon January 1855; death recorded in **M.T.G.** (1855), 2:269.
117. **Keevil**, 4:151.
118. James Elliott (?-1855); M.R.C.S., L.S.A.; joined as assistant-surgeon 1848; surgeon November 1854.
119. **M.T.G.** (1855), 2:74.
120. **Ass. Med. J.** (1855), 1136-1137.
121. **Lancet** (1855), 2:594.
122. For general accounts of this visit, see E.T. Cook **The life of Florence Nightingale** (London, 1913), 7:254-263; I.B. O'Malley, **Florence Nightingale 1820-1856** (London, 1931), 302-309.
123. Cook, (**Life**), 1:255.
124. Ibid.
125. H. Morris **Portrait of a chef** (Cambridge, 1938), 156.
126. C. Woodham-Smith, **Florence Nightingale 1820-1910** (London, 1950), 219.
127. Bonham-Carter, **Surgeon**, 175.
128. Henry Hadley (1812-1874); M.D. Edinburgh 1834; joined as assistant-surgeon 1834; surgeon 1845; served in the East April 1855 - March 1856; retired as D.I.G. 1861 (**Drew**).
129. Woodham-Smith, **Nightingale**, 221.
130. Ibid., 221-222.
131. Cook, **Nightingale**, 1:259-260.
132. Woodham-Smith, **Nightingale**, 221-222.
133. O'Malley, **Nightingale**, 313-314.
134. **Med. Surg. Hist.**, 1:532-534.
135. R. Roxburgh, 'Miss Clough, Miss Nightingale and the Highland Brigade', **Victorian Studies**, 13 (1969), 71-151. The late Sir Ronald Roxburgh, who had seen 30 letters written by Miss Clough, kindly sent me a revised version of this paper and the quotations which follow are from the typescript.
136. John Furlong (1823-1884); M.R.C.S.I. 1844; M.D. Aberdeen 1847; joined as assistant-surgeon 1847; served in the East May 1854 - June 1856; retired 1883 as S.G. (**Drew**).
137. The contemporary newspapers abound with advertisements for passages to war area.
138. Z. Alexander and A. Dewjee, eds., **Wonderful adventures of Mrs. Seacole in many lands** (Bristol, 1957), a reprint of Mrs. Seacole's original account published, with a preface by W.M. Russell, in 1858, the editors providing a short biography of Mrs. Seacole.
139. Bonham-Carter, **Surgeon**, 157.
140. This and the graves of other such women are described in detail in Colborne and Brine, **Last of the brave**.
141. John Ogilvy (1831-1899); M.B. Aberdeen 1853; joined as assistant-surgeon 1853; served in the East for the duration; M.D. St. Andrews 1859; retired 1883 as D.S.G. (obituary B.M.J. (1899), 2:1818; **Drew**).
142. **M.T.G.** (1855), 1:141.
143. **B.M.J.** (1899), 2:206.
144. **Kinglake**, 9:267-269.
145. Joseph Prendergast (1810-1895); L.R.C.S.Ed., M.D. Edinburgh, 1835; as assistant-surgeon 1836; surgeon 1846; staff-surgeon (First class) March

1854; served in the East April 1854 - July 1855, October 1855 - July 1856; retired 1863 as I.G. (obituary **B.M.J.** (1899), 2:1054; **Drew**). Prendergast went to England in H.M.S. 'Caradoc' with the body of Raglan.

146. "Abstract of the case of Field Marshall Lord Raglan G.C.B. commanding the Forces in the Crimea. Disease Diarrhoea", a report signed by Prendergast and dated 29 June, 1855, among the Raglan Papers in the National Army Museum, Chelsea.
147. S.M. Mitra, **Life and Letters of John Hall** (London, 1911), 381-382.
148. Letters of Prendergast to his brothers and sisters, December 1854 to July 1855, in the National Army Museum, Chelsea.
149. C. Hibbert, **The destruction of Lord Raglan** (London, 1963), 342.
150. **Kinglake**, 9:284-287; Hibbert, 338-342.
151. Alexander and Dewjee, **Mrs. Seacole**, 199.
152. **Kinglake**, 9:287.
153. T. Gowing, **A soldier's experience: a voice from the ranks** (2nd edition, Nottingham, 1903), 139-142.
154. H. Clifford, **Henry Clifford V.C.: his letters and sketches from the Crimea** (London, 1956), 228.
155. Ibid, 229.
156. N. Bentley, ed, **Russell's Despatches from the Crimea 1854-1856** (London, 1966), 225.
157. Letters of Prendergast.
158. O'Malley, **Nightingale**, 355.13

CHAPTER XIV

THE SCUTARI HOSPITALS (APRIL 1855 TO JUNE 1856)

THE FIRST PERIOD - APRIL TO SEPTEMBER 1855

It has been recorded how, after the terrible experiences of the winter, conditions in the base hospitals had begun to improve by the end of March 1855. The position by the end of April, one month later, was summarised by an independent witness in the Medical Times and Gazette.[1]

> The numbers in the hospitals here have received a considerable addition within the last week. With few exceptions the invalids are from the Crimea. Of these, 180 have been sent to the General Hospital, and as many probably may have been admitted to the Barrack Hospital. The diseases seem to be of a much more mitigated and less dangerous form. For the very heavy losses in the hospitals our medical men have been very much blamed, but such censure is unmerited. The men came down here with constitutions so horribly broken up as to be beyond all medical skill; their death was only a matter of time. We consider the internal arrangements for the sick to be approaching a high degree of excellence; but we cannot speak in such a flattering manner of those of an external kind. The complete recovery of the convalescents would be very much accelerated by facilities of obtaining sun and air. For this purpose the space within the quadrangle of the Barrack Hospital should have been preserved; it has, however, been blocked up in a considerable measure by sheds, cooking-houses, and work-shops, all of which not only destroy the amenity of the quarter, but limit the ground for the men to take exercise on. Another evil to which the convalescents are exposed is the multitude of grog-shops near the main entrance to the Barrack Hospital. The consequence often is, that many of the men have relapsed and are sent back to their wards.

This is probably a fair comment, perhaps exonerating the doctors rather generously, but making sound observations on the causes of the high death rate in the winter. There is no comment on the influence of Miss Nightingale or of the Commissioners. Quite clearly a lot had still to be done to establish anything like adequate conditions.

To assess just how much the base hospitals did improve in the spring and summer of 1855 it is first necessary to study the rates of admission of patients in these months, the pattern of diseases treated and, in particular, the mortality rates. For the purposes of comparison, the tables below include the figures for the earlier months of January to March 1855.

In the six months between April and September 1855, 13,193 patients were admitted to the Scutari hospitals.[2]

Of these 509 died (3.9 per cent). Although the admission rates remained fairly high until the end of September the fall in the mortality ratio after March was dramatic. From the hospital transport records it appears that, while in the three winter months 6,415 patients survived the passage to Scutari (averaging 2,138 a month), in the next six months only 7,718 patients reached Scutari (averaging 1,286 a month).[3]

Table I

Admissions to Scutari Hospitals
(January to September 1855)

	Admissions	Deaths
January to March	10,283	3,354 (33%)
April to June	5,544	342 (6%)
July to September	7,649	167 (2%)
Totals	23,476	3,863 (16%)

Of the 13,193 admissions in April-September 1855 the vast majority were medical, only 610 wounded being admitted, together with a small number of general surgical cases. Bowel diseases accounted for 35 per cent of the medical cases, fevers 32 per cent, rheumatic conditions 8 per cent, and chest conditions 6 per cent. The residue was made up by a wide variety of other conditions.

The total number of admissions for BOWEL DISEASES, once more listed mainly under Diarrhoea and Dysentery, was 4,508, of which 224 died (5 per cent).[4] This compares with 2,996 admissions in the three winter months, with 1,638 deaths (55 per cent). By months, 295 were admitted in April with 80 deaths (27 per cent), 1,181 in July with 16 deaths (1.4 per cent), 1,141 in August with 54 deaths (5 per cent) and 865 in September with 34 deaths (4 per cent). The fluctuations in mortality are difficult to explain.

Table 2

Admissions to Scutari Hospitals for Bowel Diseases
(January to September 1855)

	Admissions	Deaths
January to March	2,996	1,638 (55%)
April to June	1,381	120 (9%)
July to September	3,127	104 (3%)
Totals	7,504	1,862 (25%)

Nothing new is recorded about the nature of these bowel diseases or the treatment applied. As in the Crimea in the spring and summer, the large number of admissions in July and August with a very low mortality rate (i.e. deaths/admissions) seems to indicate relatively minor types of diarrhoea from dietary causes or hot weather. Those patients who were transferred from the Crimea to Scutari with bowel diseases are likely to have had serious relapsing or chronic states which had proved resistant to all forms of treatment. Of those patients who survived prolonged treatment in Scutari a large proportion were invalided for further care in the home hospitals, and relatively few were sent back to duty.

The total of FEVER cases admitted in this period was 3,733, of which 153 died (4 per cent).[5] In comparison, the total admission rate for the three winter months had been 2,587 (averaging 862 monthly), of which 594 died (23 per cent). In March the mortality rate had been 17 per cent, but it was more than halved in April, when 734 cases were admitted, of which only 48 died (6.5 per cent). From May to August the admissions averaged 567 per month with the mortality rate fluctuating between 2 and 4 per cent. In September the admissions for fever fell to 370, with seven deaths (1.8 per cent). As in the winter the majority of cases were listed as continuous fever. Only 40 cases were specifically recorded as typhus.

Table 3

Admissions to Scutari Hospitals for Fever
(January to September 1855)

	Admissions	Deaths	
January to March	2,587	594	(23%)
April to June	2,182	104	(5%)
July to September	1,551	49	(3%)
Totals	6,320	747	(12%)

The marked reduction in the mortality rate for fevers reflected the general improvements in the base hospitals and, perhaps most of all, the reduction of overcrowding. This cut down the incidence of cross-infection and permitted of better nursing care. It is likely that the fevers in the spring and summer were less virulent than those in the winter months. No new ideas of treatment emerged during this period. Segregation of contagious conditions was easier to achieve as overcrowding diminished.

The number of patients with RHEUMATIC CONDITIONS admitted between April and September, 1855, was 1,002, of which eight died (0.8 per cent).[6] About a tenth of these cases were listed as acute and the rest as chronic. In addition "diseases of joints" and "lumbago" were specified. In September 178 cases of lumbago were recorded but simultaneously only 17 general cases of rheumatism. This suggests a certain confusion in the diagnostic nomenclature. There is no clinical analysis of these cases in the post-war medical history. The incidence in the winter months had been double that in the spring and summer, as would have been expected. Between April and September there were 782 admissions for CHEST DISEASES, of which 35 died (4.5 per cent).[7] The average admission rate per month in the winter had been 230, with a much higher mortality (19 per cent). These conditions were again listed under nine headings. There were 98 admissions for phthisis or haemoptysis, and the mortality rate for this group was high, with 22 deaths (22 per cent). The total of cases of CHOLERA admitted was only 59, of which 21 died (36 per cent).[8] Cholera cases were not normally transferred from the Crimea in this period. The incidence of the disease in the base hospitals and in the camps and barracks in the vicinity seems to have been much less than in the Crimea. The mortality rate at Scutari in these months was the lowest recorded during the campaign.

Turning to the SURGICAL admissions, the wounded have been calculated from April to October, 1855 (many September casualties in the Crimea were not transferred to Scutari until October).[9] Of 610 transferred only 19 died in the Scutari hospitals (3 per cent). Relatively few wounded were transferred from April to July, 265 in August, and 321 in September and October. The low mortality rate at Scutari confirms that patients with serious wounds were well on the way to recovery before being evacuated. No special comment need be made on the treatment of the wounded in the base hospitals. Most of the problems must have been due to chronic sepsis and a few secondary amputations were necessary. Few general surgical cases of major types were admitted to the Scutari hospitals in this period, apart from fractures and septic lesions. Among the miscellaneous surgical conditions only those for eye diseases and for "phlegmon and ulcers" ever exceeded ten a month.

There can be no doubt that conditions in the Scutari hospitals changed greatly for the better in the spring of 1855. The improvement started in April when there were 1,629 admissions compared with 2,833 in March. This reduced overcrowding in the hospitals, a significant factor in lowering the mortality rates. Popular opinion at home, however, tended to ascribe the favourable changes to better nursing standards. Undoubtedly Miss Nightingale had exerted great influence for good in many directions but it can hardly be said that better nursing care affected mortality rates greatly. For one thing, in April there were only about 60 female nurses available in the Scutari hospitals (and often fewer because of the high rate of sickness amongst the nursing staff). As Miss Nightingale herself had to admit, the proportion of really competent nurses was quite small. These nurses were needed for some 4,000 beds. Allowing two shifts of nurses there was potentially only one nurse to every 130 beds (in the unlikely event of all the nurses available being fit for duty). Today the prescribed ratio for British hospitals is one nurse for every three beds! In fact, since the female nurses were deployed so that there were at least two in a ward, this meant that many wards had no nurses at all.

There were many other positive reasons for improvement. By better management and because of effective repairs to the buildings the hospitals could be kept much cleaner. The reorganisation of toilet facilities and laundry services combined with the reduced occupancy made it possible to maintain much higher standards of hygiene. The replanning of kitchens by Soyer transformed the patient's diet and the distribution of meals. With the improvement of the weather, windows could be opened and ventilation improved. Thanks to the pressures of the Commissioners and of Miss Nightingale, work had been done to improve the defective drains of the hospitals, floors had been relaid, new windows had been fitted which could be opened, supplies of drugs and medical equipment had been greatly increased (as had bedsteads and bed-linen), and extra comforts now poured in, almost in embarrassing quantity. Hence, if there were some reports reaching home in which there were reservations concerning the conditions of the hospitals (like the report quoted at the beginning of this chapter), the flood of criticism in the lay and medical press had now greatly diminished.

The medical staff continued in this period under the command of Cumming. He remained neither imaginative nor enthusiastic over reforms. McGrigor and Cumming did not get on well together, the former working in close co-operation with Miss Nightingale, the latter often obstructive to her. The staff-surgeons and junior medical officers were frequently changed but the numbers were now sufficient for the demands upon them. Many newly appointed assistant-surgeons served briefly at Scutari before being sent to regiments in the Crimea. A relatively small group of civil surgeons was still attached to the Scutari hospitals; many had served through the winter. A few of the medical staff appointed to Renkioi worked for a short time at Scutari until the new hospital was opened. The observations of some of the civil surgeons on the Scutari hospitals have already been quoted. Many had sensed the atmosphere of jealousy amongst the senior medical officers, and at times relations between the regulars and the civilians were strained. Hall records in his diary - "McGrigor v. Rowdon, a man of the most violent temper who has been misconducting himself with everyone".[10] Hall continued to express objections to the civil element - "It was a great mistake mixing up these civil practitioners to the extent they have done here (Scutari)".[11] For instance Hall did not like Bryce, "a most disagreeable person"[12]; but he did approve of Pincoffs, "most intelligent"[13], and he did acknowledge that some of the civilian surgeons transferred to the Crimea from the Civil Hospitals had been of great assistance to him. All in all, it cannot be said that, as far as the doctors were concerned, the base hospitals were altogether happy hospitals.

Between April and September, 1855, three doctors died in the Scutari hospitals, all of whom had attachments there. Assistant-Surgeon Harvey Ludlow[14] died on 4 April "of the prevalent fever". Before he joined the army as an acting assistant-surgeon in October 1854 he had attracted attention by his surgical writings and was appointed Surgeon to the Metropolitan Free Hospital. He served at first in the Crimea and then worked at Scutari, and was commended for his service in the hospital transport 'Trent', in which he made one voyage, in November 1854. Assistant-Surgeon Robert Simons[15] died at Scutari on 18 April "of fever". Staff-Surgeon James Wishart[16] died at Scutari on 25 May. After serving as a staff officer in Bulgaria, he did not land in the Crimea as he was sick on board ship. He then sailed in the transport 'Kangaroo' and was able to help with the casualties. On arrival at Scutari he was retained on the staff there, working mainly in the Barrack Hospital, but was seconded for three voyages in the hospital transport 'Brandon' between January and March. He gave evidence to the First Commission in which he denied the alleged shortage of lint and sheets at Scutari.

MISS NIGHTINGALE AND THE NURSES

When Miss Nightingale returned to Scutari from the Crimea she spent a short time in a small house which the Bracebridges had prepared for her, near the Barrack Hospital. She then continued her convalescence in the Ambassador's house at Therapia. She was impatient to return to duty. By July she resumed her correspondence and by August she was again actively engaged in the administration of the hospitals. Mr. and Mrs. Bracebridge went home at the end of July, both now exhausted by their labours. Mrs. Bracebridge had become increasingly muddled in dealing with the gifts and Mr. Bracebridge was now exceedingly tactless with the medical staff. Indeed, after he returned home he was to make a public speech at Leeds in which he condemned the Medical staff at Scutari for failing to take advice from the French physicians as to how medical cases should be treated, alleging that as a result of their obstinacy many soldiers died unnecessarily. There were further petty accusations, for example, that a superior medical officer took away butter from the sick (butter provided by Miss Nightingale) on the grounds that it was an unnecessary luxury. **The Times** reported Mr. Bracebridge's lecture, enlarging on the obstinacy and harshness of the army doctor.[17] Miss Nightingale was furious. She had spent almost a year trying to build up good relations with the senior army doctors, tolerating them despite their faults and always seeking to get their co-operation in reforms. She wrote to Mr. Bracebridge indicating that neither he nor she was qualified to judge whether or not the treatment adopted by the French was superior to that of the English.

Not surprisingly Hall thought that Miss Nightingale had briefed Mr. Bracebridge to attack the medical service. Hall wrote to Smith about Bracebridge's remarks.

> When one reads such twaddling nonsense as that uttered by Mr. Bracebridge and which was so much lauded in **The Times** because the garrulous old gentleman talked about Miss Nightingale putting hospitals containing three or four thousand patients in order in a couple of days by means of the **Times** fund, one cannot suppress a feeling of contempt for the man who indulges in such exaggerations and pity for the ignorant multitude who are deluded by these fancy tales.[18]

Miss Nightingale wrote to her aunt - "my cause has been destroyed by everyone - ruined, destroyed, betrayed by everyone, alas one may truly say excepting Mrs. Roberts, Reverend Mother and Mrs. Stewart ... Dr. Hall is dead against me, justly provoked but not by me".[19]

Despite the unfortunate lecture at Leeds, Miss Nightingale greatly missed the support of Mr. and Mrs. Bracebridge and remained on affectionate terms with them. When Mr. Bracebridge died in 1872 and Mrs. Bracebridge in 1874 she wrote of them - "He and she have been the creators of my life ... I cannot doubt that they leave behind them, having shaped many lives as they did mine, their mark on the century."[20] As well as the Bracebridges Miss Nightingale had lost the local support of Raglan and she had little encouragement from his successor. In the late summer her relations with the senior medical officers deteriorated, and even her favourite McGrigor seemed to have come under the influence of Cumming and Lawson, with whom she was never on good terms.

Many other troubles heaped upon her. A Miss Salisbury was appointed to replace Mrs. Bracebridge but proved a complete failure.[21] She wrote letters home accusing Miss Nightingale of neglecting her patients, of wasting the free gifts, and even of having been responsible for the death of Miss Clough. When she began to steal food, drink, and free gifts she was soon detected. General Storks, who had replaced Lord Paulet, supported Miss Nightingale and they quietly dismissed Miss Salisbury and sent her home to avert a scandal. When she reached England she said she had been unfairly treated and, with the connivance of Miss Stanley, she complained to the War Office. Mr. Hawes, the leader of the anti-reform party (always antagonistic to Miss Nightingale), wrote to both Storks and Miss Nightingale, not inviting their opinions but demanding justification for the dismissal of Miss Salisbury. The affair dragged on with "partisan intrigue, petty thwartings, irritations and discourtesies". In time Miss Salisbury's guilt was clearly proven. This was a trying affair for Miss Nightingale and it was a great relief when at the end of September her 'Aunt Mai' (Mrs. Smith) arrived to become her confidante and general support. Although as late as August Miss Nightingale maintained full authority over her nurses she was now less often seen in the wards. There were still sectarian problems, lapses of discipline, and dismissals. Miss Nightingale found most of the Sisters reliable but later in the year when asking Mrs. Herbert to send out more nuns she wrote - "But just not the Irish ones".[22]

Problems seemed to have mounted from all sides and in her debilitated state in this hot summer Miss Nightingale was almost overwhelmed. She had enough worries in Scutari but longed to return to the Crimea where she felt she was needed most, to complete the work she had begun in May. Her friends at home worried about the additional strains which she was incurring. Late in July Lady Canning wrote to Lady Stratford -

I am quite unhappy about Miss N. keeping her authority while so ill. She ought to have wholly given it up for the time ... If Miss N. were to divide between Scutari and Balaclava and not keep both - I am sure when she is well she is the best head .... but when she is ill she ought not to attempt to carry it all. I believe real change of air is what she ought to have to depute someone to take her place. I cannot believe it is now so very difficult. I mean only the managing of nurses - I feel I am sure I could do it - purveying is quite another matter and ought never to be in female hands.[23]

But Lady Canning underestimated the indomitable spirit of Miss Nightingale. At this stage she was certainly not going to relax her grip on affairs or to allow her work to be undone. Not only had she come back to take full charge of the nursing organisation (and to maintain her authority over the distribution of gifts and comforts) but now she was working at other ideas for the general benefit of the serving soldier.

It is clear from a letter written by Miss Nightingale early in May 1855 that she had begun to see that there were new fields to conquer beyond the reform of the hospitals and the administration of the nursing service. To her the horrors of the war were not only those of wounds and disease but "intoxication, drunken brutality, demoralisation and disorder on the part of the inferior: jealousies, meanness, indifference, selfish brutality on the part of the superior!"[24] Drunkenness appalled her almost more than anything else. She saw two ways of curbing this, first by the education of the soldiers and secondly by providing facilities for them to remit their pay, or a part of it, to their dependents. She herself established a money order office through which the soldiers could save and so have less to spend on alcohol. In January 1856 the Government took over this novel scheme. She was able to open reading rooms and to start classes at Scutari for the soldiers. Her confidence in them was rewarded, for they responded by treating her with great respect, by drinking less, and by behaving with the utmost politeness and good manners. Many of the officers thought she was 'spoiling the brutes', but General Storks gave her great support in these activities. Furthermore, she continued her work on the medical statistics of the war, foreseeing that she could use these in a telling manner, when the war ended, to bring home to the authorities the gross defects of the medical organisation before and during the campaign, and perhaps to pin the blame on specific persons.

Sectarian problems never quietened down completely. Miss Nightingale had won the confidence of most of the Roman Catholic Sisters who remained at the Barrack and the General Hospital, particularly the group under Mother Clare, "her greatest comfort after Mrs. Bracebridge".[25] The "Reverend Mother", as Miss Nightingale called her, stayed on until April 1856, when she had to return home after a serious illness. It was a tribute to Miss Nightingale's tact and diplomacy that when Mother Clare left she asked her to take charge of the Roman Catholic Sisters. At Koulali the Roman Catholic element remained troublesome. Miss Stanley had set a pattern of revolt against Miss Nightingale, and when Miss Stanley went home (to spread derogatory reports about her former friend) her replacement as superintendent proved ineffective. Miss Nightingale, as earlier in the year, did not visit Koulali very often.

Many nurses had to be dismissed for bad conduct. But others were invalided for sickness, and at least seven died between April 1855 and the end of the war. Those who died and were buried at Scutari were Sophia Barnes, "nurse", on 4 April, 1855; Sophia Walford, "Matron of the Barrack Hospital", on 30 August; Mary Marks, "nurse at the Palace Hospital", in October; and Mrs Willoughby Moore, "Hyder Pasha - Superintendent of Officers Ward", in December. Most of these nurses died of cholera.[26]

THE LATER PERIOD (OCTOBER 1855 TO JUNE 1856)

Between October 1855 and June 1856, 6,029 patients were admitted to the Scutari hospitals (The Barrack, the General and Koulali).[27] The mortality rate for the whole period was 4.6 per cent. In the first four months it was 7.3 per cent and in the final five months only 1 per cent. The highest mortality was in November, 15 per cent: this was due to the cholera epidemic in that month (see below). The lowest mortality rate was in May, 0.2 per cent, only one death following 586 admissions. The remarkable differences in admissions and deaths between the first and second winters are noteworthy. Comparison of February 1855 and February 1856 is particularly dramatic. In that month in the first winter there were 2,688 admissions with 1,386 deaths (52 per cent) but in the second winter only 179 admissions with seven deaths (4 per cent). The transports carried only about 2,800 patients from Balaclava to Scutari in this whole period (46 per cent of all admissions to Scutari, a lower proportion than in the earlier months).[28] The mortality rate on board the transports in the nine months was low, only three patients dying on passage.

Medical cases predominated in this period. Fevers and bowel conditions were the most frequent and a severe outbreak of cholera in November was the only significant epidemic.

1602 cases of FEVER were admitted in this period, of which 36 died (2 per cent).[29] The highest monthly mortality was in February, 1856 (11 per cent), and there was only one death between May and June. Most cases were listed as febris continua communis. Typhus was very rarely recorded. Many of the fever cases must have been relapsing or persistent conditions for which the patients were transferred from the Crimea. The contrast in the admission and mortality rates for fever between the two winters need not be emphasised.

The admissions for BOWEL CONDITIONS were mostly recorded under the headings Acute and Chronic Dysentery, while the term 'diarrhoea' was now seldom used. In the whole period, 307 cases of "acute dysentery" were admitted, with 33 deaths (11 per cent).[30] There appear to have been sporadic cases of a serious type in January and February, but it is not known whether these cases were transferred from Balaclava or brought in to the Scutari hospitals from adjacent camps. A total of 930 cases of "chronic dysentery" was admitted, with 23 deaths (2.5 per cent). There were no deaths in the last three months. Because of the different patterns of diagnosis in the second winter, (particularly the almost complete exclusion of diarrhoea), it is not possible to make a direct comparison with the first winter, but the marked fall in the admission and mortality rates in the second winter is very obvious.

In the first three months of this period, 218 cases of CHOLERA were admitted with 138 deaths (63 per cent).[31] Seven cases were recorded in October, 207 in November, and four in December. By this period, there was no cholera reported in the Crimea but a few sporadic cases had been recognised in the villages around Scutari. On 2 November a wing of the Barrack Hospital was taken over by the German Legion and by some other drafts which had just arrived from England. Two cases of cholera had been reported in the transport carrying the German Legion, and after arrival at Scutari 150 cases occurred amongst the army personnel, mostly in the German Legion. The epidemic was thought to have been influenced by the bad ventilation of the wing occupied by the German Legion and, in addition, by the humid atmosphere in November. Although there were suggestions that the disease was not contagious, sixteen medical orderlies were attacked (the mortality rate is unknown) and three army medical officers died. There were some unusual features of the epidemic.[32] In almost every case the onset was very sudden, unheralded by the premonitory diarrhoea so often seen in

earlier months. "In a great many cases ... the sufferer was at once seized with great prostration of strength, with pains in the legs, vertigo, cramps, and vomiting, and generally last of all, purging: the disease in many cases running its course in a few hours." For instance,
> Dr. Wood, acting assistant-surgeon and Mr. Beveridge, dispenser of medicines had been on duty at the hospital up to 3 a.m. on the morning of the 17th and both returned to their quarters nearby. Soon after 4 a.m. Dr. Wood was found lying on the bed, with his clothes on and said he would come immediately.[33]

A short time later he was found suffering from cramps and he collapsed and died. Mr. Beveridge also died very quickly.

The epidemic was managed by evacuating the fit army personnel from their quarters in the Barrack Hospital and encamping them two miles away. No further cases broke out in the camps. Meanwhile those with cholera were nursed in segregated wards in the Barrack Hospital, and a few were sent to the General Hospital. The epidemic had burnt out by the beginning of December. The mortality rate, at 63 per cent, speaks for the virulence of the disease. It is stated that half the deaths occurred within twelve hours of onset. The rapid subsidence of the epidemic may have been in part due to the colder weather, but the segregation of cases was also probably of importance. The usual varieties of treatment were given with as little success as in former outbreaks. It was observed that "the calomel treatment, with the continued application of external heat, had the most happy results, but in many instances nothing could arrest the fatal tendency of the disease, less characterised by the violence of its symptoms than the profound prostration of vital energy from the first".

The incidence of RESPIRATORY TRACT DISEASES was remarkably small. Most cases were labelled acute or chronic catarrh. The more serious chest conditions were rare in the second winter. Pulmonary tuberculosis accounted for 56 admissions over the nine months, with five deaths (9 per cent).

As for SURGICAL conditions, after October few men wounded in action were transferred to Scutari, and general surgical cases of any serious nature were rare. Between December 1855 and May 1856 21 cases of frost-bite were admitted, of which three died. These figures confirm that there were few serious cases of frost-bite in the Crimea for which major amputations were required.

Three army medical officers died in the Scutari Hospitals in this period. It is convenient also to list at this point two doctors and one dresser who died shortly after arriving home as invalids. Deputy Inspector-General Alexander MacGrigor[34], after serving briefly at Scutari and then in Bulgaria, was appointed to the Barrack Hospital early in September 1854. It has already been recorded how he fulfilled this difficult assignment successfully, how he collaborated with Miss Nightingale, and how, by her influence, he was promoted Deputy Inspector-General in February, 1855. MacGrigor died of cholera on 16 November, 1855, during the outbreak at Scutari. Assistant-Surgeon H.W. Wood[35] and Assistant-Surgeon J. Mayne[36] both died of cholera, on 18 and 19 November, 1855, respectively, during the epidemic.

Little is known of either except that each served at Scutari from June 1855. Assistant-Surgeon T.O. Mitchell[37] died at Scutari on 29 December, 1855, while Assistant-Surgeon Andrew McKutcheon[38] died in Edinburgh on 3 November, 1855, of fever "caught at Scutari", he having served at there from March 1855 until invalided home late in October. Assistant-Surgeon Alexander Johnston[39] who had served in the Crimea with the 68th Regiment and probably was invalided home in June 1856, died at Portsmouth on 25 June, 1856. Finally, John Flewitt[40], a Dresser, died "seven days after arrival from the East", on 16 June, 1856. He had served at Scutari and Abydos before being invalided home.

While we must accept that the pressures on the Scutari hospitals in the second winter of the war were much reduced, the low mortality rates in this period (except for the inevitably high figure for cholera) nevertheless suggest that the sanitation and general management reached much higher standards than ever before. In March 1856 a correspondent wrote as follows. "Our hospitals at Scutari continue in the best possible state containing scarcely any patients; and so seldom do they arrive that the medical men actually struggle to obtain the few that come from the Crimea. This is all the more gratifying, when we consider the condition of our poor allies the French, in their hospitals across the Bosphorous." The contrast between March 1855 and March 1856 was remarkable in every respect.

Despite the improvements, even after October 1855 there was still criticism of the hospitals from many sources, although not so much of the clinical work as of the administration. In October Panmure sent out Colonel John Lefroy[41], an adviser in scientific matters to the Secretary of War, to investigate and to report privately on the true state of the hospitals.[42] Lefroy was at once greatly impressed by Miss Nightingale's work and influence. He supported her claim that she should have control of all the nurses in the East, and reported that Hall had obstructed Miss Nightingale in the Crimea.[43] Up to this time Panmure had not shown much interest in Miss Nightingale, indeed she had continued to write to Herbert rather than to Panmure with her plans, advice and her criticisms of individuals. No doubt it was one of Lefroy's briefs to investigate the competence of the senior medical staff. Cumming was still in command in October 1855. He had found his duties onerous and for more than a year had expressed the wish to give up his post. On 25 January, 1856, he was relieved by Linton, now promoted to the local rank of Inspector-General. Staff-Surgeons Gordon and Hadaway were promoted Deputy Inspectors-General, and Staff-Surgeon Mouat was given the local rank of Deputy Inspector-General of Hospitals in Turkey. Throughout these months there was ample medical staff in the Scutari hospitals. The basic numbers were augmented by many newly appointed assistant-surgeons, attached for varying periods before given regimental appointments or sent elsewhere on staff duties. Some of these young doctors who arrived late in the war served all their time at Scutari.

At the suggestion of Dr. Pincoffs, one of the civilian doctors attached to Scutari, a Medical Society of Constantinople was formed on 15 February, 1856.[44] Pincoffs appealed to the medical men in the Allied armies, and to the practitioners in Constantinople, to join. On 1 March Dr. Baudens, Inspector-General of the French Hospitals, was elected President, Dr. Linton, Inspector-General of the English Hospitals, Vice President, Dr. Fauvel, Professor of Medicine in Constantinople, General Secretary, and Dr. Pincoffs, Special Secretary. About 80 members were enrolled. On 28 March Dr. Casselas, a French physician, opened a discussion on typhus. His description was somewhat confusing. He considered that typhoid fever and typhus were due to the same cause, "identical in their bases, typhus and typhoid fever only differ in forms".[45] Only one other item of news of this Medical Society appeared in the medical press. In an anonymous letter dated 25 March it was stated that the Society continued to have well-attended meetings, but no details were given. Judging by the meagre reports it seems likely that this group did not survive for long. No doubt many of the members began to disperse in the spring of 1856. There is no indication of the degree of support given by the British medical officers.

MISS NIGHTINGALE AND THE NURSES AND ORDERLIES

When Miss Nightingale returned from the Crimea in November 1855, Linton wrote to Hall - "Miss N. is now flitting, I am told, about the wards less and less, as yet I have not made her acquaintance".[46] The worst of the cholera epidemic had subsided when she reappeared at Scutari. She was still very much involved in the management of the nurses, and there were increasing problems to deal with, on matters of discipline or concerning the transfer of nurses to the Crimea. She was still greatly occupied with the distribution of stores and the 'Free Gifts' which accumulated in great quantity. But most of all she was intent on improving the general conditions for the soldiers, whether sick or well, by providing educational facilities and recreation rooms, and by trying to encourage the men to save money and give up excessive drinking. At Scutari she found General Storks a willing supporter in the organising of such innovations. After her third visit to the Crimea Miss Nightingale returned late in June 1856, to clear up her affairs in Scutari. The hospitals were now closing down rapidly and there was little to do except to dispose of her private stores. She left for England on 28 July, refusing a quick passage in a naval vessel but returning slowly overland.[47] Miss Nightingale was now the recipient of widespread adulation. The country was preparing to receive her as a heroine and to give her a tumultuous reception. She evaded all publicity and slipped away to her home at Lea Hurst. She was exhausted and greatly needed rest and seclusion. Whatever the world thought of her achievements she herself was depressed and felt she had failed in many aspects of her self-imposed task. But there was a firm determination to ensure, by all means possible to her, that the sacrifices of so many lives in the war, from what to her were preventable causes, were not forgotten, and that the lessons learnt should be acted upon urgently.

In these months, although the strain on the nurses had obviously lessened it seems that there was more dissension among them than in any previous period. The atmosphere was aggravated by continued attacks at home by Miss Stanley and Miss Salisbury, attacks directed largely at Miss Nightingale's management of the nurses. In the Crimea, the antagonism of Mrs. Bridgeman and her staff, perhaps encouraged by Hall, made for distrust and also, as Miss Nightingale was to discover, inefficiency and neglect in the running of the hospital controlled by Mrs. Bridgeman. Before she finally left the Crimea in April 1856, Miss Nightingale and her assistants spent three days cleaning up the Balaclava General Hospital. She wrote tartly - "the patients were grimed with dirt, infested with vermin, with bed sores like Lazarus (Mother Bridgeman I suppose thought it holy)".[48] Hall denied these accusations (which were not the only example of Miss Nightingale's exaggerated statements and vituperative asides) and took them as a slur on himself and his purveyor, Mr. Fitzgerald.

On the credit side there were some nurses and sisters who did have exceptional ability. This was recognised increasingly by many of the doctors. Miss Nightingale still had the greatest trust in nurses such as Mrs. Roberts, Miss Morton, and Mrs. Shaw Stewart (although she retained some reservations about the last-named). Of the sisters, 'Reverend Mother' (Mary Clare) had been her greatest support, and she expressed very great regret when this excellent woman was ordered home by her Bishop at the end of April 1856.[49] It was to Miss Nightingale's credit that all the religious bickerings, so often involving the Roman Catholic Sisters, did not prevent her from recognising and publicising the good qualities of individuals such as the 'Reverend Mother'. As the hospitals began to close down she took great pains to ensure that the return home of her staff was well planned. There was no problem in the disposal of the sisters for they inevitably went back to their original religious establishments but the future of the so-called professional nurses was less easy to foresee. Those such as Mrs. Roberts were earmarked for responsible posts in the hospitals at home, for already Miss Nightingale saw her future involvement in reorganising the civil nursing establishments. However, many of the nurses had proved, at the best mediocre, while a few were grossly incompetent, were inclined to drink, or had behaved irresponsibly. Miss Nightingale sent to Lady Cranworth (who had succeeded Mrs. Herbert as the convener of the committee for nurses) brief notes about the characters and abilities of all these women, stressing their virtues rather than their shortcomings. She described some of them as "the poor despised, and I fear too often exposing themselves to be despised, nurses". But she insisted that they had all "except a few humbugs" done good service."[50] There was no suggestion at this stage that any of the female nursing staff should remain attached to the army and serve in the home military hospitals. Although a few army officers who had worked with female nurses during the war were convinced of their value, it was to be long before a well-trained and well-organised military Nursing Service was established. On the other hand some of the doctors in Smyrna and Renkioi carried back to civilian life a conviction that nursing services in the hospitals at home should be reformed and expanded.

The post-war Royal Commission made scant reference to female nursing staff. Dr. Sutherland in his evidence commented that in foreign hospitals female nurses had been of great benefit in the wards and "the same observation was made by all the medical and other officers connected with the civil and military hospitals abroad".[51] Miss Nightingale in her evidence had this to say. "I think great sanitary civil reformers will always tell us that they look to the woman to carry out all their sanitary reforms ... She has a superior aptitude in nursing the well quite as much as the sick."[52]. Miss Nightingale maintained that female nurses might be introduced into general military hospitals at home and in the field, but not in regimental hospitals, and that they should be under a female head.[53] As questions had been put to Miss Nightingale before the Commission met and as she had sent written answers in advance, there was no occasion to question her in detail on her ideas, or to discuss in depth the place of female nurses in the army medical services.

In an attempt to provide a higher standard of hospital and ambulance orderlies to replace the regimental orderlies who had proved so unsatisfactory, a contingent of 300 men was sent to Scutari in November 1855.[54] Some were civilians recruited in England, some were N.C.O's unfit for active service, and some had been transferred from the Land Transport Corps. This mixed lot of men was graded, according to their education and experience, as stewards, wardmasters, cooks, washer-men, issuers, barbers or hospital orderlies. Hall demanded half of the contingent for ambulance and other duties with the regiments in the Crimea, but presumably the other half stayed in Scutari. There is no account of the activities of these men in the hospitals. That the new corps was a failure is suggested by the fact that it was abolished late in 1856. Miss Nightingale had recommended a similar "medical staff corps" as early as 8 January, 1855, in a letter to Herbert.[55] Many of her suggestions were taken up at this later date, but she does not appear to have taken any interest in this belated innovation. The project failed, most likely because discipline was poor, because there had been no preliminary medical training, and because the Corps did not have its own officers. A new 'Army Hospital Corps' was established in 1857.[56] This was a slight improvement, as the selection of personnel was done more carefully and the Corps had its own officers to maintain discipline. The post-war Royal Commission made little reference to the inadequacy of the regimental orderlies or to the new Medical Staff Corps. However Miss Nightingale was asked how orderlies should be recruited and she recommended, "discharged soldiers and civilians of good character ... who can read or write".[57] She argued that male orderlies should be under the head nurse of a ward as far as nursing duties were concerned, but under the wardmaster for general discipline.

Although in November 1855 the Barrack Hospital had been required to provide accommodation for a large number of troops (to cope with the cholera epidemic in that month), by the end of June 1856 there were few patients left in the hospital, and the last was evacuated on 16 July. The General Hospital was probably closed about the same date. Koulali Hospital was closed at the end of November 1855. Linton wrote joyously to Hall in that month - "Ladies of Koulali are going home - the attempt on the part of Lady Stratford to keep them not accepted".[58] Miss Nightingale was glad to be rid of the Koulali nursing staff which had remained largely independent of her authority but which had been a special interest of the

Ambassador and his wife. Indeed she had come to resent the interference of Lady Stratford in hospital affairs. The Haidar Pasha Hospital also closed before the end of 1855, being given over for barracks accommodation.

CONCLUSION

The larger hospitals at Scutari had functioned from June 1854 to June 1856. In these two years the total of admissions was 43,208, with 5,432 deaths (12.6 per cent). The highest mortality rate was in February 1855 (52 per cent). If the statistics for January to March 1855 - the months of exceptional overcrowding - are excluded, we are left with a mortality rate of only 6 per cent for the remaining 21 months. This figure compares very favourably with those of the best hospitals in Great Britain at the time. The exceptional mortality rates in the first three months of 1855 were explicable, not only in terms of the gross overcrowding but also in terms of the exceptional virulence of the diseases and the poor general condition of the soldiers brought from the Crimea. Faced with the same conditions, a civilian hospital in Britain would have been unlikely to have done better than the Scutari hospitals.

This is not to say that the criticisms of the Scutari hospitals, which reached a peak between November 1854 and March 1855, were unjustified. The outcry against shortages of medical comforts, medical equipment, bedding, bedsteads and hospital clothing was valid, but these shortages could not be blamed on the doctors on the spot, since they arose from failures of distribution of supplies which in fact had reached the East in large quantities. There was less excuse on the part of the medical staff for the inadequacy of the kitchens and the poor diet of invalids and bad cooking. Granted that it was difficult for the doctors to improve these conditions because of their limited executive powers, they could have broken through red tape and corrected some defects rather than have left this to the Sanitary Commissioners and to Miss Nightingale. The same arguments apply to the very slow improvement of the laundry facilities, and to the correction of the effects of drainage, water supply and ventilation in the hospitals. The senior medical officers were in many instances slow to recognise that it was desirable and possible to treat the sick or wounded soldier with more humanity. Too often they were content to express the view that conditions in the hospitals (even at their worst) were never as bad as in the Peninsular War. It was the war correspondents, Miss Nightingale, and those influential civilians who visited Scutari, who forced the medical officers to accept that after an interval of forty years it was necessary to have new attitudes and to realise that public opinion was now much more powerful and better informed. Yet in conclusion it must be emphasised that, in the light of contemporary civilian practice at home, the military doctors could not be adversely criticised on professional grounds. Their skills were scarcely inferior to those of practitioners at home; their devotion to duty and their self-sacrifice were often exceptional. Many worked to the limits of physical endurance and some worked to death.

NOTES

1. **M.T.G.** (1855), 1:533.
2. **Med. Surg. Hist.**, 2: after p.480, "General Hospital Returns. I. Hospitals in the Bosphorous".
3. Ibid., 471-475, "Vessels which arrived at Scutai etc."
4. Ibid., 2: after p.480, "General Hospital Returns". In September 1855 the additional label "Colica" was introduced (but not repeated) and this category accounted for 531 admissions of bowel disease, with one death. This temporary use of a purely symptomatic diagnosis is not readily explained.
5. Ibid.
6. Ibid.
7. Ibid.
8. Ibid.
9. Ibid.
10. 'Hall Diary', 4.8.1855.
11. Ibid.
12. Ibid., 22.9.1855.
13. Ibid., 7.4.1855.
14. Harvey Ludlow (1827-1855); M.R.C.S. 1849; F.R.C.S. 1852; joined as acting assistant-surgeon October, 1854; served in the East from November 1854 until death; buried at Scutari (obituary **M.T.G.** (1855), 1:402; **Platt**).
15. Robert Simons (1829-1855); joined as acting assistant-surgeon December 1854; served in the East from May 1854 until death; buried at Scutari.
16. James Wishart (1820-1855); M.D.Edinburgh 1843; joined as assistant-surgeon 1854; surgeon October 1854; served in the East from May 1854 until death; buried at Scutari (**Drew**).

17. **The Times**, 16.10.1855; **M.T.G.** (1855) 2:399-400; E.T. Cook, **The life of Florence Nightingale** (2 vols., London, 1913), 213,227-288; I.B. O'Malley, **Florence Nightingale 1820-1856** (London, 1931), 381-383.
18. C. Woodham-Smith, **Florence Nightingale 1820-1910** (London, 1950), 230-231.
19. Ibid., 231.
20. Cook, **Nightingale**, 2:236.
21. O'Malley, **Nightingale**, 321-328 (referring to Miss Salisbury as 'Miss X.'); Woodham-Smith, **Nightingale**, 236-237.
22. Woodham-Smith, **Nightingale**, 229.
23. 'Canning Letters', 20.7.1855.
24. Cook, **Nightingale**, 1:276.
25. O'Malley, **Nightingale**, 238.
26. Burial records from J. Colborne and F. Brine, **The Last of the Brave** (London, 1857).
27. **Med. Surg. Hist.**, 2: after p.480, "General Hospital Returns. I. Hospitals in the Bosphorous".
28. Ibid., 471-475, "Vessels...".
29. Ibid., 2: after p.480, "General Hospital Returns...".
30. Ibid.
31. Ibid.
32. Ibid., 2:81-83.
33. Ibid., 2:83.
34. For McGrigor, see note 31 to Chapter VI.
35. H.W. Wood (d.1855); joined as acting assistant-surgeon June 1855; served in the East from June 1855 until death; buried at Scutari (**Med. Surg. Hist.**, 2:83).
36. Probably John Mayne (d.1855); M.R.C.S. 1839; L.S.A. 1840; joined as acting assistant-surgeon May 1855; served in the East from May 1855 to death. Mayne's name is on the memorial at Scutari.
37. Possibly Thomas Oak Mitchell (d.1855); L.S.A. 1828; L.R.C.S.Ed. 1831; M.D. Edinburgh 1853; joined as acting assistant-surgeon; served in the East July 1855 - December 1855 (**Directories**)
38. Andrew McKutcheon (d.1855); M.D. Edinburgh; joined as acting assistant-surgeon January 1855; served in the East March 1855 until death.
39. Alexander Johnston (1832-1854); M.D. Edinburgh 1854; joined as assistant-surgeon September, 1854; served in the East September 1854 - June 1856 (**Drew**).
40. John Flewitt (1837-1856); joined as a dresser December 1854; served in the East December 1854 - December 1855. (**Med. Surg. Hist.** 1:523, "List of Dressers"; **M.T.G.** (1856), 1:128).
41. For Lefroy and his mission, see **Autobiography of John Henry Lefroy**, edited by Lady Lefroy and privately printed c.1895; **DNB**.
42. Cook, **Nightingale**, 1:297-298.
43. O'Malley, **Nightingale**, 367-8.
44. **M.T.G.** (1856), 2:123-8.
45. Ibid.
46. 'Hall/Linton Letters', ?.11.1855.
47. For an account of Miss Nightingale's last weeks at Scutari, see Cook, **Nightingale**, 1:299-303.
48. Woodham-Smith, **Nightingale**, 252. See also Miss Nightingale's later statements (**Royal Commission**, 379).
49. O'Malley, **Nightingale**, 387-388.
50. Ibid., 391-392.
51. **Royal Commission**, 224.
52. Ibid., 379.
53. Ibid., 376.
54. **Cantlie**, 2:171.
55. Cook, **Nightingale**, 1:224-229.
56. **Cantlie** II, 233.

57. **Royal Commission**, 233.
58. 'Hall/Linton Letters', 26.11.1855.

CHAPTER XV

THE NAVY IN THE BALTIC AND BLACK SEAS (1855-1856)

THE BALTIC FLEET 1855

The Baltic Fleet refitted in the winter of 1854.[1] Napier, whose leadership in that year had been greatly criticised, was replaced by Rear-Admiral Dundas who had previously commanded the Black Sea Fleet. It was complained that there had been no positive plan of action in 1854 and that little had been achieved. The hope was expressed that a more positive attack would be made on Russia in 1855. By a combined operation Kronstadt, or even St. Petersburg, might be taken. In fact no more was to be achieved than the routine blockade of the Russian Baltic ports, and the destruction of Sveaborg and of two minor forts in the Gulf of Finland. Part of the Fleet did penetrate within fifteen miles of Kronstadt but Dundas decided that an attempt to capture the port should not be made. In this decision he was supported by the Admiral of the French Fleet which was in company. The bombardment of Sveaborg took place on 11 August. Thereafter the mortar vessels were withdrawn and it was clear that the role of the Fleet was reduced to a blockade alone. The correspondent of **The Times** wrote in October - "Our presence has obliged the Emperor to maintain in a state of inactivity an enormous army ... along the coasts of Bothnia and Finland while the food, clothing, luxuries, and all manufactures of countries more civilised than his own, have been rigidly withheld from approaching his shores ... His mercantile marine has ceased to exist; it is calculated that we have made prizes of, burnt, or sunk some 80,000 tons of shipping in the Gulf this summer."[2] But it was the general feeling that the British Navy had achieved little to hasten the end of the war, or to have influenced Russian strength in the Crimea. With the approach of winter the Fleet left for Kiel and returned to England. It was announced that the allies, "at the head of an immense armament", would re-enter the Baltic in the spring of 1856. There were ambitious plans to destroy Kronstadt and to land at St. Petersburg with 80,000 men. But all was rendered abortive by peace being declared.

The Baltic Fleet in 1855 comprised some 86 vessels of which 20 were 'ships of the line'. All ships were in steam, for in 1854 it had been found that those in sail were tactically useless. This formidable force was manned by approximately 18,000 officers and seamen.

DISEASES AND SURGERY

The sick rate throughout the year varied in different ships from 2.6 to 6 per cent. Medical conditions predominated. Although the total at risk was greater in the Baltic Fleet than in the Black Sea Fleet, the number of men dying from disease was less in the former than in the latter. In 1855 there were 144 deaths from disease, but only 118 of these can be traced in the reports recording individual diseases. A total of 144 deaths out of some 18,000 officers and men was not an excessive rate and suggests that the health of the Baltic Fleet was remarkably good in 1855. It is not possible to give complete figures of those reporting sick. At least 1,900 were listed as sick, but in the post-war report for some diseases the sick rate is not given.[3]

To begin with FEVERS. It was stated - "The febrile diseases which prevailed in the Fleet during 1855 were with few exceptions of so mild a character as hardly to deserve notice." Minor epidemics of a catarrhal nature were not uncommon. There were in the whole period 425 cases of "Continued and Remitting Fever", of which 19 were fatal (4.5 per cent). "Eruptive Fevers" included smallpox, scarlatina and measles. There were 10 cases of scarlatina and 81 of measles, of which one was fatal. (Measles did not appear in the Black Sea Fleet.) But there were 135 cases of smallpox in 1855. An epidemic broke out in H.M.S. 'Duke of Wellington' before it left Portsmouth, and three cases were sent ashore to Haslar Hospital. When the ship reached the Gulf of Finland on 8 May the disease spread rapidly. Cases totalled 58, of which three were fatal. "The number of cases having considerably increased ... the Commander-in-Chief put to sea en route for Faroe Sound, for the purpose, if possible, of preventing the spread of contagion by landing and placing in tents, those affected with the epidemic."[4] This timely isolation of the smallpox cases in a temporary hospital proved successful in controlling the epidemic. Many of the cases were mild, particularly in those men who had been vaccinated previously, but of four unvaccinated men two died. There were 49 cases in H.M.S. 'Arrogant', with one death, and again the infection was brought on board before the ship sailed from England. These patients also were isolated in the hospital at Faroe. H.M.S. 'Amphion' had eight cases, with no deaths, and the total was made up by another 20 cases occurring sporadically in the Fleet, without any fatalities. The total mortality rate, four out of 135 cases (3 per cent) was remarkably low. This suggests that vaccination had been done quite effectively in the Navy by this date.

Turning to OTHER CONDITIONS, only 21 "Inflammatory Attacks of the Alimentary Canal" were reported, diarrhoea and dysentery being seldom mentioned. Cholera was very rare in 1855. Of three cases in H.M.S. 'Colossus' all recovered, but single cases in three other ships all died. Diseases of the respiratory tract were more common. Under the heading "Inflammatory Affections of the Lungs and Pleura" there were 478 cases, of which 17 were fatal (4 per cent), and 126 cases of "Haemoptysis and Consumption" were reported, of which 39 were fatal (31 per cent). In an unspecified total listed under "Diseases of the Skin etc." there were 162 cases of erysipelas, of which five were fatal. Many skin conditions seem to have been due to secondary infection of ulcers or wounds. It was believed that the incidence of these lessened greatly when oranges and fresh vegetables were in good supply. This raises the possibility that some skin conditions were associated with scurvy. Scurvy is not referred to directly in the post-war report but "ulcer", affecting the lower leg in particular, which was frequent in some ships, may well have been scorbutic in origin. Both ulcer and erysipelas seem to have affected mostly new recruits of poor physique, "whose constitutions were impaired by previous disease or by want and the privations incident to a life of destitution". As far as is known there was a routine issue of lemon juice to the Baltic Fleet in 1855 and the victualling system was reasonably good, with fresh meat and vegetables brought from England regularly.

Under the heading "WOUNDS, accidents, and drowning" there were 63 deaths, of which 23 were due to falls from the rigging or other ship-board hazards, 11 from wounds in action, two from "poison", and 27 from drowning. The total incidence of wounds in action is uncertain. Included in the deaths were those of five men who died of gun-shot wounds, "in a murderous attack made by the enemy on a boat's crew who were landing several of their own countrymen [i.e. Russians] under a flag of truce at Hango".[5] At the same time four men were seriously wounded. The medical officer in the party was Surgeon R.T. Easton, who was at first reported killed; but subsequently it was learnt that the Russians had taken him prisoner and then released him unhurt.[6] Little surgery was done in this period. Of the small number of men who died of wounds on board the warships most were inoperable. A few wounded were transferred to the hospital ship 'Belleisle'.

The 'Belleisle' entered the Baltic in the Spring and was in the Gulf of Finland in August. Surgeon Robert Beith[7] is known to have done most of the operating. He published a report of a successful case of excision of the head of the humerus following a gun-shot wound of the shoulder. Beith advocated local resection of shattered bone rather than amputation, particularly for injuries of the upper limb.[8] Not a great deal is known of the types of cases admitted to the 'Belleisle' in 1855. In general those with medical conditions were kept in their own ships (with the exception of smallpox cases). It is likely many of the admissions were quite quickly sent to England, where they were taken to Yarmouth Naval Hospital or Haslar. The accommodation and staffing of Yarmouth had been greatly increased in 1854, since it was more conveniently placed than Haslar for the reception of casualties from the Baltic Fleet.[9]

MEDICAL STAFFING

The shortage of medical officers, particularly assistant-surgeons, which had caused concern in 1854, still persisted. It was calculated that the Baltic Fleet was well below the appropriate war-time complement of assistant-surgeons.[10] To counteract this shortage, the Admiralty notified all the teaching hospitals in Great Britain that medical students would be employed as dressers.[11] They were to serve in the Baltic from April to October, so that they could return to their medical studies in the winter. They were required to have reached an advanced stage in clinical instruction and to sit an examination. Pay was at six shillings a day in the rank of acting assistant-surgeon.[12] A gratuity of £25 was to be paid on completion of service. Medical schools and medical students had already expressed strong views concerning the conditions under which qualified assistant-surgeons served. There had been a strong indication that in most schools students on qualification would not volunteer to serve in the navy.[13] At mass meetings of students there was general rejection of the Admiralty plans.[14]

However, according to one report, as many as 67 dressers served in the Baltic Fleet in 1855.[15] No official list has been traced. Despite the resolutions passed in most of the medical schools many individuals saw these posts as an exciting challenge. The introduction of students awarded the rank of acting assistant-surgeon was greatly objected to by the assistant-surgeons already in the navy, since the latter were fully qualified and had often held the rank for many years. Three dressers who attained some eminence have been traced. Christopher Heath[16], eventually a Professor of Clinical Surgery, and President of the Royal College of Surgeons, served as a dresser on board H.M.S. 'Impérieuse' from March to September 1855. William Swain, later a distinguished surgeon in the West of England, served as a dresser on board H.M.S. 'Exmouth' during 1855.[17] Robert Lewer[18], later a Deputy Surgeon-General in the Army, also served as a dresser in the Baltic Fleet in 1855.

No record has been found of any death in action or from disease of a medical officer or dresser serving in the Baltic Fleet in 1855.

THE BLACK SEA FLEET 1855-1856

In 1855 the command of the Black Sea Fleet was taken over from Dundas by Admiral Lyons.[19] The main base was still the crowded harbour of Balaclava. The landing facilities were now much better organised, and included a separate wharf for the hospital transports. Consideration was given to transferring the facilities to Kazatch Bay, adjacent to the French naval base at Kamiesh. Lyons did not pursue this idea which, had it been realised, would have shortened the distance between the British camps and the base at which supplies were landed. The British did, however, use Kazatch Bay increasingly as an anchorage during 1855. The construction of the railway from Balaclava to the camps did much to improve the delivery of stores from the ships. By now, with most of the Russian Fleet scuttled or disarmed in the harbour of Sebastopol, and with nearly all the Russian sailors brought ashore to man the defences, the Allies had full command of the Black Sea. A blockade of the Black Sea ports could be enforced, shipping was controlled at the mouth of the Danube, and supplies to Sebastopol brought through the Sea of Azov were intercepted.

It has already been described how the first expedition to Kertch, early in May, had to be recalled for political reasons. Three weeks later, in a combined operation planned largely by Lyons, a powerful force was landed at Kertch and Yenikali. Many store-houses and their contents were destroyed, and much shipping was sunk in the Sea of Azov. An army of occupation was left at Kertch for the rest of the war. Casualties in the operation were minimal. By this action, reinforcements and supplies for Sebastopol had henceforth to come almost entirely by the slow and difficult land route. The success of the expedition raised the morale of the Allies considerably.

As far as the siege was concerned, in 1855 the Fleet took relatively little part. In April a limited naval force supported the land attack by moving inshore under cover of darkness, but the attack was unsuccessful and the warships were soon withdrawn. On 15 August, small mortar-vessels were sent in to shell the Russian positions. This tactic was repeated in the Final Bombardment of 8 September. Each mortar-vessel carried a single gun firing a 13 inch shell, and was manned by a crew of twelve. Usually about six mortar-vessels operated together. Cree (surgeon to H.M.S. 'Odin', the parent ship of the mortar-vessels) stated - "While we were firing either I or Hamilton, my assistant, is on board one of the vessels in case of accidents".[20] This was a hazardous duty for the medical officers, since the unprotected mortar-vessels came under heavy fire. The last naval operation of any importance was the attack on Kinburn, 40 miles to the west of Odessa.[21] The object was to block communications between Odessa and the rivers Bug and Dnieper. A bombardment of Kinburn was carried out early in October by seven British warships and mortar-vessels, assisted by the French. The forts were soon taken and casualties on the British side were minimal.

The Black Sea Fleet largely maintained a passive role in 1855. Its presence and its complete domination over Russian sea-power was of great importance. By the maintenance of the blockade, by the rapid transfer of troops by sea from one sphere of operation to another, and by the organisation of transport for all forms of supplies and for the sick, much was achieved. The naval organisation worked efficiently in this year not only in these routine duties but in the maintenance of the Naval Brigade and the marine force in the Crimea. Hence, the experience of the Crimean War sowed the seed for the development of combined operations in future wars. The last duty of the Black Sea Fleet was to take home the part of the army awaiting transport in June and July 1856. There was much clamour at home for the quick return of the soldiers, a clamour supported by Queen Victoria who insisted that the Fleet need not lie idle abroad.

DISEASES AND SURGERY

It is not easy to extract accurate sick rates and mortality rates for the different diseases encountered in 1855.[22] In such reports as are available it is not always clear if the Fleet tables include statistics of the Naval Brigade and the marine force ashore (the personnel of which were derived from the war-ships). The total complement of the ships in 1855 seems to have varied between 14,000 and 16,000, according to the demands made for reinforcements in the Crimea. The average sick rate was 4.3 per cent, lower than in 1854, and the lowest figures were in the smaller ships. It is not possible to calculate the percentage of those reporting sick in their ships who were subsequently sent to hospital ships or base hospitals. Medical conditions accounted for the vast majority of men reporting sick. From the post-war reports it is possible to give only general pictures of the diseases encountered and detailed statistical analyses cannot be produced.

FEVER was used only as general descriptive term. There was little attempt to divide cases into the categories employed in the army tables. The post-war report states - "Febrile diseases prevailed with various degrees of severity in the respective vessels, although the crews of the larger seem to have suffered most". Epidemics occurred in only a few ships. In H.M.S. 'Hannibal' there were 76 cases of fever from July to September and 65 from October to December. The mortality rates are not stated.

> The disease was of a low type ... the great majority of these [cases] assumed a typhoid form with a characteristic eruption and usual bowel complications: in all cases more or less diarrhoea preceded or accompanied fever. Delirium existed in all cases; sometimes it was furious but more frequently of a low muttering kind ... As the fever was evidently of a typhoid character, if not true typhus, its continuance may safely be ascribed to infection, as evidenced by its attacking the sick attendants in greater numbers than any class of men in the ship.

In H.M.S. 'Royal' 69 cases of fever occurred between April and September. "In some the fever was not severe, but in all there was more or less irritability of the bowels." Clearly there was confusion between bowel diseases and the specific fevers. It remains therefore very uncertain as to the true nature of the fevers reported from these two ships. A total mortality rate for fevers cannot be calculated for 1855.

Turning to BOWEL CONDITIONS, under the general heading of "Stomach and Bowel Diseases", diarrhoea and dysentery were diagnosed quite frequently. Epidemics were rare but H.M.S. 'Tribune' had 110 cases labelled diarrhoea or dysentery between July and September. "The principal feature observable in the dysenteric attacks being a decidedly remittent type, the accessions were as regular and well marked as they are in many forms of that kind of illness (ague)." Again the confusing overlap between fevers and bowel conditions is revealed. In a few warships patients with bowel conditions of some severity were recorded. Most of these had been transferred from the camp of the Naval Brigade. In H.M.S. 'Algiers', out of 85 cases, "nearly all had been sent on board from the camp before Sebastopol ... they were in a wretched state of exhaustion". Of these 85 cases, 8 died (9 per cent), and 15 had to be sent to Therapia to recover. In H.M.S. 'Rodney', H.M.S. 'Albion', and H.M.S. 'Queen', throughout the year 20 men died from dysentery or diarrhoea, mostly contracted while serving ashore. It has been remarked in previous chapters that very few cases of serious bowel disease were reported from the Naval Brigade and that there were few deaths. In fact it is clear that some serious cases did occur, but that the policy of transferring men with early or mild symptoms back to their ships (as recommended by Dundas in November 1854) meant that these cases did not appear in the records of the Naval Division. Nevertheless, neither in the Naval Brigade nor in the warships did bowel conditions ever give rise to the very high admission and mortality rates experienced by the army.

CHOLERA was listed somewhat vaguely under the heading "Stomach (e.g. Cholera)". In consequence it is difficult to assess the true incidence in 1855. All we have is a confusing statement. "Cholera did not acquire epidemic force in any vessel throughout the year. There were only 71 cases entered in the sick returns of the fleet ... but there were 80 deaths. This discrepancy can only be accounted for by cases of diarrhoea terminating in cholera after they had been entered (as diarrhoea) in the sick reports." If there were indeed 80 deaths ascribed to cholera, this would represent at least a 50 per cent death rate, and so the admission rate must have been about 160. One thing is certain, that, compared with the situation during the summer of 1854, cholera was a negligible threat to the strength of the Black Sea Fleet in 1855.

SMALLPOX appears in the post-war report under the heading "Eruptive Fevers (e.g. Small-Pox)". There were at least 68 cases in the Black Sea Fleet in 1855 with three deaths (4 per cent). In H.M.S. 'Curacoa', between November 1855 and January 1856 there were 17 cases. The outbreak was thought to have originated from a soldier who embarked with the disease in England. Although he was sent ashore at Portsmouth, occasional cases appeared until the ship anchored in the Bosphorous. "In every case where the vaccination marks could be observed, the disease was slight and modified, but it was invariably severe where the safeguard had been neglected." More detail is known about an outbreak of smallpox in H.M.S. 'Jean d'Acre'. This ship left Cork crowded with troops. Initially an epidemic was thought to be due to varicella, a less dangerous condition than smallpox, and not until the ship anchored off Sebastopol was smallpox recognised. The surgeon of the ship observed - "The general protective influence of vaccination must be admitted when it is considered that of 870 individuals crowded into a small space only 42 were attacked and two died".

This epidemic in the 'Jean d'Acre' was reported in some detail in the diary of Captain Keppel (then commander of the ship, and later commander of the Naval Brigade). His observations throw considerable light on the management of smallpox on board ship. He does not mention the outbreak until 21 March, 1855, when "a man died from a virulent attack of smallpox". A week later he recorded - "Another case of smallpox. Admiral suggested our getting under weigh, by way of cutting off communication. Thought it advisable to have mids and youngsters vaccinated; having the necessary lymph on board, they were ordered to my cabin. Some seeing doctor's preparations, rather hesitated, on which I requested the surgeon to perform on me first, when all went smoothly." On 3 April, Keppel recorded - "Nineteen cases of smallpox. Took surgeon with me to the Admiral and got permission to land on a small uninhabited island and build huts." Next day Keppel went to Balaclava to get huts from Admiral Boxer (in charge of supplies in the harbour). He was given an order for the huts immediately and had them sent to Kazatch. The same day he wrote - "Returned to Kazatch, selected ground, marked out sites, and had two houses up by sunset. Yellow flags hoisted and regular lazaretto established." On 5 April he noted -

> Thirty-nine cases of smallpox. Hospital establishment creditable to designer. Patients doing well. Landed band in afternoon to cheer them. At suggestion of surgeon, walked through my newly erected hospital, airy and clean. The smallpox room was a trial. Having obtained the names, I endeavoured to say something consoling to each. Their heads were swollen into the shape and appearance of huge plum puddings, eyes closed - their own mothers would not have known them. Prompted by the doctor I was enabled to say something cheery to them and could see by a short movement of their heads that it gave pleasure.[23]

Keppel's account illustrates the close involvement of the commanding officer of a warship in a medical problem, and his personal care for his men. Regimental commanding officers seldom showed the same interest and initiative. For Keppel to acquire the materials for huts, to transport these across the Crimean Peninsula, and to erect them within twenty-four hours was a remarkable achievement. This was done without any need to get permission at a high level, or to get involved with the red tape of officialdom. From five other ships nine sporadic cases of smallpox were reported. There were no deaths in this group.

CHEST DISEASES were frequent in many ships and attributed to climatic conditions or dampness in the sleeping quarters. There were 312 cases of "Inflammatory Infections of the Lungs", with 21 deaths (7 per cent). The exact nature of these conditions is unknown. In addition there were 59 cases of "Phthisis or Haemoptysis", with 32 deaths (54 per cent). This high incidence of what was probably pulmonary tuberculosis was attributed largely to defective ventilation in the ships, a justifiable assumption.

Despite positive efforts to prevent SCURVY, by supplying regular lemon or lime juice and fresh vegetables, the disease appeared in some ships. In H.M.S. 'Hannibal', in February 1855, the surgeon reported that "nearly the whole of the ship's company exhibited symptoms of scurvy ... the gums were swollen, livid or ulcerated, and bled on being slightly rubbed or pressed. In others there were brown spots on the legs, or unhealthy looking ulcers with general debility. By the use of lime-juice, however, a marked improvement took place in the general health." Scurvy appeared also in H.M.S. 'Odin', in December 1855. The supplies of fresh provisions had been limited but lemon-juice had been issued daily. "By a more liberal supply of fresh meat and vegetables, together with oranges for the sick, all the scorbutic symptoms vanished." H.M.S. 'London' had a particularly high incidence of "ulcer". Out of 73 cases, 11 had to be sent to Therapia. Ulcer was most likely often associated with scurvy. A remarkably high incidence of scurvy is surprising in view of the awareness of the naval doctors of the risk of the disease at sea, and the acceptance of the necessity for the use of prophylactic lime or lemon juice. It may be conjectured that some of the supplies of the anti-scorbutic agents were, as in 1854, wrongly prepared, or else that they had deteriorated because of storage at high temperatures.[24]

From the post-war report it is not possible to give exact figures for the incidence of wounds or accidents in 1855. There is uncertainty whether or not in some tables the casualties in the Naval Brigade were included. In the actions of 1855, four men of H.M.S. 'Dauntless' were killed by the bursting of a gun during the bombardment of Sebastopol, in April. Naval casualties were few on the expedition to Kertch in May, and accidental rather than from enemy action. During the bombardments by the mortar-vessels, Cree mentions only one serious wound in action. At the reduction of Kinburn there were few wounded. Many of the accidental deaths were from falls from the rigging, boiler explosions, and drowning. The total of these deaths during the whole war is given in a comparison below of the figures of the Black Sea Fleet and the Baltic Fleet.

MEDICAL STAFFING

The senior medical officer of the Black Sea Fleet was Inspector of the Fleet David Deas who was accommodated in the flag-ship H.M.S. 'Rodney'.[25] Deas conducted medical affairs in the Fleet in a competent manner. Inevitably the success or failure of the naval medical service depended greatly on the more junior doctors, the surgeons and assistant-surgeons, often working in isolation for long periods. The experiences of Edward Cree are typical. After service in the Baltic Fleet in 1854, his ship, H.M.S. 'Odin', was laid up for the winter. He rejoined her in 1855, and the ship anchored off Sebastopol on 28 May. In the following weeks Cree was in a good position to view the activities of the siege and to participate in the attacks made by the mortar-vessels. He went ashore frequently to visit his friends in the Naval Brigade. At the final assault in September he regretted that the 'Odin' was not allowed to take part in the bombardment. He offered to go ashore to assist with the wounded after the attack on the Redan, but his offer was refused. On 10 September Cree went into the smoking ruins of Sebastopol. "What a sight was there, the wounded had all been removed but most of the killed were still lying in heaps: the smell was horrid and the sights heart-rending ... We then came down in the Russian Hospital which although cleared of all the living, exhibited signs of what it had been and smelt - oh, how it smelt." In October H.M.S. 'Odin' sailed on the Kinburn expedition. Once more the ship's company was responsible for the mortar-boats. Cree had to attend to only two wounded marines. He went ashore to inspect the damage and learned that despite the very heavy bombardment the Russian casualties numbered only 45 killed and 187 wounded. On 6 February, H.M.S. 'Odin' returned to the anchorage at Kazatch. Next day Cree wrote in his journal - "I am feeling weak and ill, the old Chinese dysentery has troubled me for the last month or more, so I applied for a medical survey. The result was that I should be sent home by the first opportunity."[26] He went home in the transport 'Andes', to stay in the Navy until 1869, when he retired as a Deputy Inspector-General.

The medical complement of the warships was never up to strength, particularly at assistant-surgeon level. In addition medical officers had to be sent ashore to serve with the Naval Division or the marines in the Crimea. The failure of recruitment was because of the slowness with which the Admiralty dealt with the complaints of the junior doctors. Numerous memorials were forwarded drawing attention to the inadequate accommodation on board ship, to the poor pay and status of the assistant-surgeons as compared with those in the army, and to the recent employment of medical students as dressers in the Baltic Fleet. It was announced in July that most of these complaints had been dealt with appropriately.[27] It was soon noticed however that assistant-surgeons were to have cabins only "whenever the service will admit". For this and similar reasons dissatisfaction persisted in the Fleets until the end of the war.

In the whole campaign only four deaths of naval medical officers are reported. This is a surprisingly low mortality rate considering the hazards of cholera and other infective conditions in the confines of a ship. No naval doctor was killed in action. Surgeon Percy Chapman died in camp in August 1855, while serving with the Naval Brigade.[28] Surgeon John Corbett died of cholera on 1 December, 1855, while serving as Surgeon to H.M.S. 'Jean D'Acre'.[29] Surgeon Edward Derriman died in hospital at Therapia on 5 October, 1855.[30] He had been attached to the Marines at Balaclava. Assistant-Surgeon Terence Wall, serving in H.M.S. 'Leopard', died at Constantinople on 16 December, 1855, and was buried at Scutari.[31]

THE NAVAL HOSPITAL AT THERAPIA

The accommodation which the Navy had acquired early in 1854 for use as a hospital was in a somewhat dilapidated Turkish dwelling or Kiosk, close to the sea on the North shore of the Bosphorous.[32] The building was only three feet above sea level and the drainage system was defective. Originally there were only 40 beds in the main building but later, with the acquisition of an adjacent house, the capacity varied from 100 to 150. The hospital was well equipped and the medical staff gradually increased during 1854. Deputy-Inspector John Davidson[33] was in charge of the hospital, assisted usually by two surgeons and two assistant-surgeons. At different times other doctors who served there included Surgeon John Stewart[34], Surgeon Thomas Bellot[35], and Surgeon William Dalby[36]. At first the nursing was done by 23 naval ratings who were not very skilled. These ratings were eventually returned to their ships and replaced by Maltese who spoke no English, and were reported to be "inefficient and dishonest".[37] In November, 1854, the Admiralty, aware of the success of Miss Nightingale and her nurses at Scutari, decided to send out "tried and approved nurses".[38] As far as is known, the selection of these nurses was done independently of Miss Nightingale and of the Ladies Committee in England. Miss Nightingale probably visited Therapia on at least one occasion, when she was convalescing near the hospital after her illness in the Crimea in the early summer of 1855, but she had no influence on its management.

In the summer of 1854 numerous patients with chronic conditions or the after effects of fever, cholera, or bowel diseases were admitted to the hospital from the Fleet.[39] These patients were rapidly transferred to Malta so that as many beds as possible could be made available for the casualties expected from the siege of Sebastopol. Many wounded were admitted after the participation of the Fleet in the October Bombardment. During November and December 1854 a large number of marines on the heights above Balaclava required admission, "in an exhausted state suffering diarrhoea, dysentery, scurvy, consumption and frost-bite ... mere skeletons, covered with bed sores, and far beyond the reach of human aid".[40] While the sick and wounded from the Fleet were usually taken to Therapia in warships, in relative comfort and without undue delays, the marines and some of the casualties of the Naval Brigade had the misfortune to be carried in the hospital transports at the time when delays in embarkation and disembarkation were frequent and when conditions on board were so appalling. During 1855 the hospital worked at full capacity but was never grossly overcrowded.

The total number of cases admitted to Therapia during the whole of the war is stated to have been 1,775. In the post-war report, under specific categories the total admissions amount to 1,519. If the higher figure is correct the difference of 256 must have been made up of undiagnosed or minor cases. Of the 1,519 cases listed in detail 148 died (10 per cent).

FEVER accounted for 154 admissions, with 27 deaths (18 per cent). The most intractable cases were sent from the Crimea in the early part of 1855: "as many of the patients betrayed a scorbutic taint when admitted, they rapidly sank into a typhoid state, from which only a few were rescued by warmth, mild nutritious diet, and wine judiciously administered".[41] Of the 20 cases of SMALLPOX admitted from H.M.S. 'Albion' in December 1854 and January 1855, three died. The disease did not spread in the hospital. Of a total of 367 cases of diarrhoea and dysentery 58 died (16 per cent), but of the 91 cases treated between October 1854 and March 1855 no fewer than 36 died (40 per cent) - this being the period during which the army death rate from BOWEL DISEASES was high. It is not indicated how many of these severe cases came from the Naval Brigade, but it is likely that a large proportion were sent from the Marine camps at Balaclava, in which the pattern of disease was very similar to that in the army regiments. In addition, seven cases of cholera (included in this general heading) were admitted with six deaths. Turning to OTHER CONDITIONS, of the 72 cases of "Inflammation of the Lungs and Pleura" admitted, nine died (13 per cent); and of 79 cases of "Haemoptysis and Consumption" 19 died (24 per cent). Patients with rheumatism or bone and joint disease accounted for 186 admissions with only one death. Of 150 admissions for skin diseases, including erysipelas, three died (one from abscess and two from erysipelas). Frost-bite accounted for 25 admissions with two deaths. Although 61 cases of scurvy were admitted, in no instance was this given as the primary cause of death. Ulcers which may have been often scorbutic in origin accounted for another 80 admissions (with no deaths). Finally, miscellaneous medical conditions numbered 108 admissions, with four deaths. The largest group under this heading was for venereal disease (57 cases of syphilis and two of gonorrhoea with no deaths).

There were 230 admissions for "WOUNDS and Injuries", with 22 deaths (10 per cent). The total number of these patients wounded in action is not given. Some general reference is made to amputation cases and other wounded admitted in October, presumably from the ships engaged in the bombardment of that month. "In nearly all cases the stumps were in a sloughing state: the wounds, many of which were of a formidable character, particularly those produced by fragments of shell, had an unhealthy appearance."[42] There was apparently an outbreak of "hospital gangrene", but by isolation of the cases a serious spread was prevented.

Up to January 1855 the inadequacy of the male nursing staff caused great problems. Deas wrote - "there is great difficulty in obtaining assistance for the hospital in Therapia - but we drag on somehow".[43] The situation was corrected by the arrival on 9 January of the Reverend John Mackenzie, Mrs. Mackenzie and a small party of ladies and nurses.[44] Mackenzie was a minister of the Established Church of Scotland. Greatly moved by the sufferings of the army he and his wife had offered their help. Herbert was glad to recommend that they should go out to Scutari, but as Miss Nightingale did not want them, they were persuaded by the Admiralty to go to Therapia. Mackenzie acted as an unpaid chaplain to the hospital, offending some by his readiness to take services according to the liturgy of the Church of England (there being no Anglican chaplain). He acted also as a general assistant to his wife, who was in charge of the nursing staff. She was an experienced nurse, having trained at the Middlesex Hospital, and was assisted by three ladies, Miss Vesey, Miss Bartlett, and Miss Erskine, and by three (un-named) professional nurses. Davidson and his medical staff welcomed the nurses on their arrival. Davidson wrote to Burnett - "they render the hospital services much more satisfactory to the medical staff. I already appreciate the good they will do."[45] Mrs. Mackenzie was even made an honorary member of the Officers Mess - something that never happened to Miss Nightingale at Scutari.[46]

However, after a month Davidson seemed a little less enthusiastic, for he wrote to Burnett - "Mrs. Mackenzie and her staff are doing admirable service ... but, Sir, I do not reckon on a continuance of this. The watchful night and sombre day will, I expect, drown ere long a flame which temporary enthusiasm has lighted. The fame which has encircled Miss Nightingale may be stimulus enough to cause her to move on: but will others feel that they have an equal inducement?"[47] Davidson misjudged Mrs. Mackenzie. She ran the hospital with great efficiency, until exhausted by her efforts she had to return home in November 1855. She owed her success to her great skill in dealing with the doctors, "anxious that no offence should be given by tactless comment ... herself imaginative, sensitive and sensible, she entered into the feelings of all concerned and smoothed down ruffled feathers".[48] She managed her nurses extremely well, "keeping such a set of good, respectable women with unrestrained tempers and foolish ideas in order, and concealing their most violent rows from Dr. Davidson, who would think nothing of blowing the whole thing sky high and saying it was a failure!"[49] Mrs. Mackenzie visited Scutari soon after she started work at Therapia, but whether she met Miss Nightingale or not is uncertain. She wrote of her visit -

> I went over for one day to Scutari where I found all in a state of confusion. Miss Nightingale in bed from overwork and Mr. Bracebridge distracted. They have quantities of stores they cannot open for lack of hands. I think nothing can be done. But it is a frightful place to manage, and it would need the Duke of Wellington to cope. This [Therapia], however, is manageable.[50]

Visitors to Therapia were always impressed with its cleanliness and orderly management. Heron Watson, for example, called at the hospital in April 1855.[51] He recorded that the naval medical officers were "infinitely superior" to the army medical officers. Initially the hospital had not been so impressive. A report by the First Commission was highly critical. When Mrs. Mackenzie arrived she wrote - "We are now in the Palace of the Sultans: squalid misery it has been for some days but we are more comfortable now".[52] She found that much had to be done to clean up the hospital and, in particular, to provide an adequate laundry service. But there were no complaints about the kitchens or the supply system. When the war ended there were many tributes to Mrs. Mackenzie and her staff.

> They shrunk from no kind of employment, however dangerous or laborious, nor was there any office connected with the sick which they deemed to be low or debasing ... Mrs. Mackenzie's health at last gave way and she was compelled to return to England in November: but Miss Erskine and Miss Vesey remained behind until the termination of the war happily brought their labours to a close ... but their memories will live long in the grateful remembrance of the officers, seamen, and marines who fought before Sebastopol.[53]

No member of the nursing staff died at Therapia but in February Miss Erskine had an attack of smallpox and Miss Bartlett and two of the professional nurses "had taken the fever of the country". But all recovered and were able to return to duty.

Mrs. Mackenzie had been aware that when the Admiralty sent her to Therapia there was the intention "to make female nursing general throughout their hospitals if it is successful in Therapia".[54] Despite the undoubted success of Mrs. Mackenzie this idea was dropped after the war. Not until 1885 was a naval nursing service firmly established by the appointment of "a limited number of trained sisters of the position of gentlewomen under the superintendence, in each hospital, of a Head Sister".[55]

In conclusion, this relatively small hospital at Therapia can scarcely be compared with the large, overcrowded establishments at Scutari. The difficulties encountered by Mrs. Mackenzie in establishing her small nursing staff cannot be compared with Miss Nightingale's continual problems. Nevertheless it does appear from the statistics available and from many eye-witness accounts that Therapia was conducted with a high degree of efficiency and that the clinical results compared favourably with those in the army hospitals. It does seem that the medical officers were remarkably independent and were not subjected to excessive control by executive staff.

THE TOTAL NAVAL CASUALTIES (1854-1855)

In the post-war report there are tables giving the total number of deaths for the whole war for each disease or group of diseases.[56] Unfortunately there are no precise figures of the incidence of each disease. It is not possible therefore to give exact total mortality rates, nor to compare naval and military statistics. Much of this difficulty arises from the fact that the Navy reported the number of men off duty from sickness, while the army reported admissions to hospital for each disease. Some off-duty seamen were treated as out-patients and slept in their own quarters, some were admitted for treatment in the sick bay, some were eventually discharged fit for duty, some transferred to a hospital ship or base hospital, and some died. It was stated that the total number of deaths in the two fleets over the whole war was 2,029, and of these 1,574 died from disease, 228 from accidental injuries or drowning, and 227 from wounds in action. The deaths occurring in the Black Sea Fleet included those of the Naval Brigade and the marines in the Crimea. The total complement of the Baltic Fleet exceeded that of the Black Sea Fleet throughout the war but the incidence of serious disease in the latter was greater than in the Baltic Fleet. It is possible to indicate significant differences in the mortality rates of the two fleets and give some reasons for these differences.

"Fevers" accounted for 39 deaths in the Baltic Fleet and 133 in the Black Sea Fleet. Exact figures of the incidence of fevers are not available but it would seem that the mortality rate was much higher in the Black Sea Fleet. This is most probably accounted for by a combination of several factors: endemic fevers, often of serious types, were common on the shores of the Black Sea, the ships were often anchored near shore, and the men frequently landed for various purposes. In the Baltic there were fewer endemic fevers and the men less often went ashore. Moreover, there was greater hardship in the Black Sea Fleet than in the Baltic Fleet, with occasional shortages of essential items of diet such as fresh vegetables and fresh meat. The Baltic Fleet operated nearer the home bases and supplies arrived more regularly. This factor influenced the frequency of many diseases other than the fevers. "Eruptive fevers" accounted for 23 deaths in the Baltic Fleet and 6 in the Black Sea Fleet, most of these deaths being from smallpox. It has been noted that outbreaks of smallpox in a few ships were due mainly to infection from individuals who brought the disease on board in England, while most of the ships in the Black Sea were already stationed abroad when the war began.

"Diseases of the Respiratory Organs" accounted for 124 deaths in the Baltic Fleet and 93 in the Black Sea Fleet. The number of deaths from pulmonary tuberculosis was thought to be greater in the Baltic Fleet, and it was suggested that a higher rate of chest disease of one kind or another was due to the poor quality of the recruits, particularly in 1854, who were sickly, poorly clothed, and careless in their habits. It could be that the medical examination before entry to the navy was less stringent than in the army and that as a result men with pulmonary tuberculosis were overlooked, men who, in the adverse conditions of damp and crowding, not only themselves deteriorated rapidly but also infected others. "Diseases of the Stomach and Bowels" accounted for 127 deaths in the Baltic Fleet and 734 in the Black Sea Fleet. The higher figure in the latter is in the first instance accounted for by the fact that diarrhoea or dysentery of a serious type was rare in the Baltic Fleet. But secondly, and more importantly, cholera was included under "Diseases of the Stomach and Bowels". The deaths from cholera in the Black Sea Fleet in the summer of 1854 alone numbered 411. In the whole war there were only 103 deaths from cholera in the Baltic fleet but 522 deaths in the Black Sea Fleet. "Diseases of the Brain", "Diseases of the Heart and Blood vessels", "Diseases of the Liver", "Diseases of the Kidneys", "Diseases of the Skin and Cellular Tissue", "Rheumatism" and some unspecified conditions were the cause of very few deaths, with little difference between the two Fleets. The total incidence of these conditions is uncertain.

"Wounds and accidents" accounted for 139 deaths in the Baltic Fleet and 316 in the Black Sea Fleet. Of this total of 455, 228 were from accidental injuries, and 227 from wounds in action. The wounds in action were more frequent in the Black Sea Fleet because of the inclusion of deaths of men in the Naval Division. In a discussion at the end of the post-war report it was agreed that the mortality from wounds in action could not have been lessened, except by curbing the tendency of the sailor to expose himself unnecessarily to risk.

The report further argued that diseases arising from deficiencies in food, clothing and shelter (such as scurvy, fever, dysentery and diarrhoea) could not have been lessened, "for during the whole period of the war the fleets were well supplied with good wholesome food and suitable clothing - and as for shelter it was such as has always been found to be sufficient for British seamen, namely the decks of their respective ships". This was rather an optimistic statement for although adequate clothing was always available in the ships, supplies of fresh meat and vegetables were sometimes erratic, and the conditions on board ship, such as dampness and poor ventilation, were undoubtedly factors in favouring disease. It was agreed that the sickness rates, for example from cholera, would have been much less if the Fleet had not been required to anchor off Varna in 1854. But tactical plans demanded that such risks should be taken (if indeed the risks were foreseen).

The report's summing-up shows a degree of self-satisfaction. Nevertheless the naval health record, even allowing for the fact that as compared with the army the background conditions were always easier, suggests that the Naval Medical Service came out of the war rather better than the Army Medical Service. "Fortunate was the service which escaped such a critic!"[57] (The critic designated was, of course, Florence Nightingale.) Fortunate was the service which escaped the censures of the press (except with regard to the shortage of junior doctors). Fortunate too was the service which did not have inflicted upon it innumerable Commissions of Enquiry, during or after the war.

NOTES

1. For the background to this section, see D. Bonner-Smith, ed., **Russian War, 1855, Baltic** (Navy Records Society, London, 1944), 3-15.
2. **The Times**, 8.12.1854.
3. These figures are derived from **Medical Statistical Returns of the Baltic and Black Sea Fleets during the years 1854 and 1855. Parliamentary Report.** Page references are not given as information is scattered in an erratic fashion through the report. The statistics given in the report are only approximations, but some additional information from medical journals has been used.
4. **M.T.G.** (1855), 1:559.
5. Ibid., 1:636.
6. M.D.; surgeon 1842.
7. M.D.; surgeon 1852.
8. **Lancet** (1856), 1:207-208.
9. Ibid., (1854), 1:652.
10. **M.T.G.** (1855), 1:214.
11. **Lancet** (1855), 1:273-274.
12. **Ass.Med.J.** (1855), 265. The pay was not ungenerous for a medical student. In 1934, as a medical student ranked as Surgeon Sub-lieutenant R.N.V.R., I was paid seven shillings a day when on training!
13. **M.T.G.** (1855), 1:214.
14. Ibid., 1:298-301.
15. Ibid., 2:49.
16. Christopher Heath (1835-1905); M.R.C.S. 1856; F.R.C.S. 1860; P.R.C.S. 1895 (obituary **B.M.J.** (1905), 2:359-360; **Plarr**; W.R. Merrington, **University College Hospital and its medical school. A history** (London, 1976), 75-80). Heath returned to complete his studies and qualified in 1856. He became Assistant Surgeon in the Westminster Hospital in 1862, but in 1866 transferred to University College Hospital, where he became Professor of Clinical Surgery in 1876. He made a considerable reputation as a surgeon and teacher and published numerous text-books. His long attachment to the Royal College of Surgeon culminated in the Presidency from 1895-1896, succeeding another Crimean veteran, John Hulke.

17. William Swain (1834-1916); M.R.C.S. 1857; L.S.A. 1858; F.R.C.S. 1867 (obituary **B.M.J.** (1916), 2:859; **Plarr**). He returned to complete his studies, qualifying in 1857. He eventually settled in Plymouth, where he played an active part in issues of public health.
18. Robert Lewer (1835-1914) joined army as assistant-surgeon 1857 after his naval service; retired as S.M.G. in 1895 (obituary **Lancet** (1914), 1:1639; **Drew**).
19. For the background to this section, see A.C. Dewar, ed., **Russian War, 1855, Black Sea** (Navy Records Society, London, 1945), 3-24.
20. M. Levien, ed., **The Cree Journals** (Exeter, 1981), 257 (and illustrations of mortar-vessels).
21. Ibid., 262-265; P. Warner, **The Crimean War: a reappraisal** (Newton Abbot, 1972), 146-149.
22. See note 3 above.
23. H. Keppel, **A sailor's life** (London, 1899), 2:259-262.
24. See **M.T.G.** (1854), 2:635-636, for letters between Burnett and the Board of Trade concerning the preparation of lime juice.
25. For biographical information on Deas, see Chapter XIX.
26. Levien, **Journals**, 247-267.
27. **M.T.G.** (1856), 1:586.
28. For Chapman, see note 116 to Chapter XIII.
29. John Corbett; M.D.; promoted surgeon 1845 (**Ass.Med.J.** (1855), 1153; **Med. Directory** (1856)).
30. Edward Derriman (1817-1855), L.R.C.P., M.D.; promoted surgeon 1846 (obituary **M.T.G.** (1855), 2:432).
31. Terence Wall, qualified Edinburgh 1850; assistant-surgeon 1853.
32. M.E. Penney, 'Letters from Therapia 1855', **Blackwood's Magazine** (May, 1954), 413-422. This article contains a wealth of information concerning conditions at Therapia in general and the nursing service in particular. The letters quoted are mainly from either the Rev. John Mackenzie or Mrs. Mackenzie.
33. John Davidson; M.D., D.I. 1855.
34. This may have been the same man as John Stuart; surgeon 1852.
35. Thomas Bellot (d. 1857); M.R.C.S. 1828; joined as assistant-surgeon 1837; surgeon 1842; F.R.C.S. 1846 (obituary in **Med. Directory** (1857); **Plarr**). Bellot was an erudite writer on classical, oriental and related subjects.
36. William Dalby; surgeon 1854.
37. Penney, 'Letters', 415.
38. Ibid.
39. **Parl. Report.** (see note 3 above), 45-49, "Therapia".
40. Ibid., 47.
41. Ibid., 48.
42. Ibid., 49.
43. Penney, 'Letters', 415.
44. Ibid., 415-416.
45. Ibid., 417.
46. **Parl. Report**, 47.
47. Penney, 'Letters', 418.
48. Ibid., 420.
49. Ibid.
50. Ibid., 417.
51. 'Heron Watson Letters'.
52. Letter of 23.2.1855, in possession of Mrs. M.E. Penney, a descendant of Mrs. Mackenzie.
53. **Parl. Report**, 48.
54. Penney, 'Letters', 416.
55. **Keevil**, 4:67.
56. See note 3 above.
57. **Keevil**, 4:153.

CHAPTER XVI

THE TURKISH CONTINGENT

As early as July 1854, it was announced that a British Medical Staff for the Turkish army would be formed, and that applications were invited.[1] Already at least one doctor was giving assistance unofficially to the Turks in Bulgaria. This was Humphry Sandwith,[2] who had practised in Constantinople for a few years, and had published a useful account of the climate and diseases of Turkey.[3] Around July he was appointed "Staff Surgeon to the Turkish Force in Bulgaria", this force being under the command of a British officer, General Beatson.[4] It is not certain that Sandwith was ever officially in the Turkish Contingent but he had close contact with its officers.

The selection of doctors for what came to be known as the 'Turkish Contingent' was made by Inspector-General Duncan MacPherson[5], a senior medical officer of the Indian Medical Service on leave in England, who was put in command of the Contingent. The Army Medical Director-General approved the appointments. MacPherson did not go out to the East until late in 1855 and John Fuller[6], who had formerly been in the Indian Medical Service, was put in charge of the first draft. In the medical press the appointments were criticised. "Fuller was placed in a half-dependent and very anomalous position ... Against Dr. Fuller himself, as against Dr. Meyer, we believe there is nothing to be urged, but the appointments have been made under the old and in some respects objectionable system of private patronage."[7]

In May MacPherson started a recruiting drive in the London and provincial medical schools. He offered to take into immediate service surgeons, assistant-surgeons, and dressers (rated acting assistant-surgeons), at army rates of pay. The surgeons had to be experienced men over 30 years of age, the assistant-surgeons newly qualified, and the dressers in their second or third year of clinical study as students. MacPherson referred to "the liberal terms offered by the government", and he pointed out "the vast opportunities young men accepting would have of acquiring a practical knowledge of their profession, and the éclat that would be attached to their names during the rest of their careers".[8] It was reported that the response to this appeal was favourable. At the time the number of doctors in the Indian Medical Service was considerable and an attempt was made to induce any who happened to be on home leave at the time to be seconded for attachment to the Turkish Contingent.[9] It was thought that their experience of tropical diseases would be useful. Not very many were attracted by the rates of pay offered, but those who did volunteer were given senior posts. In 1854 and early in 1855, some regular army doctors, already in the Crimea, were loaned for short periods to the Turkish Army, but prolonged secondments were unusual.

Some doctors who joined the Turkish Contingent have been identified with reasonable certainty. Of these 44 were civilian doctors, ten were seconded from the I.M.S., and five were army medical officers detached from regimental or other duties. It is possible that the total may have exceeded 60. The first draft arrived in Turkey in March 1855. Fuller was in charge of some twelve surgeons, an uncertain number of assistant-surgeons, and a few dressers. Only 14 of this party were named in a report published in the **Lancet**.[10] Alexander Farquhar[11] served as deputy to Fuller, while Drs. Bird, Cubitt, Foote, Jenkins, Philips and Pont were sent initially to the Turkish Hospitals in Varna but later must have moved to Turkey.[12] Thomas Buzzard[13], Frederick Le Mesurier[14], Ray Millard[15], Laurence Ormerod[16], John Radcliffe[17], and one Edwards[18] were all attached initially to Omar Pasha's Army in the Crimea. Millard and Ormerod both died of cholera in the summer. Fuller remained in the East for only four weeks and was then invalided home.

The next list of doctors did not appear in the medical journals until November 1855.[19] This included one surgeon, six assistant-surgeons, and ten acting assistant-surgeons labelled "gents" (it may be assumed that these were dressers). Smaller reinforcements must have been sent out before and after November 1855.[20] From the second published list and from various other sources additional names have been traced, as follows: Walter Acton[21], Robert Boxall[22], James Brown[23],

Brudenell Carter[24], William Cattle[25], Archibald Cockburn[26], James Cowper[27], A. Czadkay[28], John Dee[29], John Elkington[30], Alexander Irvine[31], Archibald Irvine[32], James Keeling[33], Edmund Larkin[34], William MacFie[35], R. Richardson[36], Andrew Risk[37], Habib Riskillah[38], William Tate[39], W. Temple[40], Ernest Wigan[41], William Wolseley[42], Christopher Wolsten[43], George Yates[44], and four names, Dingan[45], Edsall[46], McAuley[47], and Turner[48]. Of these doctors Boxall, Edsall and McAuley died from disease on service.

A list of 25 officers of the Indian Medical Service who served in the Crimean War exists but includes service doctors who joined the I.M.S. after the war.[49] The following ten medical officers of the I.M.S. were however seconded to the Turkish Contingent, Major Ainger[50], Alexander Boggs[51], Edward Campbell[52], William Harris[53], James MacAlister[54], William McEgan[55], John MacGregor[56], Duncan MacPherson[57], James Vaughan[58], and St. George Williams.[59] None of them died during service with the Turkish Contingent. Five army medical officers have been traced as having been seconded to the Turkish contingent and it is likely that others were attached for short periods. An official list of these secondments has not been traced. The five were Richard Banbury[60], Thomas Beale[61], Cameron McDowall[62], Ferdinand Odevaine[63], and George Sutherland.[64] From the list of appointments to the Turkish Contingent in November 1855 we learn the surnames of five doctors who had been replaced - Patteson, Lewins, Littleton, Risk, and Willet. Patteson and Willet cannot be traced. Risk has already been listed as one of the civilian doctors of the Turkish Contingent. Lewins may have been Robert Lewins[65], an army medical officer, and Littleton may have been Thomas Littleton[66], a naval medical officer (but as their attachment has not been proved conclusively, they have not been counted in the total of doctors serving in the Contingent).

The number of dressers attached to the Turkish Contingent and given the rank of acting assistant-surgeon is uncertain. The names of 13 have been found. Eight are from the list of appointments in November 1855: John Carlaw, Hugh Clark, T.W. Hamilton, Patrick

Hutcheon, Cavalié Mercer, Robert Sim, Robert Stirling and William Tindall.[67] Two are mentioned in Buzzard's memoir, Charles Balding and Skinner.[68] Two are recorded on a memorial at Scutari, Sibbald and Coates (both died on service).[69] Robinson Boustead is traced from the I.M.S. list. Of these dressers only Balding[70], Boustead[71], Carlaw[72], and Mercer[73] have been found in the directories as having subsequently qualified in medicine. It is known that at least another ten dressers went out with the first party in March 1855 and it is likely that the total reached between 30 and 35. It may be assumed that these dressers had a much more difficult time than the group attached to the Scutari Hospitals. Two died and most likely several were invalided. No personal reminiscences written by the dressers have been found. The small number who have been proved to have qualified might suggest that they were discouraged by their experience from continuing their medical studies.

THE TURKISH MILITARY HOSPITALS

Most of the doctors in the Contingent served in the Turkish Military Hospitals, where the conditions were often primitive. The Turkish Medical Service was poorly trained, ill-equipped and understaffed. From the beginning of the campaign in Bulgaria it had been unable to cope with the large numbers of sick and wounded. The strength of the Turkish Army had originally been 140,000 but by the time the British doctors arrived it was reduced to 80,000. The exact mortality rates in Bulgaria are unknown.

A newspaper correspondent reporting the arrival of the Turkish Contingent described the state of the sick and wounded.

> One third have been carried off by diseases that under the circumstances no known means could arrest: the rest have been killed by the doctors, who with the aid of the pashas turned the hospitals into slaughter houses. The doctors are, with half a dozen exceptions, Italians, usually refugees ... the vast majority were impudent mountebanks, runaway bankrupts and blacklegs, escaped criminals, expelled students, forgers, coiners and what not: very few knew anything about medicine or surgery more than their patients ... Any European officer in the Turkish Service will tell you at once that if sick or wounded, he would as soon blow his brains out at once as of committing himself to the hands of a regimental surgeon ... To show you the estimate in which the authorities hold their doctors, I may mention

an incident ... several of the latter went as a deputation to Bay Pasha to ask for a payment of their salaries which were long in arrears. He instantly ordered each of them to receive fifty blows of the stick, and the sentence was executed on the spot.[74]

In August 1855 an anonymous member of the Turkish Contingent had this to say.

> The present hospitals, I believe, are conducted on the same model as the Norfolk County Hospital for the Insane, in England, and have their condition much in the same state. An ignorant man, who has risen to a certain status from subserviency in the menial offices he has filled to some of the authorities, has what is called the management: he purchases the food, selects the attendants, bullies the Medical Officers ... Indeed his object is to obtain as large a profit for himself by the various means he can employ ... As this steward supplies the Medical Officers with their rations of course if they fall in with the system they are rewarded: if not he makes it very unpleasant for them and puts them to all kinds of inconvenience, but as they are generally men of the same spirit and feeling as himself, things go smoothly - they smoke their chibouques and drink their coffee, and if the patients die, it is God's will, and they must be buried. Of course few recover ... In the Turkish Army the Medical Officers, with few exceptions, have been hitherto the most ignorant you can possibly imagine, for in Turkey the Profession is scarcely at all studied by the Turks: and as sufficient inducement is not given to educated Europeans, the state of treatment is vile in the extreme.[75]

Such reports indicate the chaotic conditions with which the British doctors had to cope. The Turkish Government had asked for medical assistance, but the cooperation between the existing medical service and the Turkish Contingent was never to prove very satisfactory. As the British doctors arrived they were split up into small parties to be sent to Bulgaria, the Crimea, and Eupatoria. In each area there were large Turkish armies. The first party which arrived in April 1855 went initially to Bulgaria and took charge of two hospitals in Varna. In four months 3,000 patients were admitted suffering from "diarrhoea, dysentery, fever, scurvy etc".[76] The British doctors had to work very hard and the climate took a considerable toll of them, for three had to be invalided.

Of those sent to the Crimea, some acted as regimental medical officers in the front line and others were employed in the hospitals. The main Turkish General Hospital was on the heights of Balaclava and was described fully by Radcliffe. It was a collection of 24 small huts supplied by the British Army, each hut holding 14 patients. Radcliffe thought the hospital remarkably clean, considering the environment. But the

Turkish soldiers were filthy in their habits and their tattered uniforms were invariably infested. The latrines adjacent to the hospital, situated between the kitchens and the slaughter house, were always in an appalling state. The water supply was grossly contaminated and the stench in the area was aggravated by the close proximity of a burial ground in which internments were superficial. The British doctors seemed to have created reasonable conditions within the hospital huts but they could do little about the environmental hazards. According to Radcliffe, the British doctors in this hospital dealt mainly with surgical rather than medical cases.[77]

In Eupatoria a large Turkish army was stationed to threaten the Russian line of supplies to Sebastopol. The hospitals were primitive and probably tented. In addition a Turkish hospital of 500 beds was established at Sinope and staffed partly by the Turkish Contingent. There were numerous Turkish hospitals in Constantinople, but the British doctors were not employed in these.

The experiences of the British doctors attached to the Turkish Army can be culled from several sources, of which the memoir written by Buzzard is of particular interest.[78] Although published many years after the War this is apparently an accurate account, and from it the movements of many medical officers in the Turkish Contingent can be traced. Buzzard left London on 24 March, 1855. He disembarked at Constantinople and was attached briefly to the Barrack Hospital on 9 April. Having purchased a horse he sailed for Balaclava in company with Le Mesurier. He spent some weeks visiting various camps and caught up with many friends who entertained him in their huts or tents. He went up to the front line on several occasions but at first had no official duties. Later with Le Mesurier he was posted to a Turkish camp near Balaclava. He took part in the expedition to Kertch in May but had little medical or surgical work to do. In September he was up at the front during the final assault on Sebastopol. Buzzard was much more fully employed when he was sent to Trebizond in Asia Minor, in October, to take charge of a large Turkish hospital of 1,500 beds. Between October

1855 and April 1856 thousands of sick and wounded were treated. Buzzard received great praise for his work, dealing in particular with severe outbreaks of dysentery and cholera. His colleague Edsall died but Buzzard escaped serious illness. He knew of Snow's views on cholera and "survived by not drinking water." He finally left Trebizond in June 1856 and returned home. His account is full of details unrecorded elsewhere. He describes how the Turkish Contingent were rather lax about their uniforms. He himself wore a tweed jacket, blue trousers with a red stripe, and a fez. Altogether he greatly enjoyed his experiences. His personal contribution was considerable and recognised by Omar Pasha with the award of a high decoration. Buzzard's experiences were probably fairly typical, with periods of inactivity punctuated by spells of exhausting work.

Another individual who gave a personal account of the work of the Turkish Contingent was Sandwith. In his narrative of the Siege of Kars there is much information concerning the Turkish hospitals and the medical problems encountered. Sandwith moved from Trebizond to the besieged town of Kars, having been appointed by General Williams to the hospitals in Kars as Inspector-General (a local appointment and not related to the Turkish Contingent). The number of hospitals must have been considerable as Sandwith had under him 50 surgeons, physicians and apothecaries, "ignorant practitioners, surgeons ignorant barbers, preferring to bleed, draw teeth and dress wounds". The medical stores were adequate but there was no ambulance service. The Pashas were corrupt, but with the help of General Williams, Sandwith was able to rectify conditions remarkably. He succeeded in controlling the spread of typhus and "no hospital gangrene broke out in the hospitals". In October cholera struck and there were 2,000 cases, the men dying at the rate of 100 a day. The siege of Kars had dragged on from June to November 1855. Relief had been expected but the half-starved garrison had to capitulate on 25 November. Most officers were made prisoner but Sandwith managed to escape, making his way to Constantinople by a long and perilous journey on foot. Sandwith had been joined at Kars by some of the medical staff of the Turkish Contingent but

CHAPTER XVI

mentions only two by name, Williams and Teasdale. Williams may have been St. George Williams, described above in the I.M.S. list. Teasdale has not been traced but may have been a dresser.[79]

From sporadic accounts which appeared in the contemporary medical press we obtain other details of the Turkish Contingent. Some accounts are anonymous. For example 'V' contributed this in July, 1855.

> A considerable number of medical gentlemen were engaged in a very short space of time, the choice, as experience is now proving, was in almost every instance very fortunate. Some of the juniors had but lately passed, and had to begin the toils of an active life, with the cares and anxieties attendant on professional avocation in a large camp, where disease, if not quickly stopped, and assiduously attended to, runs through the various stages in an incredibly short space of time ... they have shown themselves to be a body of gentlemen emulated by high and honourable feelings, a credit to the noble profession to which they belong ... they have shown themselves equal to the present emergency, and have been well tried in the commencement of their duties in the Indian sun, and, as a matter of course, not the most comfortable accommodation or covering ... it is to be hoped that our Government will not as in the case heretofore, overlook and poohpooh the claims of medical officers for rewards which they have deserved; but not having telling interest in high places, they are generally overlooked and forgotten.[80]

All reports emphasise the difficult conditions in which the doctors of the Turkish Contingent had to work. Some at once took over highly responsible duties in command of large hospitals and despite the lethargy and peculation of the Turks succeeded in effecting rapid improvements and bringing to the sick and wounded degrees of comfort and skill which had previously been completely unknown to them. There is little evidence that the Director-General or Hall took much notice of the work of the Turkish Contingent. "Chirurgicus" writing in January 1856 emphasised this isolation.

> As numerous articles have appeared in the periodicals of the day reflecting or attempting to reflect discredit on the Medical Staff of the Turkish Contingent, and the scale and working adopted by the heads of that department, and it is a matter of little doubt that these animadversions have emanated from the pen of officers of Her Majesty's army it is but fair that the following instance of timely aid, afforded by one of the medical staff of the Turkish Contingent, to an English soldier, be recorded to prove at least that our staff has been consulted with advantage, and that in all respects the Contingent can boast of as well-educated, disciplined, and sufficiently supplied a body of men as the now much improved regular staff of Her Majesty's Army.

The case mentioned was that of a regular soldier who had been seriously ill but was cured by the intervention of a medical officer of the Turkish Contingent. The letter claims, probably justly, that the military authorities at home and abroad took little interest in the Turkish Contingent. The writer went on to state -
> The stores of the Turkish Contingent are freely supplied to the [British] troops: our blankets, our medicines, our instruments are at their service, and lastly our professional aid is freely given ... Despite the difficulties of having nothing but Turkish orderlies, and the immediate increase in labour for the medical men of this force, the hospitals of the Contingent are superior in neatness, warmth, and comfort, to any in the Crimea.[81]

It does seem that after he came out in November 1855 MacPherson proved an able commanding officer. "Dr. MacPherson, on his arrival, pitched his tent with them, associated with the men, explained to them that he had been in the last twenty years with Mohammedans in the Nizan's army: that Her Majesty's Government had sent him out to take care of them and that he would treat them as his own sons. He speedily won their confidence, and he got his staff, who have proved first rate men, into a system equal to that of any other officers of Her Majesty's army, and their patients are always sending them gifts."[82] The small group of I.M.S. officers must have been a great help to the junior civilian doctors who had just qualified and found it difficult to adapt to strange surroundings and to deal with the Turkish soldiers. If the work of the Turkish Contingent was not appreciated by the regular army doctors or by the authorities at home, at least the Turks were grateful, and their commander, Omar Pasha, expressed his gratitude for their assistance publicly and awarded decorations to many individual doctors.

In February 1856 the Turkish Contingent began to be withdrawn. A dinner was given at Kertch in honour of the Inspector-General. "The health of Dr. MacPherson was given and received very enthusiastically. That gentleman acknowledged the compliment in appropriate terms and referring to the cordiality which had prevailed between the Army and the Turkish people, said that the contacts would do much to bring about a social regeneration."[83] At times relations between the Turks on the one hand and their British and French allies on the other had been strained. By their service to the Turkish soldiers the doctors of the Contingent did much to smooth over such difficulties. However, some of the doctors became disillusioned, as shown by a memorial sent to the Secretary of State for War in August 1855.[84] They complained that they had not received the allowances promised and that their salaries were lower than those of the civilian doctors attached to the base hospitals.[85] A few may have resigned over these grievances, and indeed before the end of 1855 there were rumours that the whole contingent was to return to England.

Five qualified civilian doctors, Boxall, Edsall, McCauley, Millard and Ormerod, are known to have died of disease while serving with the Turkish Contingent (about 10 per cent of those serving). At least two dressers, Coates and Sibbald, are known to have died in service. The number of deaths indicates the high risks this group faced during service. No I.M.S. medical officer or army officer on secondment appears to have died. From the whole Contingent an uncertain number of doctors were invalided, but probably in the region of 15.

The Turkish Contingent was never given a good press. In June 1856 **The Times** described it as a "hopeless mission."[86] There is no mention of it in the official medical history of the war, nor in subsequent accounts. The Royal Commission did not discuss its activities or its value. Belatedly it seems appropriate to pay some tribute to the doctors of the Contingent who, in the face of great difficulties, and at considerable risk to their lives, brought to the Turks a great improvement in medical care. If to some extent the services of the Turkish Contingent were offered initially as a diplomatic gesture, it is clear that in many ways this was to prove an humanitarian exercise, and hence one deserving considerable credit.

NOTES

Fuller biographical notes on a number of the medical officers serving in the Turkish Contingent are to be found in Appendix II.

1. **M.T.G.** (1854), 2:75.
2. Humphry Sandwith (1822-1881); M.D. (? of London), F.R.C.P. 1859 (obituary **B.M.J.** (1881), 1:868; T.H. Ward, **Humphry Sandwith: Memoir** (London, 1884); **Munk; DNB**). Surprisingly Sandwith's name does not appear in Directories. Another Humphry Sandwith, M.D. St. Andrews 1832, listed erroneously as F.R.C.P., was probably the younger Sandwith's father.
3. H. Sandwith, 'A brief sketch of the diseases of Northern Turkey', **Ass.Med.J.** (1854), 434-436.
4. **Lancet** (1854), 2:115.
5. Duncan MacPherson (1812-1867); M.D. Edinburgh (obituary **Lancet** (1867), 2:56-57 (**Crawford**).
6. John Fuller (b. 1809) (**Crawford**).
7. **M.T.G.** (1855), 1:287.
8. **M.T.G.** (1855), 1:469-470.
9. The term Indian Medical Service (I.M.S.) is used as this was common practice by 1854, although officially the East India Company Medical Service did not change its title until 1896.
10. **Lancet** (1855), 2:157.
11. Alexander Farquhar (d. 1890); L.S.A. 1833; M.R.C.S. 1838; F.R.C.S. 1856 (**Plarr**).
12. The names of these six doctors are known from the **Lancet** list. No other details such as ranks and qualifications have been traced.
13. Thomas Buzzard (1851-1919); M.R.C.S. 1855; M.B. London 1857; M.D. London 1860; F.R.C.P. 1878 (obituary **B.M.J.** (1919), 1:59-60; H.W. Lyle, **Kings and Kings' Men** (Oxford, 1935), 76-77; **Munk**).
14. Frederick Le Mesurier (b. 1813); M.R.C.S., L.S.A. 1835 (**Crawford**).
15. Ray Millard (d.1855); M.R.C.S., L.S.A. 1854 (**M.T.G.** (1855), 2:851).
16. Laurence Ormerod (d. 1855); **M.T.G.** (1855), 2:50.
17. John Radcliffe (1830-1864); M.R.C.S. 1853 (obituary **B.M.J.** (1884), 2:588).
18. Edwards listed in the **Lancet** and **M.T.G.** (1856), 1:25.
19. **Ass.Med.J.** (1855), 1021.
20. No complete official list has been found. Some names have been traced by chance discovery in the medical directories or journals. The amount of information on each doctor therefore varies.
21. Walter Acton (1826-1911); M.R.C.S., L.S.A. 1850 (obituary **B.M.J.** (1914), 2:348).
22. Robert Boxall (1831-1855); buried at Yenikale (**M.T.G.** (1855), 2:653).
23. James Brown (d. 1861); M.R.C.S. 1845; M.D. St. Andrews 1849.
24. Brudenell Carter (1828-1918); M.R.C.S. 1851; L.S.A. 1852; F.R.C.S. 1864 (obituary **B.M.J.** (1918), 1:502-503; **Plarr**).
25. William Cattle (1832-1872); M.R.C.S. 1855; L.S.A. 1856.
26. Archibald Cockburn (d. 1862); F.R.C.S.Ed. 1838; M.D. St. Andrews 1842. For Cockburn's doubtful character, see letter from Dr. Tyler Smith (**Ass.Med.J.** (1855), 1136-1137.
27. James Cowper (1826-1866); L.R.C.S.Ed., M.D. Edinburgh 1851 (J. Kinnear, 'Dundee doctors in war time', **J.R.A.M.C.**, 100 (1954), 141-146.
28. Czadkay was named in the **Ass.Med.J.** list.
29. John Dee; M.R.C.S. 1855.
30. John Elkington; M.R.C.S. L.S.A., 1855.
31. Alexander Irvine (d. 1899); M.R.C.S. 1831.
32. Archibald Irvine (d. 1903) L.R.C.S.Ed., M.D. Aberdeen 1849.

33. James Keeling (1832-1909); M.D. Edinburgh; M.R.C.S., L.S.A. 1852; F.R.C.S. 1869 (obituary **B.M.J.** (1909), 1:761; **Plarr**). See an amusing sidelight on Keeling in E. Finch, 'The song of the squirt', **Med.Hist.**, 4 (1960), 59-64.
34. Edmund Larkin (1834-18?); M.R.C.S. 1855 (**Crawford**).
35. William MacFie (d. 1859); M.D. Edinburgh 1854.
36. Richardson listed in **Ass.Med.J.** (1855), 1021.
37. Andrew Risk (d. 1862); M.D. Glasgow 1851; joined as assistant-surgeon 1854; resigned September 1854 (**Drew**).
38. Riskillah listed in **M.T.G.** (1855), 1:287.
39. William Tate (d. 1913); M.R.C.S. 1849; M.D. Aberdeen 1854; L.S.A. 1858.
40. Listed in **Ass.Med.J.** (1855), 1021, as W.F.H. Temple, but not traced elsewhere.
41. Ernest Wigan listed in **Ass.Med.J.** (1855), 1021.
42. William Wolseley (d. 1859); M.D. Edinburgh 1843.
43. Christopher Wolsten (d. 1886); M.R.C.S. 1855; M.D. St. Andrews 1875.
44. George Yates; L.S.A. 1852.
45. Dingan was named in T. Buzzard, **With the Turkish Army in the Crimea and Asia Minor** (London, 1915).
46. Edsall named in Buzzard, **Crimea**.
47. Memorial to McAuley (d. 1855) noted in J.F. Burke, 'The medical Crimean graves at Scutari', **J.R.A.M.C.**, 41 (1923), 63-68.
48. Turner named in Buzzard, **Crimea**.
49. D.G. Crawford, **A history of the Indian Medical Service** (London, 1914), 197.
50. Ainger (1820-1861); M.R.C.S. 1842; L.S.A. 1848; F.R.C.S. 1854 (**Plarr; Crawford**).
51. Alexander Boggs (1823-1890); M.R.C.S. 1856 (**Crawford**).
52. Edward Campbell (1815-1890); M.R.C.S. 1856 (**Lancet** (1855), 2:286, 474; **Crawford**).
53. William Harris (1830-1914); M.R.C.S. 1851; L.S.A. 1852; M.D. St. Andrews 1859 (obituary **B.M.J.** (1915), 1:99).
54. James MacAlister (1816-1860) (**Crawford**).
55. William McEgan (1817-1857) (**Crawford**). For McEgan, see note 67 to Chapter II.
56. John MacGregor (1820-1857); M.R.C.S. 1844 (**Crawford**).
57. Duncan MacPherson (1812-1861); M.D. Edinburgh (obituary **Lancet** (1867), 2:1433).
58. James Vaughan (1828-18??); M.R.C.S. 1841; F.R.C.S. 1856 (**Plarr**).
59. St. George Williams (1824-1859); L.S.A. 1854 (**Crawford**).
60. Richard Banbury (1830-1860); L.S.A. 1854 (**Crawford**).
61. Thomas Beale (d. 1860); joined as acting assistant-surgeon May 1855; commissioned assistant-surgeon after his service in the Turkish Contingent; died on service July 1860 (**Drew**).
62. Cameron McDowall (1832-1892); joined the army as acting assistant-surgeon (**Crawford**).
63. Ferdinand Odevaine (1836-1910); L.R.C.S.I. 1835; joined army as acting assistant-surgeon; F.R.C.S.I. 1975 (obituary **B.M.J.** (1910), 1:910).
64. George Sutherland (1833-1908); joined army as acting assistant-surgeon; L.R.C.S.Ed. 1855; M.D. Edinburgh 1857; (**Crawford**).
65. Robert Lewins (1817-1895); L.R.C.S.Ed., M.D. Heidelberg 1842; joined as assistant-surgeon 1842; surgeon March 1842; retired 1868 as S.M. (obituary **Lancet** (1895), 2:347; **Drew**).
66. Thomas Littleton (1824-1878); M.R.C.S. 1847; F.R.C.S. 1849; M.B. London 1832 (obituary **B.M.J.** (1878), 2:898-899).
67. Listed in **Ass.Med.J.** (1855), 1021.
68. Buzzard, **Crimea**.
69. Burke, **Graves**. Calder recorded on 7 July, 1855 - "Sibbald of Edinburgh died of cholera" ('Calder Diary').

70. Charles Balding; M.R.C.S. 1856; L.S.A. 1857.
71. Robinson Boustead (1832-1916); M.R.C.S. 1858; M.D. St. Andrews 1866; F.R.C.S.Ed. 1866; retired from I.M.S. 187980 as S.M. (**Crawford**).
72. John Carlaw; L.R.C.S.Ed.; joined army as assistant-surgeon 1858; retired 1878 as S.M. (**Drew**).
73. Cavalié Mercer was a Syrian doctor and subsequently qualified L.F.P.S. Glasgow in 1859.
74. **M.T.G.** (1855), 1:378-379.
75. Ibid., 351-352.
76. Ibid., 2:276.
77. J.N. Radcliffe, 'The Turkish Hospital at Balaclava', **Lancet** (1855), 1:7-9.
78. Buzzard, **Crimea**.
79. H. Sandwith, **A narrative of the siege of Kars** (London, 1856).
80. **Lancet** (1855), 2:62.
81. Ibid. (1856), 1:136.
82. **M.T.G.** (1856), 1:77.
83. **Ass.Med.J.** (1856), 224-225.
84. **M.T.G.** (1855), 2:2149-250; **Lancet** (1855), 2:286.
85. **Lancet** (1855), 2:287.
86. **The Times**, 8.6.1856.

CHAPTER XVII

STALEMATE AND WITHDRAWAL FROM THE CRIMEA (OCTOBER 1855 - JULY 1856)

The fall of Sebastopol did not bring an immediate end to hostilities.[1] The Russians, after setting fire to buildings, and destroying great quantities of stores had retreated to establish themselves to the North but still within artillery range of the Allies, now in the ruined town. Their main lines of communication with the heart of Russia were still intact. In October the French were ready to conclude a peace treaty, but England with her colonial and commercial interests wanted to humble the Russians more completely. France had fewer of these interests and was more concerned with European politics, moreover France had borne very heavy losses in the war, the sickness rates in her army towards the end of 1855 far exceeding those in the British forces. Again, the French had been more active and successful in the later months of the siege and were content to rest on their laurels, while the British after Inkerman had achieved little militarily. Hence Queen Victoria, **The Times**, and a large majority in parliament demanded that the Russians should be driven out of the Crimea completely.

A British army of about 50,000 men was still in the Crimea, soon to be commanded by Codrington, replacing the ineffectual Simpson. It was a well trained and now a remarkably healthy force. "The men were well-fed, well-sheltered ... a great contrast to those of the previous winter; no one would have taken the smart clean troops on the plateau of Sebastopol in January 1856 to have been the same race and nation as the care-worn, over-worked, and sickly soldiers guarding the trenches in January 1855."[2] The British put forward innumerable plans of attack, to destroy the Russians or at least push them back. One plan involved a second landing in Eupatoria and a second battle of the Alma, another plan called for a flank march along the route taken in October 1854, but this time from the South to the North. In practice, the only major attack finally agreed on by both nations was an expedition to capture Kinburn, which took place successfully early in October. The earlier attack on Kertch, the occupation of Kars, and the Kinburn expedition were the only major incursions into Russian territory outside the Crimea during the whole war. After September 1855 the war entered a long period of stalemate. The forces occupying Russian territory had to remain in a state of readiness until March 1856, on the remote chance that the Russians might counter-attack in strength. But on 14 March an armistice was agreed, on 30 March the final peace treaty was signed in Paris, and during the next three months the Allied armies were evacuated from the Crimea. A few British regiments left in May but the majority in June. The last of the French forces had gone by 4 July and the last of the British by 12 July, whereupon the Russians immediately reoccupied the whole peninsula.

By the terms of the Peace Treaty, Sebastopol, Balaclava, Kamiesh, Eupatoria, Kertch, Kinburn and all other occupied areas were restored to Russia, while Kars was returned to Turkey. The Black Sea was neutralised, no naval bases or arsenals were to be maintained on its shores, and ships of war were denied passage through the Bosphorous. The Danube was declared an open waterway. The Russians ceded only a small area of Southern Bessarabia to the Porte, while Turkish sovereignty in the Danubian principalities was to be restored. Turkey agreed that conditions for Christians in the Ottoman Empire would be improved, but there was no mention of the guardianships of the holy places, ostensibly the casus belli. For all the blood and sweat the gains to the allies seemed trivial.

MEDICAL AND SURGICAL CONDITIONS

Between October 1855 and June 1856, 58 British regiments served in the Crimea, most for eight to nine months but a few for shorter periods. Of these, 51 were infantry regiments, with strengths varying from 650 to 900 men. In the earlier months of the war the cavalry regiments had lower sickness and mortality rates than the infantry regiments, because the latter were living and working under the more difficult conditions. But after September, 1855, conditions were much the same for each group and in consequence the sickness and mortality rates were now equalised. The total number of admissions to the regimental hospitals in the final months was 25,392 and the deaths numbered 460 (1.8 per cent).[3] The figures were highest between October and December and fell considerably in the later months. Analysis of these statistics need not be so detailed as the analyses of those for the more active periods of the campaign. But it is informative to note the contrasts between the winter of 1854/1855 and the winter of 1855/1856, not only in the admission and mortality rates but also in reference to conditions such as frost-bite. Fevers and bowel conditions amounted to almost a quarter of all admissions, but this was a much smaller proportion than in the earlier months. The astonishingly low mortality rates for medical conditions (other than cholera) stand out very clearly. Yet again medical conditions far exceeded surgical conditions.

In the nine months there were 3,050 admissions to the regimental hospitals for FEVER, with 63 deaths (2 per cent). The average monthly admission rate was about 340 and the average monthly death rate about 7. The admission rate was highest in October and then fell in November and December. After January the numbers admitted were very low. The highest mortality rate occurred in the 82nd Regiment - of 106 admissions from October 1855 to January 1856, eight died (8 per cent), but in December of only seven admissions three died, which if such low figures have any meaning might suggest a virulent fever. The 82nd Regiment had throughout the winter a bad health record, attributed to various causes. The regiment did not arrive in the Crimea until late in September 1855, but the surgeon reported that the camp site was unhealthy, and further, although not in action the regiment was engaged on heavy fatigue duties. The surgeon referred "to the habitual carelessness of the men in not changing their clothes on returning to their quarters ... and to the facility which increased pay afforded to their indulging in excesses ... the severity of fatigue duties and the necessary exposure which their performance implied were no doubt prejudicial to young and unseasoned men". In contrast, most other regimental reports indicate that, after October 1855, the fevers presented relatively minor problems, the admission rates falling rapidly and the mortality rates always low. In the regimental tables the fevers were evenly divided between Febris Intermittens and Febris Communis Continua. Despite the very severe outbreaks of typhus in the French camps, very few fever cases were so designated in the British records. In the review of the fevers in the post-war history there is nothing to suggest that any new observations or therapy were forthcoming in this period.

In the nine months there were 3,556 admissions for BOWEL DISEASES with only 23 deaths (0.6 per cent). The average monthly admission rate was about 410, and the average monthly death rate less than three. As with the fevers, the highest numbers of admissions were in October, November and December, with a gradual fall to very low figures by the end of the period. Most cases were listed under the general heading of Diarrhoea. There was no severe epidemic in any regiment.

The virulence of these conditions was much less than in the previous winter. This is very clear from the fact that at least 28 regiments serving throughout the full period had no deaths from bowel diseases. In the survey of bowel diseases in the post-war medical history there is little mention of these conditions from October 1855 onwards, a remarkable contrast to the detailed analysis in the winter of 1854/1855, when bowel conditions of all kinds presented such major problems. New observations on these diseases or new therapy were not reported in this period.

The total number of admissions for RESPIRATORY TRACT DISEASES was quite large but the majority were labelled acute or chronic catarrh, representing minor conditions. The mortality rates for all respiratory tract diseases were remarkably low. It can be assumed that patients with acute bronchitis, pneumonia, or suspected tuberculosis were transferred to the general hospitals, and that those who died there were not necessarily included in the regimental tables. A comparison of the major lung conditions occurring in the two winters can be made from the figures quoted for the whole army (figures which most probably reflect fairly accurately, despite the variations in the strength of regiments, the situation in the Crimea). In the first winter, between November and April, 125 cases of pneumonia were admitted to hospital, with 79 deaths (63 per cent). In the same period of the second winter 257 cases were admitted with 43 deaths (17 per cent). The higher mortality in the first winter is readily accounted for by the poor general conditions prevailing and by the fact that these were often cases with associated scurvy, dysentery, or other debilitating disease. The higher admission rate in the second winter is surprising but can be attributed in part to the extreme cold and to "the frequent exposure to which the patient had previously been subjected while under the influence of drink". The incidence of pulmonary tuberculosis remained surprising low in the winter of 1855/1856. Acute bronchitis doubled in the second winter, but the mortality fell to 2 per cent, as compared with 28 per cent in the first winter. The more serious respiratory tract diseases reached a peak between December 1855 and March 1856, during the coldest weather.

Between October 1855 and February 1856 there were 240 admissions for CHOLERA to the regimental hospitals, of which 143 died (60 per cent). Few regiments escaped sporadic cases but the highest number of admissions in a regiment seldom exceeded 10 a month. About two fifths of the cases occurred in October, three fifths in November and one fifth in December. There were only ten cases in January and February 1856, and one in March. Thereafter the disease did not reappear in the Crimea. In the survey of the disease in the post-war medical history the cases which continued throughout the winter were regarded as representing a continuation of the Second Epidemic.[4] No comment is made on the fact that no regiment suffered a major epidemic. It can only be supposed that improved hygiene in the camps and possibly the progressive installation of piped water supplies accounted for this freedom from serious outbreaks. Nevertheless the 143 deaths contributed 31 per cent of the total mortality in the regimental hospitals from October 1855 to June 1856. Most medical officers considered that the newly joined young recruits were the most likely to be attacked by the disease. During this period no new ideas on the treatment of cholera were advanced.

Between October 1855 and May 1856 there were 340 admissions to the regimental hospitals for FROST-BITE. In October there were five cases. in November 22, in December 178, in January 54, in February 22, in March 22, in April 12, and in May five. Only one patient with frost-bite is reported as having died in a regimental hospital (0.3 per cent). In contrast, 1,518 cases were admitted in the first winter with a mortality of 8 per cent, so there was a dramatic drop in the admission and mortality rates in the second winter.

CHAPTER XVII

Yet the second winter was at least as severe as the first and possibly more severe. Meteorological records were kept at the Castle Hospital from April 1855 to June 1856.[5] Although these cannot be systematically compared with the sporadic readings taken in the first winter, it is clear that during the six months from November 1855 to March 1856 there were many days on which the temperature fell well below freezing point, and on a few days temperatures were as low as 15-25 degrees F. Such figures do suggest a harder winter than that of 1854/1855. In the post-war history the following comment is made. "The cause which induced gangrene in the winter of 1855 and 1856, was almost exclusively the application of severe, intense cold ... a large proportion of the cases this winter occurred on the 19th and 20th December ... the exceedingly low temperatures occurred suddenly and surprised the troops and it would appear that in many instances the necessary precautions were not adopted in time."[6]

In general, these cases were relatively minor, the frost-bite affecting only the ears or the hands. While amputations of the fingers are described there is no reference to severe conditions of the feet so often requiring major amputation such as occurred in the first winter. The 4th Regiment reported 14 cases in December. "All the cases occurred on the same day (the 19th) the sufferers belonging to a fatigue party at Balaclava. In consequence of the insufficient protection afforded by the caps served out to the Corps, the ears of all fourteen were frost-bitten". Other causes were summarised in the post-war survey.

> Some of the cases this winter occurred to men who during the exposure were employed in carrying timber from Sebastopol or Balaclava: others were affected with frost-bite while engaged in carrying water, or serving out rations of pork to the troops and again it was noticed as an effect of handling iron chains, pick-axes etc. Further many men suffered the affection from omitting to wear gloves and ear-lappets to their caps ... Dr. Hall observes that all the fatal cases and a large proportion of the severe, occurred among men who remained exposed while in a state of drunkenness.[7]

Although only one fatal case of frost-bite is listed in the regimental records, a few deaths were recorded under the heading "Exposure to Cold". Amongst the cases of frost-bite transferred to Scutari there were no deaths, confirming that in the second winter there were probably no lower leg amputations in the Crimea with subsequent septic complications, and no lower leg gangrenes which required secondary amputation in Scutari. The frost-bite cases in the second winter were therefore very different from those in the first winter. Warm clothing, improved foot-wear, hutted accommodation, better diet, better general health and the absence of trench duties all contributed to the low mortality rate. More particularly the frost-bitten patient in the first winter had often been exposed not only to a low temperature but also to excessive damp, frequently sleeping in wet clothes and frequently failing to remove tight, ill-fitting and wet boots at night.

Turning to the SURGICAL admissions, some cases of wounded from September were carried forward to the October and November records. The Russian guns established to the North of Sebastopol bombarded Sebastopol sporadically. A correspondent in January reported - "At present there is but little doing, except an amputation occasionally from shell wounds in Sebastopol; they sometimes fire rather heavily from the north side."[8] The exact number of wounded after September 1855 is uncertain and a full analysis of these cases has not been possible. It is not always clear from the regimental reports whether the wounds reported were caused by direct enemy action or were as a result of clearing the large amount of live ammunition from the battlefields. General surgical conditions in this period were mostly minor.

On 19 November, 1855, men from several regiments sustained severe injuries following a massive explosion in a large ammunition dump close to some of the British camps. This is described vividly by an anonymous medical officer.

> I was almost a mile away from the spot when that awful explosion took place in the French camp ... the earth positively writhed under the shock and the air was so tumultuously driven about by the concussion that my tent pole bent and quivered like a reed in a storm. It was a fearful sight and the wounds were much worse than would have been received in action ... I could go on for an hour giving you a rough sketch of many of the mangled bodies that were brought into hospital, some dead, many of them dying, and many others only to die.[9]

Hall in his weekly report specified that it was the reserve magazines of the French and English right attacks which exploded. He recorded that "of the British one officer and 20 men were killed and 5 officers and 135 men wounded, many of them seriously indeed."[10] He described how hospital huts came down like a pack of cards and shells passed through hospital marquees. "Considering the quantity of powder, shells and rockets exploded we have reason to be thankful our loss is so small. I believe that of the French is considerably greater than ours."

We come now to the General Hospitals in the Crimea. Between October 1855 and June 1856 the General Hospital at Balaclava admitted 1,363 patients and there were only 27 deaths (2 per cent).[11]

Fever accounted for 313 admissions with six deaths (2 per cent). In May and June there was an exceptionally high admission rate for intermittent fevers, 59 and 78 respectively, but with only one death each month. Out of 14 cases diagnosed as typhus between December 1855 and June 1856, five died (36 per cent). In earlier months cholera cases were sent to this hospital frequently, but between October 1855 and January 1856 only 14 cases were admitted, of which six died (43 per cent). There were 218 admissions for other bowel conditions, with two deaths (1 per cent). The Camp General Hospital admitted 466 patients with 37 deaths (8 per cent).[12] In October and November 118 wounded were admitted (most likely problem cases from the regimental hospitals with wounds which had been inflicted in September). Of these, 22 died (19 per cent), which accounts for the relatively high total mortality in the nine months. The medical admissions were mainly for fevers or bowel conditions. Only one case of cholera was admitted and was fatal. The Castle Hospital admitted 550 cases in the nine months and 15 died (3 per cent).[13] In October 158 wounded were admitted, of which 11 died (7 per cent). Only four patients died therefore of the remaining 391 medical cases, these being mainly fevers and bowel diseases (1 per cent). In June, 129 eye cases were transferred from the Monastery Hospital.

The Monastery Hospital, originally opened for convalescents, admitted 559 patients in the nine months, of whom 11 died (2 per cent).[14]

From December 1855 onwards more than two thirds of the admissions were for EYE CONDITIONS, and so the establishment may be seen as the first specialist hospital run by the army during a campaign. Unfortunately there was no post-war survey of the eye conditions treated during the war. In most regimental reports these were recorded under the general heading of Morbi Oculorum. It can be conjectured that various types of conjunctivitis of a severe or chronic nature provided the majority of cases. Very few eye injuries following facial wounds were recorded during the war and there is no mention of trachoma. In June most of the eye cases were transferred for a short period to the Castle Hospital. Here it may be noted that 473 men with eye conditions were invalided to England during the whole war (these too were under the general heading Morbi Oculorum).[15]

Four medical officers died in the Crimea in this period. The exact cause of death in two cases is unknown, one died of fever and one committed suicide (the only suicide recorded of a doctor during the campaign). Staff-Surgeon Christopher Bassano[16] died "of fever" at Balaclava on 1 February, 1856. He had served in the Crimea as a staff officer until his death. Assistant-Surgeon Nathaniel Farley[17] died in the Crimea on 24 June, 1856; Assistant-Surgeon John Gilborne[18] of the 71st Regiment died in the Crimea on 25 January, 1856; Staff-Surgeon Nicholas O'Connor[19] died at Balaclava on 7 June, 1856. There is evidence that the last-named committed suicide. He came out to serve in the Barrack Hospital in October 1854, but later became P.M.O. of Koulali Hospital and was said to have been over-worked. It is not clear why he had gone to the Crimea.

To sum up the medical conditions of this period. The low sickness rate is readily explained. Although the army was kept in a high state of readiness there was immediate relief from exhausting trench duties, from the desperate assaults on almost impregnable fortifications, and from the perils of intense bombardments or sniping. There was hard physical work in maintaining the camps, bringing up supplies, and clearing up the debris of previous battles. But no longer did the soldier have to return to restricted rations, and wet sleeping accommodation. Most of the regiments were now in huts. In the early winter Sebastopol had become a favourite place for foraging. Russell records - "Sebastopol gradually came up piecemeal to the Camp. Doors, windows, locks, hinges, fire-places, stoves, pictures, chains, tables, beams of wood, roofing, floors, sheet lead, rolled copper, cut stone, crockery and innumerable articles of every description, were brought up by carts, horses, ponies and by men every day in great quantities, and were found most useful in the construction and ornamentation of our huts."[20] With time on their hands officers and men were able to make their winter quarters very comfortable.

Although, as has already been noted, it was a hard winter, the effects of this were largely neutralised by the high standard of general fitness of the men, the lavish supply of warm clothing, the increased fuel supply, and the improved kitchens and adequate rations. The railway up to the camps was working effectively and the roads were so much improved that there was no repetition of the terrible problems encountered in the first winter. There was of course a danger that discipline would slacken, that boredom would supervene, and that the drink problem would increase. Alcoholism did in fact become a major problem, as with any army of occupation. If the soldiers who had served for all or most of the war were impatient to get home, nevertheless morale remained remarkably good, and at no time were there any mutinous tendencies.

For the medical officers the strain of the previous months had now gone. No longer were they overworked, shortages of drugs and medical equipment were now corrected, the regimental hospitals and the general hospitals were never again to be overcrowded, and the conditions in which the sick were nursed were greatly improved. The grievances of the doctors now came to the fore. Between July 1855 and April 1856 three memorials were sent to the war office by the army medical officers. The assistant-surgeons pressed for more pay, more rapid promotion, and better terms for retirement. The surgeons pressed for equality with the fighting men, particularly with regard to the distribution of honours in times of war; and they also asked for active service to be reckoned in claims for promotion as worth three times the same period of peace-time service. They objected to the employment of civil practitioners and to the higher rates of pay which the latter were accorded. Before the end of the war promises to remedy these grievances were made, but in the event nothing was done until much later.

There was now also considerable discussion as to whether the system under which the primary loyalty of medical officers was directed towards their regiments should continue. With the experience of nearly two years of active service in brigade and divisional formations, a number of medical officers believed that this loyalty should in future be primarily towards the Medical Department. However, some of the older men, including Hall, thought that the co-operation between the commanding officer and the regimental surgeon was one of the most important requisites for the care of the sick. Nevertheless Hall agreed that a more independent departmental attitude would improve morale. Despite this undercurrent of criticism and insistence on reform, the number of medical officers who resigned in this period was not great, anxious as most of them were to return home to enjoy a well-deserved leave.

During these months Hall stayed on the Crimea, attending to every detail of his command with his customary industry and care. Yet even in this relatively quiet spell he did not apparently think fit to visit the base hospitals. From 1854 Hall had been obsessed by the notion that Raglan was conspiring to have him replaced by Deputy Inspector-General James Barry[21], who was serving in Cyprus. Barry was a curious character, not surprisingly, since 'he' is generally believed to have been a female, or at the very least a pseudo-hermaphrodite.[22] Of small stature and effeminate appearance he had a powerful personality. Barry came to the Crimea some time in the autumn of 1855 on an unofficial visit. In his diary Hall makes several references to his dislike and distrust of Barry. In October, Cumming wrote to Hall warning him of Barry's arrival.

> I may as well warn you that you are to have a visit from Dr. Barry. He called on me yesterday and as I never met him before his appearance and conversation rather surprised me. He appears to me in his dotage and is an intolerable bore ... He will expect you to listen to every quarrel he has had since coming into the service, you probably know that they are not a few.[23]

Dr. Barry had met Miss Nightingale in Scutari and she recorded - "I never had such a blackguarding in my life ... he behaved like a brute. After he was dead I was told she was a woman. I should say she was the most hardened creature I ever met."[24] With eccentrics like Barry around, with persistent criticisms of his management of the medical service throughout the war, and facing accusations from all sides, the sensitive and now exhausted Hall soldiered on for these last months with an increasing sense that he had been unjustly treated.

By now both Hall and Smith were only too well aware that recriminations would continue after the war was over. Smith wrote to Hall on 24 December, 1855 - "You and I must leave some records behind us that shall be useful to posterity ... The Board which I have formed in this office will work in concert with those in the East and I see no reason, if men are zealous, that something creditable should not be produced."[25] This was the germ of the idea for a medical history of the war which was eventually published in 1858. Quite clearly Hall and Smith intended to put the record straight and by doing so defend themselves from persistent critics. In this same letter Smith expressed his continued confidence in Hall. "You will be satisfied that you will have every support I can give you. Keep up a hot line in reference to anything which I consider has relation to the health of the army."[26]

THE CRIMEAN MEDICAL SOCIETY

On 3 January, 1856, twenty medical officers met at the medical headquarters of the First Division to discuss the formation of a Medical Society.[27] Deputy Inspector-General James Williams[28] took the chair and expressed the hope that the project "would tend to benefit, not only the medical officers of the Division but trusted would also raise our position as Military Medical Officers: thus showing to our Professional brethren at home that we are alive to our present position, anxious for the advancement of science, and are not behind the Civil branches of the service, either in experience or successful practice ... A cloud appears to have hovered over us: let us dispel that cloud, and obtain the rights justly due, for we do not think we have always been fairly treated." He proposed that the society should be called "The Military Medical and Surgical Society, First Division, British Army, Crimea". There may have been feelings that the civil medical staff at Smyrna, by the publicity given to their medical society, had somewhat stolen the limelight. Surgeon Robert Thornton[29] of the 9th Regiment was elected Secretary.

The first meeting was held on 10 January.[30] Dr. Hall was in the chair and he recommended that a general rather than a divisional society should be formed. French and Sardinian medical officers were made honourary members. Surgeon George Blenkins[31], of the Grenadier Guards presented the first clinical paper, on two cases of scorbutic ulceration and sloughing of wounds, and there was a long discussion in which Hall took a prominent part. Thornton then gave an account of delayed union of the tibia after a gun-shot wound. On 17 January Staff Surgeon Robert Bowen of the Rifle Brigade[32], discussed amputations for frost-bite of the hands with gangrene. A lively discussion ensued which revealed that differences of opinion persisted over early or late amputation, hence over the dependence on late spontaneous separation of gangrenous tissue - on balance, late amputation was favoured by most of the British surgeons present and by their French colleagues.[33] Surgeon Daniel Barry[34] read a paper on frost-bite. Assistant-Surgeon L. Herbert demonstrated his own mutilated hand, having lost two fingers while in the Crimea during the second winter.[35] On 24 January Barry read a paper on diarrhoea in the Crimea. He disagreed with Lyons, the civilian pathologist, who considered that diarrhoea in the Crimea was a variety peculiar to that area.[36].

On 31 January Assistant Surgeon Henry Lawrence of the Grenadier Guards[37], gave a paper on cholera. He favoured treatment with small doses of calomel, but in the discussion which followed there was little unanimity concerning the cause or the treatment of the disease. Bowen accepted that the gastro-intestinal mucous membrane was the "focus morbi" of cholera.[38] Dr. Hume (probably Deputy-Inspector Thomas Hume[39]) was realistic. "If attacked with cholera he would rather be left alone. He considered that patients were 'death-struck' and all our efforts unavailing. He believed that those patients who recovered got well in spite of treatment." On 7 February Assistant-Surgeon Francis De

Chaumont[40] read a paper on fever complicated with thoracic affections.[41] On 28 February Staff-Surgeon Edward Menzies[42] discussed amputations. On balance he was in favour of primary amputation, but had reservations concerning a strict rule that all cases of compound fracture of the femur should be amputated early. A long discussion took place in which personal experiences of single cases were brought forward in favour of different theories of management.[43] No long series of cases were presented to support either primary or secondary amputation (or local resection as a more conservative measure).

On 13 March Dr. Sclaveroni, of the Sardinian Army, read a paper on the diseases of the Sardinian troops in the Crimea. This was a somewhat vague presentation, mainly about fevers. The Editor of the **Medical Times and Gazette** politely published it. "The style of Dr. Sclaveroni's paper is rather obscure owing to the fact of its being delivered in a language not perfectly understood by the author." Dr. Hall and the other British doctors were extremely generous about the contribution.[44] If the substance was somewhat confusing the cordiality generated by this participation by Dr. Sclaveroni was considerable. About this date the Society changed its title to "The Medical and Surgical Society of the British Army", and it was now reported in the medical journals as "The Crimean Medical and Surgical Society".

On 20 March Thornton read a second paper, on local excision of bone or joints after gun-shot wounds. After describing three cases he presented a list of 54 major excisions done during the campaign, of which 36 were in the upper limb, 14 in the lower limb, and four "miscellaneous". Two of the upper limb cases and seven of the lower limb cases died. Thornton suggested that the operation was a useful alternative to amputation (although the results in the lower limb were very poor). In the discussion there was general support from most of the surgeons, based very largely on very limited experience of the operation. Macleod, the Civil Surgeon, was much more cautious about the application of the technique in military surgery.[45]

On 19 April a discussion, perhaps the most important held by the group, was initiated on the use of chloroform in military surgery. It was opened by Mouat, who recalled how Hall had introduced a note of caution concerning its use early in the campaign and had incurred unfair criticism for this. Hall was chairman of this meeting and perhaps some medical officers thought it wise to support his original directive! Mouat set out to answer two questions. First, "Is the administration of chloroform, in the severe depression consequent on large gun-shot injuries, fraught with danger?" Secondly, "Are we justified in a moral point of view, in giving a dangerous remedy for such trifling operations as the removal of a finger or toe, or the extraction of teeth, or bullets lying near the surface?" He proposed less dangerous alternatives such as Arnott's technique of local anaesthesia by freezing, or Esdaile's mesmerism. He quoted numerous cases and was disposed to answer his first question firmly in the affirmative and his second question firmly in the negative. In the discussion, in which eleven doctors took part, of those who gave firm opinions three supported Mouat in the first question and four disagreed with him. Two supported Mouat in the second question and three disagreed with him. The most outspoken critic of Mouat's cautious attitude was Macleod. Mouat answered his critics and stated that - "He was an advocate for the administration of chloroform, but not for its indiscriminate use". He admitted that it was not always easy to be certain that chloroform had been a primary cause of death.[46]

On 1 May the arguments concerning chloroform were continued with a paper by Macleod. He reviewed the theories on the action of chloroform and the experience of its use in civilian practice. He "emphatically denied that there was anything in gunshot wounds which make the use of anaesthesia in these less beneficial than in the same accidents of civil life: and he contended that as the pain and suffering in these cases were very great, so much the more necessity existed for its use". Macleod suggested that the number of deaths ascribed to chloroform was exaggerated and that these could be prevented by more careful techniques. Mouat was not present to take part in the discussion. Of the small number attending all four who spoke supported Macleod's views strongly.[47] The last recorded meeting was held on 8 May. There was further discussion on the use of chloroform but the details were not reported.[48] The regular meetings were terminated as the medical officers and medical establishments were now beginning to be dispersed.

The Society had flourished for nearly six months. Hall acted as chairman at most meetings and gave the medical officers every encouragement to attend. On 10 January he had announced that the Director-General had called for reports on the Crimean diseases and had promised immediate promotion to whoever should produce the best essay or treatise.[49] As usual with most medical societies the proportion of eligible doctors who attended was small, and it was the same limited group who contributed to the discussions at each meeting. The attendance varied from 15 to 40 and was augmented from time to time by French or Sardinian medical officers. The proceedings have been given in some detail to bring to light some of the topics which concerned the army doctors. In addition, it is of interest to know which of the army doctors were possessed of clinical curiosity and the desire to advance medical knowledge from their experiences. If no epoch-making discoveries were announced at these meetings the enterprise was profitable to all who participated.

As a repercussion, a general meeting of army medical officers was called in London on 15 October, 1856, for the purpose of re-establishing the Crimean Society. It was agreed that the Medical and Surgical Society of the Army established in the Crimea, "found so beneficial in its results", be transferred to London as "The Medical and Surgical Society of the British Army", and that all officers of the Medical Department on full and half pay should be invited to become members. A provisional council was elected to plan the activities and rules of the society.[50] Sadly it does not seem that the new society flourished.

THE LATER VISITS OF MISS NIGHTINGALE TO THE CRIMEA

On 9 October, 1855, Miss Nightingale left Scutari for her second visit to the Crimea.[51] She was still viewed with suspicion and her authority was questioned. Mr. Bracebridge's attack on the army doctors still rankled, and Hall remained antagonistic. As Herbert had written in 1854 - "Dr. Hall resents offers of assistance as being slurs on his preparations".[52] Hall wrote of "a system of detraction against our establishments kept up by interested parties under the garb of philanthropy".[53] The Deputy-Purveyor-General in the Crimea was equally suspicious of Miss Nightingale's further visit, and he wrote to the War Office criticising the nurses in the Crimea and arguing against Miss Nightingale's claim to have authority over these nurses. It was not until 16 March, 1856, that Panmure, the Secretary of War, finally defined Miss Nightingale's position in General Orders.[54]

> It appears to me that the Medical Authorities of the Army do not correctly comprehend Miss Nightingale's position as it has been officially recognised by me ... Miss N. is recognised by Her Majesty's Government as the General Superintendent of the Female Nursing Establishment of the military hospitals of the army. No lady, or Sister, or nurse, is to be transferred from one hospital to another, or introduced into any hospital, without consultation with her. Her instructions, however, require to have the approval of the Principal Medical Officer in the exercise of responsibility thus vested in her. The Principal Medical Officer will communicate with Miss Nightingale upon all subjects connected with the Female Nursing Establishment, and will give his directions through that lady.

(It may however be thought that the second last sentence in this statement is ambiguous). This attempt at clarification of Miss Nightingale's position came too late to ease relationships between her and Hall.

In October 1855 there was a particularly difficult crisis.[55] A group of Roman Catholic sisters under their Reverend Mother, Mrs. Bridgeman, had been transferred from Koulali to the General Hospital at Balaclava. Since the move had been arranged by Hall without consultation, Miss Nightingale saw this as an usurpation of her authority. She did not think that the work of this Irish group of nurses was efficient. However, some observers thought that Miss Nightingale was exhibiting a petty and sectarian attitude. Hall was greatly impressed by Mrs. Bridgeman and her nurses and would not allow them to be moved from Balaclava. When Panmure's final edict came through, Hall advised Mrs. Bridgeman to resign rather than to become subservient to Miss Nightingale, and Mrs. Bridgeman and her sisters did in fact leave the Crimea at the end of March. Before they left Miss Nightingale did her best to persuade them to stay, affirming that all she wanted was to make some reforms in their administration. This long drawn-out quarrel caused Miss Nightingale great vexation. In her letters to Herbert and others she complained that by such actions Hall was "attempting to root her out of the Crimea". Herbert, although not now officially involved in the control of medical affairs in the army, was still the one who received all Miss Nightingale's complaints. More and more he had begun to realise that she exaggerated some of her reports. He beseeched her to write with less vehemence and irritation. "You attribute motives to those whose misstatements you may disprove and whose misconduct you may expose."[56]

If Miss Nightingale was unhappy about the nursing situation in the Balaclava Hospital she found some solace in her visits to the Castle Hospital. There the nursing staff was efficiently run by Mrs. Shaw Stewart, energetic and devoted to her work, albeit a difficult person to deal with at times. But Miss Nightingale's second visit to the Crimea was cut short in November when news reached her that cholera had broken out in Scutari.

She arrived for her third and last visit to the Crimea on 24 March, 1856.[57] Rather to her surprise, she had received a letter from Hall asking her to send ten nurses for the Land Transport Corps Hospital, the sickness rate in the Transport Corps having become one of his greatest problems. She was well received by the medical officers of the Transport Hospital, but found that Hall and Fitzgerald (the Deputy Purveyor, who had been a constant thorn in her flesh) were still, in her opinion, conspiring against her. The state of the patients in the Transport Hospital reminded Miss Nightingale of the first winter of the war. For a short time she nursed the sick herself and reorganised the kitchens. With the departure of Mrs. Bridgeman early in April Miss Nightingale then had to take over the management of the Balaclava General Hospital. She found it in a neglected state, confirming once more her distrust of the Irish nurses, but with the help of some trustworthy and able nurses from Scutari she rapidly improved conditions. She found time to visit the French hospitals in the Crimea and although flattered by the attention of the senior doctors, she was critical of the younger doctors, believing that they tended to experiment on their patients with new forms of treatment.[58] She was particularly interested in the French record system and their use of statistics. One of her main preoccupations at this period was with the deplorable state of the British sick records, an administrative weakness she was determined to correct. She finally left the Crimea at the beginning of July, to spend a short time winding up her affairs in Scutari. Miss Nightingale regarded this third visit to the Crimea as one of the most profitable periods of her service abroad. At last she had been able to deploy her nurses to her own satisfaction.

NOTES

1. For an account of the political situation at the end of the war, see J.S. Curtiss, **Russia's Crimean War** (Durham N.C., 1979), 472-529.
2. D. Judd, **The Crimean War** (London, 1975), 181.
3. **Med. Surg. Hist.**, 1, with statistics from the regimental tables as before.
4. Ibid., 2:72-88.
5. Ibid., 2:399-464.
6. Ibid., 2:190.
7. Ibid., 2:190.
8. **Ass.Med.J.** (1856), 75.
9. Ibid., 75-76.
10. **M.T.G.** (1855), 2:585.
11. **Med. Surg. Hist.**, 2: after p.480, "General Hospital Returns. III. Balaclava".
12 Ibid., "V. Camp Hospital."
13. Ibid., "IV. Castle Hospital."
14. Ibid., "VI. Monastery Hospital."
15. **Med. Surg. Hist.**, 2:229.
16. Christopher Bassano (1824-1856); joined as assistant-surgeon 1848; surgeon August 1855; served in the East from October 1855 until death (**Drew**).
17. Nathaniel Farley (d.1856); acting assistant-surgeon 1855; served in the East from August 1855 until death (**Drew**).
18. John Gilborne (1833-1856); acting staff assistant-surgeon 1854; served in the East from January 1855 until death (**Drew**).
19. Nicholas O'Connor (1814-1856); M.B. Dublin 1834; joined as assistant-surgeon 1839; staff-surgeon (1st. class) May 1855; served in the East October 1854 until death (**Drew**).
20. N. Bentley, ed., **Russell's despatches from the Crimea 1854-1856** (London, 1966), 268.

21. James Barry (1799-1805); M.D. Edinburgh; joined as hospital assistant 1813; assistant-surgeon 1815; D.I.G. 1851; retired 1859 as I.G. (**Drew**); **DNB**). For this episode see **Cantlie**, 2:413-417; I. Rae, **The strange story of Dr. James Barry** (London, 1958).
22. B. Harwitz and R. Richardson, 'Inspector General James Barry M.D. : putting the woman in her place', **B.M.J.** (1989), 299-305.
23. 'Hall/Cumming Letters', 11.10.1855.
24. **Cantlie**, 2:416.
25. 'Hall/Smith Letters', 14.12.1855.
26. Ibid., ?.11.1854.
27. **M.T.G.** (1856), 1:152.
28. James Williams (1805-1885); joined as assistant-surgeon 1846; D.I.G. July 1855; served in the East October 1855 - June 1856; retired 1863 as D.I.G. (**Drew**).
29. Robert Thornton (1822-1884); M.R.C.S. 1844; L.S.A. 1846; joined as assistant-surgeon 1846; surgeon April 1855; served in the East from April 1855 - June 1856; retired 1877 as D.S.G. (**Drew**).
30. **M.T.G.** (1856), 1:175, 218-219.
31. George Blenkins (1813--1895); M.R.C.S. 1840; joined as assistant-surgeon 1837; F.R.C.S. 1852; surgeon October 1854; served in the East for the duration of the war (obituary **B.M.J.** (1894), 2:789; **Plarr**; **Drew**).
32. Robert Bowen (1817-1895); M.R.C.S. 1840; joined as assistant-surgeon 1841; surgeon 1851; served in the East for the duration of the war; F.R.C.S. 1861; retired 1877 as S.G. (**Plarr**; **Drew**). Bowen was a survivor of the disastrous ship-wreck of the troop-ship 'Birkenhead' in 1852.
33. **M.T.G.** (1856), 1:248-249.
34. Daniel Barry (1825-1901); M.R.C.P.I., M.R.C.S., 1846; joined as assistant-surgeon 1846; served in the East June 1855 - June 1856; retired 1867 as S.M. (obituary **B.M.J.** (1901), 1:683; **Drew**).
35. Herbert was an acting assistant-surgeon who served in the East October 1855 - June 1856.
36. **M.T.G.** (1856), 1:322-324.
37. Henry Lawrence (b. 1830); joined as assistant-surgeon February 1854; served in the East for the rest of the war; retired 1885 as B.S. (**Drew**).
38. **M.T.G.** (1856), 1:374-375.
39. Thomas Hume (1807-1888); joined as hospital assistant 1826; assistant-surgeon 1827; D.I.G. June 1855; served in the East January - April 1855, December 1855 - June 1856; retired 1865 as I.G. (**Drew**).
40. Francis de Chaumont (1833-1888); M.D. Edinburgh 1853; joined as assistant-surgeon April 1854; served in the East November 1854 - June 1856; F.R.C.S.Ed. 1864; S.M. 1865; Professor of Military Surgery at Netley 1875 until death (obituary **Med.Pres.** (1888), 1:447; **Drew**).
41. **M.T.G.** (1856), 1:423-424.
42. Edward Menzies (1820-1904); M.R.C.S. 1841; joined as assistant-surgeon 1841; surgeon 1855; served in the East October 1854 - January 1856; retired 1870 as D.I.G. (**Drew**).
43. **M.T.G.** 1856, 1, 495-497.
44. Ibid., (1856), 2:47-50.
45. Ibid., (1856), 2:273.
46. Ibid., (1856), 2:225-227, 252-254.
47. Ibid., (1856), 2:376-378.
48. Ibid., (1856), 2:378.
49. Ibid., (1856), 1:175.
50. Ibid., (1856), 2:454.
51. For accounts of this visit, see E.T. Cook, **The life of Florence Nightingale** (2 vols., London, 1904), 1:283-289; I.B. O'Malley, **Florence Nightingale 1820-1856** (London, 1931), 331-337.
52. Lord Stanmore, **Sidney Herbert, Lord Herbert of Lea: a memoir** (2 vols., London, 1906), 1:368.

53. Cook, **Nightingale**, 1:288.
54. Ibid., 292-293.
55. Ibid., 289, 293; O'Malley, **Nightingale**, 374-389.
56. Stanmore, **Herbert**, 1:416-420.
57. For an account of the last visit, see O'Malley, **Nightingale**, 374-389.
58. O'Malley, **Nightingale**, 383, 388-390.

CHAPTER XVIII

EPILOGUE: POST-WAR CONSEQUENCES

MORTALITY OF ARMIES AND DOCTORS

There is uncertainty concerning the total of deaths in the British Army during the whole of the war. In the post-war medical history a figure of 18,058 deaths is given, of which 16,297 were from disease and 1,761 from wounds.[1] In 1922 Garrison quoted a total of 21,827 deaths in the whole campaign, with 17,225 from disease.[2] He estimated that a total of 97,864 officers and men were deployed: this gives a mortality rate of 22 per cent.

The mortality rates of the other armies involved in the war are uncertain, and an accurate comparison with the British Army is not possible. Garrison estimated that the French deployed 309,268 officers and men and that 72,415 died (23 per cent).[3] Of these deaths 59,815 were from disease, 8,250 were killed in action, and 4,354 died of wounds. The mortality rates of the Russian Army are the most uncertain of all. At one extreme, Garrison stated that 324,478 officers and men were deployed during the whole war and that the deaths numbered 73,125 (23 per cent), of which 37,454 were from disease, 14,671 "died of wounds" and 21,000 were "killed in action".[4] In contrast Seaton has suggested (from Russian sources) that as many as 100,000 officers and men were killed in action and that the "whole casualty list through exposure and disease, typhus in winter and cholera in summer, was nearer half a million men".[5]

From a variety of sources the names of 720 medical officers who served in the Army of the East in the war, for varying periods, have been traced. These officers held full commissions or acting rank. The figure may be a slight underestimate because of the difficulty of tracing all the acting assistant-surgeons who joined after February 1855. We have traced a total of 52 army medical officers who died during the war. This comprises two deputy-inspectors-general, eleven staff-surgeons, eight surgeons, 20 assistant-surgeons and 11 acting assistant-surgeons. With 52 deaths out of 720 serving officers the mortality rate was 7 per cent. This rate may be compared with a peace-time one: in the year before the Crimean War 22 medical officers out of a total of 556 employed died of disease, that is, 4%.[6] During the war one doctor was killed in action, one was drowned, one was accidently shot and the remaining 50 died of disease. In the Turkish Contingent five deaths occurred. In addition one Civil Surgeon on the official list, two civilian doctors serving unofficially, two civilian doctors serving in hospital transports, and five naval medical officers died during the war. The total of medically qualified men lost in the whole campaign was therefore 65.

It is difficult to find the exact number of deaths in the French medical service. It is recorded that during the war as many as 70 doctors died of typhus alone, and again that 64 died between November 1855 and June 1856, mainly of typhus.[7] The likelihood is that well over 120 French doctors died during the whole of the war. The French did not call for assistance from civilian doctors or from foreign doctors.

The number of deaths of Russian medical officers is not known but was almost certainly higher than that of the allies. The Russians were short of trained doctors and not only enlisted German doctors (and many German medical students as dressers) but also a group of 30 Americans of whom ten died of typhus.[8]

THE POST-WAR SANITARY COMMISSION AND ITS RESULTS

As recorded in Chapter XI, in 1856 the Chelsea Board met and in a white-washing exercise overthrew the reports of the Supplies Commission for which McNeill and Tulloch had been responsible. Only brief mention need be made of the Second Parliamentary Select Committee which met in 1856. The terms of reference of this Committee, appointed in April 1856, were to enquire into the organisation of the Medical Department and the grievances which the army medical officers had expressed in their memorials to the Secretary of State.[9] The

Chairman of the Committee was Augustus Stafford M.P., who had visited Scutari in 1854. Of the witnesses who came before this committee, Smith, the Director-General, was the one "upon whom the heavy artillery of irrelevant questions was chiefly brought to bear". The most important discussions concerned the rates of pay of medical officers. In the end this committee made some useful recommendations, but the government shelved the report as it was soon clear that the Royal Sanitary Commission would deal with the same questions more completely.

By far the most important enquiry was that conducted by the Royal Sanitary Commission, for this had far-reaching effects on the Army Medical Service. The pressure on the government to establish a Royal Commission to enquire into the sanitary state of the army and all aspects of the medical service came from two individuals, Miss Nightingale and Sidney Herbert. Miss Nightingale was determined that major reforms should be made urgently, so that there would be no repetition of the calamities of the Crimean War. Herbert too was an idealist, but as a politician he realised that caution was needed and that reform could not take place quickly. Herbert was out of office at the end of the Crimean War and the support of his successor, Lord Panmure, had to be gained. This was achieved in due course by Miss Nightingale. After some delay, Herbert was appointed President of a Commission of eight. Miss Nightingale had considerable influence in selecting the members, three of whom were regular army medical officers, Alexander, Balfour, and Smith.[10] Herbert and Miss Nightingale worked tirelessly to prepare for the enquiry, inspecting army establishments and preparing statistics, and Miss Nightingale had a large share in the selection of witnesses. There was considerable discussion as to whether or not Miss Nightingale herself should appear as a witness. The compromise was reached by which she was permitted to provide written answers to written questions (which put her at some advantage).

The terms of reference were "to inquire into the organisation, government and direction of the Medical Department of the Army".[11] First, the terms and conditions of service of the medical officers were to be considered. Secondly, the existing regulations "to prevent disease in the army" were to be investigated (this included matters concerning barracks, clothing and rations). Thirdly, the state of military hospitals was to be assessed. Fourthly, the system of invaliding oficers and men was to be reviewed. Fifthly, the organisation of the Medical Department was to be investigated. In the terms of reference there was no specific suggestion of an enquiry into the working of the medical service during the Crimean War. But in the Report it is clear that much information was derived from the findings of the numerous Commissions and Committees of Enquiry conducted during and immediately after the War. Inevitably many of the witnesses called had been involved in the East.

Between May and July 1857, 51 witnesses were examined, and finally Miss Nightingale's written evidence was presented. Among the witnesses were two serving Medical Directors-General, Andrew Smith of the Army and John Liddell of the Navy, and seven army medical officers who had served in the Crimean campaign: Thomas Alexander (soon to succeed Smith), George Beatson[12] a staff-surgeon then on half-pay, James Gibson, later to become Director-General, John Hall, Senior Medical Officer in the East, Henry Mapleton, once Raglan's personal physician, James Mouat V.C., a staff-surgeon, and John Taylor[13] formerly a staff officer in the Crimea and now Deputy-Inspector-General in charge of Fort Pitt Hospital. Three civilian practitioners who had served in the East, John Meyer, Edmund Parkes, and Henry Rowdon also gave evidence.

Over 10,000 questions were put to the witnesses and their answers were sometimes very lengthy. One contemporary review of the proceedings noted - "The result of the enquiries is a mass huge, and we had almost said, indigestible ... The diligent student of the Report and Evidence will find that to reach important and positive facts and to secure for himself matter for practical thought, he must search through a quarry containing much formless and pretentious rubbish." For an historian of the Crimean War, however, the Report and

Evidence contain much material which throws light on many aspects of the medical service and on its performance in the Crimea in particular.

Smith had inflicted upon him the longest session in the witness box. No fewer than 623 questions were put to him.[14] He was asked his opinion on every aspect of the medical service. His answers were clear and he showed an extraordinary grasp of detail. The criticism that emerged in the Report was less of him than of the system which he had inherited.

The written answers of Miss Nightingale deserve close study.[15] It appears that she herself had set the questions! After giving her interpretation of the Scutari mortality rates she made important observations on the mortality of the army at home as compared with that of the same age groups in the civilian population. She demonstrated that if the army was as healthy as the population from which it was drawn the soldiers "would die at one-half the rate they die now". This statement astonished and shocked many people and was a powerful condemnation of the conditions under which soldiers lived.

When the Report of the Royal Commission appeared in 1858, together with recommendations, complete records of the evidence and numerous appendices, the whole publication amounted to 700 pages. A full analysis cannot be presented here. It is sufficient to state briefly the recommendations and to indicate to what extent and how effectively they were implemented. The Report noted the insanitary and overcrowded state of the army barracks and called for urgent attention to the problem. As far as army camps were concerned, it recommended that medical officers, preferably sanitary experts, should in future be consulted on their siting. Strong recommendations were made about the provision of uniforms appropriate to different climates. The mode of construction of army hospitals should be changed, adopting the pavilion system and improving sanitation, and adequate medical transport should be provided. The statistical methods used in the army required to be revised. New proposals were made for the selection of army doctors and for increases in pay. The establishment of an Army Medical School was recommended.

Implementation of these recommendations was slow. On Herbert's suggestion, four sub-commissions were appointed, the first to arrange improvements in hospitals and barracks, the second to draw up a plan for a statistical branch in the medical service, the third to establish an Army Medical School, and the fourth to deal with hospital regulations and the conditions of service of medical officers.[16] During the next five years, despite many setbacks, most of the recommendations were implemented. Although the final report from the Barracks Sub-Commission did not appear until 1861, considerable improvements had already been made in the conditions of the buildings. The Sub-Commission on Statistics reported in June 1858, and by the time its report was printed (not until 1861) a military statistical department was working well and was far in advance of any similar organisation in Europe. The Sub-Commission concerned with Conditions of Service - the pay and promotion of medical officers -met more obstruction than any other of the sub-commissions, probably because the War Office did not really understand the necessity of improving the status and training of the medical officer as a means of improving the health of the army. The work of the Sub-Commission on the Establishment of a Medical School, although also subject to many delays and obstructions, had positive results.

Before the war had ended Smith had laid plans for a new hospital of 1,000 beds to replace the inadequate Fort Pitt Hospital.[17] The plans were lavish, and among many others Miss Nightingale disapproved of the lay-out.[18] Nevertheless, the hospital was built, at Netley overlooking Southampton Water, and was to serve the army well from 1863 until it was demolished in 1973. An Army Medical School, inaugurated at Fort Pitt in March 1860, was moved to Netley in 1863.[19] Initially Thomas Longmore was appointed as Professor of Surgery, Henry Parkes as Professor of Hygiene, and William Aitken as Professor of Pathology. Significantly, all three had served in the Crimea - and all were sponsored by Florence Nightingale. Newly joined medical officers could at last be trained in specialised subjects such as hygiene, tropical diseases and war surgery.

On balance it can be said that the Royal Commission of 1857 did produce many beneficial effects. Had it not been forced through by the efforts of Herbert and Miss Nightingale it is arguable that the reforms which were most urgently needed in the Medical Service would have been delayed indefinitely. The Commission was a direct consequence of the Crimean War and its subsequent influence must be seen as one of the most important gains of a campaign in which so much went so completely wrong.

CLINICAL LESSONS OF THE WAR

It is not easy to judge to what extent the intensive clinical experience in medicine and surgery gained during the war was assimilated, and whether or not any real advances were made which influenced practice either in service or civilian life. To make any judgement we must look at official clinical reports, at relevant articles in the medical journals, and at the military texts produced after the war.

The most important official document is the massive work of 1,637 pages entitled, **Medical and Surgical History of the British Army which served in Turkey and the Crimea during the War against Russia in the years 1854-1855-1856.**[20] This was published in 1858. Volume I consists mainly of the medical histories of the 66 regiments which served in the campaign, for periods varying from one to 17 months. These histories appear to have been derived largely from the routine monthly reports furnished by the regimental surgeons (usually unnamed). Almost all the reports were edited by Staff-Surgeon William Hanbury[21] and Staff-Surgeon Thomas Matthew, who were in Smith's Department. The value of the regimental reports is greatly enhanced by standard statistical tables. Four-fifths of this volume is given over to these regimental reports and tables. The remaining fifth consists of an "Appendix" with a variety of records. The reports provided early in 1854 by Dumbreck, Linton, and Mitchell on the climate, medical topography, and diseases of areas in which the campaign was expected to take place, are given in detail.[22] Of value is the "Return showing the Names and Periods of Service of all officers who served in the hospital staff with the armies of Her Majesty", listing 418 individuals, both acting and commissioned medical officers.[23] Ranks and Christian names are not given, and deaths are not indicated, but periods of service at each "Station" are recorded. In a few instances there are additional notes about invaliding or temporary leave to Britain. Other lists of medical personnel follow. Dates of service and stations are given for 53 apothecaries and dispensers and 43 hospital dressers[24], and 30 "Civil Surgeons" are noted as serving at Scutari, Koulali, or in the Crimea.[25] The civil surgeons serving at Smyrna or Renkioi are not listed, except for a few of those who worked for a short time in Scutari or in the Crimea.

Long lists are provided of "Medical Comforts shipped for the use of Hospitals in the East."[26] The names of the transports, dates of arrival, and ports of arrival are given, as are the totals of medical comforts provided between February 1854 and March 1856. The supplies sent seem lavish but no estimate is given of the proportion that ever got to the hospitals. A "List of Hospital Stores sent to the East" is as elaborate.[27] Of special value is the "Return showing Medical and Surgical Stores forwarded from Feb. 11th 1854 to March 18th 1856".[28] This list includes drugs of all kinds, dressing materials, and surgical equipment. Note must be taken of the quantities of important drugs such as quinine, opium derivatives, and chloroform, in view of the repeated accusations of serious shortages of these drugs. It may be concluded that initial shipments of these three important drugs were just adequate, but that delayed unloading or diversion to Varna accounted for temporary shortages after the battle of the Alma and for the next three months.

The first section in Volume II deals with the "Topography and Climate of Bulgaria and the Crimea".[29] These observations relate to the conditions in the camps and the incidence of diseases. There is a short description of the hospital at Varna. Sections follow on specific diseases or groups of diseases.[30] But little is recorded of the clinical work in the base hospitals, except for some account of the cholera epidemic at Scutari in November 1855. A long section follows concerning the mortality rate in the army from disease,[31] and another section records invaliding and discharge from the service consequent on disease.[32] The section on wounds and injuries is detailed,[33] and finally shock and general anaesthesia are discussed.

Tables are printed of the "Return of Vessels which arrived at Scutari etc., with Sick and Wounded".[34] From these a complete account of all the voyages of the hospital transports from the Crimea to the Base Hospitals can be obtained, 212 passages being reported. The details include the name and tonnage of the ship, the number of sick and wounded officers and men carried, the sailing date from the Crimea, the mortality rate on the voyage, the arrival date and the disembarcation date. The names of the medical officers on each voyage are given. At the end of Volume II are tables recording the work in the hospitals at Scutari, in the Crimea, at Abydos, at Varna, at Smyrna, and at Renkioi.[35] From these tables can be obtained complete statistics of admission and mortality rates.

The value of the **Medical and Surgical History** as a source for the present study is considerable. Yet, despite the mountain of details, the reader looks in vain for a discussion of the problems in the Scutari hospitals - the overcrowding, the poor accommodation and the shortages of medical stores in the first winter of the war. If the table of admissions and deaths in the Scutari Hospitals at the end of Volume II had not been printed this aspect of the medical history of the war would have received no recognition at all. Equally there is no discussion of the appalling conditions of the transports in the first months of the war. No guidance is offered as to the success or otherwise of the Civil Hospitals at Smyrna and Renkioi, an experiment which was surely worthy of some record. Their existence would be unknown to the reader but for the tables of admissions and deaths and the records of the hospital transports. The name of Florence Nightingale nowhere appears, nor is there any mention of the attachment of female nurses to the hospitals. The influence of the various Commissions reporting during the war receives no comment.

Apart from the official Medical History, little else was written contemporaneously concerning the diseases encountered during the war. Radcliffe, who served in the Turkish Contingent, published in 1858 a monograph on the problems encountered in the care of the Turkish Army.[36] The only important text-book was Parke's **Manual of Practical Hygiene ... for use ... in the army**, published in 1864.[37] This text reflected the urgent need to instruct the army doctor in military hygiene, in order to prevent a repetition of the gross neglect of this branch of medicine in the camps and the hospitals.

It might be expected that numerous articles on debatable medical topics relating to the war would have been produced, but in fact this did not occur. No doctor other than Hanbury (in the official medical history) attempted to survey the experience of cholera during the campaign. Since at the time theories of the cause and spread of cholera were still the subject of great argument, it would have been of value to have investigated how army experience measured up to Snow's theory of transmission by water supply. With regard to the common bowel disorders and fevers there was admittedly little new to be said. In the immediate post-war period many clinicians took refuge in the general descriptions "Crimean Dysentery" and "Crimean Fever". For instance, in a paper on cases invalided from the Crimea and observed in the Military Hospital at Portsmouth, a Dr. Burgess used these heading quite indiscriminately.[38] In the medical journals there was some slight interest in reports from the French Medical Service. We find Dr. Milroy reading a paper to the Epidemiological Society on sickness and mortality rates in the French Army.[39] Among several papers by French authors there was reprinted a useful study of scurvy in the French Army.[40]

We find more enthusiasm for recording the Crimean experience in the field of surgery. The surgical section in the Medical History is informative but lacks the imprint of personal experience. Longmore did considerable research into the mortality rates in different campaigns and was especially interested in the effects of the new types of projectiles. His **Gunshot Injuries**, published in 1877, was his main work and much of the material was derived from his wide experience in the Crimean War.[41] The contribution of George Macleod was more practical than that of Longmore, albeit in his first publication he blithely and insensitively expressed regret that the war had ended just when there had begun to be marked improvements in the management of war wounds.

> It is, I have no hesitation in saying, a very great loss to the advancement of surgery, that this war has so soon come to a close. We were just beginning to forge ahead of the difficulties which beset its commencement, and a new era, during which much might have been accomplished, was beginning to dawn. As it is, little has, I fear, been added to the lessons taught by the experience of former wars.[42]

His observations and opinions had appeared in a series of four articles in the **Edinburgh Medical Journal** between 1855 and 1856.[43] These articles were expanded and published as a text in 1858, **Notes on the Surgery of the War in the Crimea**.[44] Macleod understood the influence of the new Minie rifle and the conical ball in producing by high velocity much more serious injury to soft tissue and splintering of bone than had occurred in earlier campaigns. In his text he devotes considerable space to compound fractures from gunshot wounds. He recognised that even if conservative treatment was adopted and there was initial survival, death was common later from prolonged infection or secondary haemorrhage. His analysis of the methods used in the Crimean War, his wide personal experience, his understanding of the conditions in which the surgeon had to work, and his appreciation of the influence of associated medical conditions on the survival or otherwise of his patients combined to produce one of the most intelligent surgical reviews of the period.

Lesser contributions came from Assistant-Surgeon Flower on amputations,[45] from Dr. Patrick Fraser on chest injuries (Fraser was one of the few against venesection in such cases),[46] from Dr. Charles Kidd on late complications of amputation,[47] from Assistant-Surgeon George Lawson on wounds of the chest,[48] and from

Assistant-Surgeon Jeffery Marston[49] on hospital gangrene.[50]

THE MEDICAL SERVICES IN LATER WARS

Between 1857 and 1860 Britain was involved in the Indian Mutiny and in the Second and Third China Wars. Until May 1858 Smith was Director-General and responsible for the army medical organisation in these wars, thereafter he was succeeded by Alexander. The Indian Mutiny broke out in May 1857.[51] Thus the campaign came too soon for the medical service to be greatly influenced by either its experience in the Crimean War or by the observations of the Royal Commission. The Crimean War had been fought over foreign soil, but the engagements of the Mutiny were fought on British territory. At the outbreak of the Mutiny there were already some 20,000 British troops East of Suez, although those were scattered widely over India, Persia and Burma. A medical organisation operated on a regimental basis, with small tented hospitals set up when needed and only a few fixed hospitals situated in or near the larger barracks or depots. An established supply system existed and there were considerable reserves of equipment of all kinds. Across a very wide area of India the British forces were engaged in major siege operations (for example, at Lucknow and Cawnpore), in long forced marches (in intense heat), and in frequent skirmishes and ambushes along the lines of communications. In such a campaign it was inevitable that there should be dependence largely on a regimental medical service, very few general or base hospitals being established.

As in the Crimea, fevers and bowel conditions headed the disease list. Heat-stroke, seldom recorded in the Crimea, accounted for a very large number of admissions and a total of 791 deaths.[52] There is little precise information concerning the frequency or the management of wounds. At times the conditions under which operations were done were primitive in the extreme, a description by Munro suggesting the eighteenth-century surgeon in action.[53] Clearly the only significant gain to the army medical service in India from the Crimean experience was the presence of a large proportion of regimental medical officers who had seen active service recently, who had learned to act independently, and who had had some experience of the immediate care of the wounded. Out of 300 army medical officers who served during the Mutiny approximately 110 had gained experience on active service in the Crimea.[54] The senior medical officer was Inspector-General William Linton. He had been one of the three officers sent out by Smith early in 1854 to investigate conditions in the East, and he had then served in responsible posts in the field and in the base hospitals.

Of the five awards of a V.C. to army doctors in the campaign, two were won by medical officers who had previously served in the Crimean War. Surgeon Anthony Home of the 90th Regiment was gazetted "for noble conduct at Lucknow in defence of the wounded".[55] Assistant-Surgeon William Bradshaw of the same regiment was gazetted "for distinguished bravery and devotion to the wounded".[56] At least four army medical officers were killed in action or died of wounds. One of these, Assistant-Surgeon Stuart Moore[57] had previously served in the Crimea. At least five died of disease, of whom three had previously served in the Crimea. These were Surgeon William Dumbreck[58], Assistant-Surgeon William Irwin[59], and Assistant-Surgeon Charles Nelson.[60]

As in the Crimea, a Naval Brigade was landed in support of the Army.[61] Some 750 officers and men from two ships were landed at Calcutta. Only three naval medical officers came ashore and these were all assistant-surgeons. Details of sickness and mortality rates are unknown. As in the Crimea, the Naval Brigade adapted well to their unaccustomed surroundings.

No female nurses worked in the army hospitals during the campaign. Miss Nightingale, although in poor health, wanted to go to India in 1857. She wrote offering her services to Lady Canning, who was now in Calcutta with her husband, the Viceroy of India. Lady Canning in a letter home gave her opinion.

> Miss Nightingale has written to me. She is out of health and at Malvern, but says she would come at twenty-four hours notice if I think there is anything to do 'in her line of business'. I think there is not anything

CHAPTER XVIII

here, for there are few wounded men in want of actual nursing ... The up-country hospitals are too scattered for a nursing establishment, and one could hardly yet send women up."[62]

In any case Herbert did not wish Miss Nightingale to go, for he needed her help in the work of the Royal Commission.[63] In February 1858 a leader in the **Lancet** pressed for nurses to be sent out to India, not "the ladies who did their ministering so gently and tenderly that poor fellows kissed their shadows as they passed ... but the homelier working women to whom nursing was a business and means of subsistence but whose aid and presence were vast comforts to soldiers lying wounded or dying in a strange land".[64]

The Indian Mutiny was swiftly followed by the China Wars.[65] Between 1858 and 1860 14,000 British troops were landed in China. The Principal Medical Officer was Deputy Inspector-General William Muir[66], who had served in the Crimea and was later to be Director-General. A generous number of medical officers was provided, one of whom, Staff Surgeon William Rutherford[67], was appointed specifically as a Sanitary Officer, the first occasion on which such an appointment was made. A considerable proportion of the medical officers had served in the Crimea. As in the Mutiny, the medical officers with Crimean experience must have made a major contribution towards the efficiency of the medical service during the campaign. An important feature of the expedition was the immediate provision of two 200-bedded hospital ships, the 'Mauritius' and the 'Melbourne', well-equipped with operating rooms and "all the latest appliances". Since transport was largely by river or sea, the hospital ships largely replaced field hospitals. Muir proved an able P.M.O. It appears that Cantlie's comment is well justified: "a successful campaign noteworthy for the excellence of its medical arrangements and the high standard of health which was maintained throughout. The troops were well fed and suitably clothed".[68] It appears that the mortality was little more than 3 per cent per annum.[69] Apparently some reforms had already been put to the test and had proved their worth.

EPILOGUE

POST-WAR CAREERS

The earlier career of Andrew Smith was described in Chapter II. At the end of the Crimean War he might have hoped for some relief from his worries and responsibilities. In the immediate post-war period there were strong hints from his critics that he should be removed from office, but he was able to ignore this pressure. He was determined to see out all the enquiries and to justify his actions as completely as possible before he retired from the scene. He was encouraged by the support of the majority of the medical profession. Many influential bodies gave him honorary degrees and passed votes of confidence in him. In August 1856, for instance, the Royal College of Surgeons of Edinburgh elected Smith an Honorary Fellow. To crown the many academic honours he had already received, in 1857 Smith was elected a Fellow of the Royal Society. This was awarded for his pre-war studies in zoology and comparative anatomy.

In May 1858 he resigned, and in July he was appointed K.C.B. Many of his critics had now been silenced but **The Times** made yet another scathing attack on him. "He is to be shelved at last, and to be consigned to a splendid insignificance ... It is the fault of injudicious patrons and friends if they have thrust upon him honours which he has neither wanted nor earned."[70] Exhausted and prematurely aged (he was now only 61) by the strain of his position, and by chronic ill-health, Smith retreated from public life. After the death of his wife in 1864 he became a recluse, and he eventually died, aged 75, in 1872.

The obituaries in the medical journals were relatively short, only summarising his career and making little of his versatility.[71] The **Lancet**, however, concluded its obituary with the following tribute. "He was an excellent representative of the class to which Sir James MacGrigor, Sir William Burnett, and other equally energetic Scotsmen belonged. A class not without its foibles or its failings, but distinguished by its sterling ability, high sense of duty, and exemplary suit and service to crown and country." Few men in high position had been subjected to such bitter and exaggerated attacks. In fact, in the face of great administrative difficulties and of divided loyalties to many masters, and although ill-paid and with meagre staff, he emerges as an able Director-General.

The career of Hall before 1854 was described in Chapter II. He served in Bulgaria from June 1854, landed in Eupatoria in September, and remained in the Crimea for 22 months. When he returned home in July 1856 it may be presumed that he served on the staff of the Director-General and that he assisted in the preparation of the medical history of the war. However, in the introduction to this work Smith makes no acknowledgement of help from Hall. Before leaving the Crimea Hall had been awarded the K.C.B. This was the result of a strong recommendation to Lord Panmure from Smith, who wrote of Hall as "possessing an iron frame, an aptitude and ability for work, and a mental capacity which falls to the lot of few. The public has made Dr. Hall an object of vengeance and although the Director-General is far from believing for one moment that the Government has in any way countenanced this endeavour, the omission of his name in the recognition of services rendered in the field gives his traducers to infer that he has merited the obloquy so profusely cast upon him." Continuing his eloquent appeal, Smith "earnestly implores, nay prays, that some step may be taken to sweeten the bitter cup that officer has been called to drink, and that Dr. Hall and his friends may not have the mortification of thinking that a first rate medical officer should have been on the Director General's recommendation sent to the Crimea, there to lose what is dearer than life itself, a good name which till then the public service had secured for him". In their correspondence throughout the war Smith had always expressed admiration for Hall's work and had realised that he had been criticised unjustly. This plea on behalf of Hall was generous, for Smith himself had to wait rather longer for his K.C.B. Cantlie has recorded that Miss Nightingale sent a polite note of congratulation. But her true feelings were expressed in a letter to Herbert soon after she heard of Hall's honour. "We in the Crimea know it, and we know and knew at the time, what filled the Crimean graves last winter. K.C.B., I believe, now means Knight of the Crimean Burying

Grounds."[72] It is perhaps unlikely that Hall heard of this malicious remark, but he was soon to realise that any ambition on his part to succeed Smith as Director-General was certain to be thwarted by Miss Nightingale.

Hall retired on half-pay in January 1857. He spent his remaining years attempting to vindicate his actions during the war and to answer all his critics. Before he returned to England he had sent a long letter to Smith correcting many errors printed in the final report of the Commission headed by McNeill and Tulloch. In April 1856, he sent an even longer document to Smith, placing in one column quotations from the Commissioner's report and in the opposite column his own interpretation of the facts.[73] This document gives convincing evidence that Hall was well justified in defending his reputation. Letters and pamphlets of this nature continued to flow from Hall's pen for several years. In his last years Hall travelled abroad in an attempt to cure his chronic ill-health.[74] He finally settled in Italy and died at Pisa in 1866.

The medical journals published only brief accounts of Hall's career,[75] with no hint of the criticisms to which he had been subjected, with no suggestion that he had been faced with an exceptionally difficult task in the Crimea, and with no admission that if he had faults he also had many virtues. Perhaps it was inevitable that because Hall was so closely involved during the whole of the campaign he should be attacked even more harshly than Smith, who could at least plead some ignorance of the state of the medical services because of the distance which separated him from events. Despite the efforts of Mitra, his rather partisan biographer, and of Barnsley, his more recent protagonist, Hall has not been given fair recognition for his work. Particularly in some of the biographies of Florence Nightingale, Hall comes in for excessive condemnation. This is not least the case in Woodham-Smith's 1950 biography. A critic has drawn attention to many erroneous statements in this work.[76] For instance, it greatly exaggerates Hall's involvement in the scandal of the Hounslow flogging case; it suggests wrongly that Hall had no medical qualification prior to 1845; it misinterprets Hall's directive on anaesthesia; and it paints a picture of Hall as a ruthless disciplinarian, even sadistic and cruel, all on the most slender evidence. In fact, Hall's letters show that he was a sensitive and caring doctor throughout his career. There is a revealing passage in a letter to his wife, sent when he was in South Africa. A woman under his care died in child birth and Hall was with her at the end. "All these things are painful and though doctors are generally accused of being insensible to such scenes, I must confess I have never been able to surmount the unpleasant feeling they create in my mind. I suppose nature never intended me for the profession I have, by some accident, selected." There were periods of doubt and depression when he was, without warning, transferred from Bombay to the East. Most of all he hated the long separation from his wife and child. "God only knows when I shall see you all again ... I go on this service with a heavy heart and without the expectation of reward of any kind."

An entry in Hall's diary in November 1854, following the accusations of negligence in the 'Avon' case, records the strain under which he had to work and a tendency amoting to almost a persecution mania on his part.

> This day Lord Raglan issued a severe general order censuring Dr. Lawson and blaming me for not having the ship properly found. I put the Inspector's report into his own hand for it was ample for everything ... it is quite evident he is preparing for enquiry and his intention is to throw as much discredit on the Medical Department as he can and to make a scapegoat for other mismanagements and I it will be, I dare say, as the weakest always goes to the wall and we have no friends to protect us.[77]

This and other evidence suggests that in November 1854 Hall was near breaking point. It is to his credit that he remained at his post and faced his difficulties.

As senior medical officer to the British Army in the East Hall had found himself in a very difficult position. The medical department was considered the least important in the army as far as stores, transport, staffing and accommodation were concerned. Miss Nightingale's first biographer, in a very fair assessment, wrote - "Dr. Hall was the victim of a false position. He had been appointed Medical Inspector-General in the Crimea when he was still in India, and he did not arrive on the scene in time to think out the preparations properly".[78] Hall had little executive power. Raglan, the Commander-in-Chief, had scant appreciation of the problems of the medical service, observing and then intervening only in relation to the most trivial matters. The machinery by which changes or reforms could be effected was time-consuming and highly complicated, always involving a heavy load of paper work. It is remarkable how Hall stood up to all the problems he encountered. He did not, like some senior officers, take the easy way out and contrive to be invalided.

To many observers Hall appeared somewhat weak and lacking in imagination. Longmore described him as "a theorist, all his faith seems pinned in returns, I have seen no evidence of his being a practical man".[79] Hall laid himself open to harsh criticism because he visited the base hospitals at Scutari only once after the fighting started in the Crimea. In his dealing with Miss Nightingale he could have been more understanding and co-operative. But he was not alone in believing that she had been sent as an informer who was to report directly to Herbert and others of influence at home. In addition, Hall was of a generation which did not accept readily that a woman should be given such authority and power.

Hall died a disappointed man. He was not chosen to succeed Smith. Not a great deal of notice was taken of the numerous pamphlets and letters in which he had tried to justify himself. To quote a later epitaph -

> Thus passed away ... an honourable and upright servant of the Queen, one whose keen sense of duty upheld him through all vicissitudes of his long and arduous military career. For forty-one years he served his country in various parts of the globe, and during this time he proved a hard worker, a strict disciplinarian, a man not of words but of action ... the medical profession can count many a distinguished name on its roll of honour, but none whose success has been more nobly and worthily attained.[80]

To this day a picture is given, quite unfairly, of a stupid, incompetent and stubborn person. No one can say that Hall was a great man, yet some recognition should be afforded to him for the way in which he laboured to correct the formidable situation that overwhelmed the army medical service.

Six army medical officers, all of whom had served in the Crimea, each in turn became Medical Director-General of the Army. All six had qualified in Scotland, and all were

Scotsmen except Crawford, who was from Ulster. No one was more interested in these appointments than Miss Nightingale. On the resignation of Smith, she was determined that Alexander should be chosen as Director-General, for she believed that he would support her in all her projected reforms. The early death of Alexander while in office was a great blow to Miss Nightingale. She did not approve of the selection of Gibson as his successor, knowing that he was likely to be influenced greatly by those less committed to reform.

Thomas Alexander[81] landed with the original expeditionary force and in Bulgaria was attached as a staff-surgeon to the Light Division. In January 1856 he was given the local rank of Inspector-General in Turkey. When he came home he was almost at once sent to Canada, but largely through the influence of Miss Nightingale he was brought back to England to serve on the Royal Commission. He became Director-General in June 1858. During his short tenure of the office, Alexander appeared at first to be highly successful. He had much to do with a Royal Warrant greatly improving the status and terms of service of medical officers and increasing the powers of the Director-General. His unexpected and sudden death in 1860 was a great loss.

James Gibson[82] had been a staff-surgeon in the Crimea and was personal physician to the Duke of Cambridge. In 1860 largely by the inflluence of the Duke of Cambridge (now Commander-in-Chief), Gibson was appointed Director-General. During Gibson's term of office the progress of reform was slow and the Medical Department stagnated. In 1867 Thomas Logan[83] became Director-General. He had served with distinction in the Crimea as P.M.O. of the Highland Division. He filled the post of Director-General with great ability. When in 1874 William Muir[84] took office the Medical Service had improved beyond recognition. Muir had served as a regimental surgeon in the Crimea. His directorate was seen as "one of the most formative" in the development of the department. Muir was succeeded in 1882 by Thomas Crawford[85], who also had served in the Crimea as a regimental surgeon. He was a competent Director but fell foul of various committees particularly over alleged defects of the medical organisation during the war in Egypt in 1882 and over a fall in the recruitment of medical officers. However he resisted all attacks and protected the interests of the army doctors. William Mackinnon[86], who took office in 1889, had served as a regimental assistant-surgeon in the Crimean War. A man of great character, less interested in administration than in surgery, he retired in 1896 leaving a service, following this succession of directors-general, substantially reshaped and improved to face the new century.

As well as the Directors-General, reference must be made to Thomas Longmore[87], who served for most of the Crimean War as Surgeon to the 19th Regiment. He was an outspoken critic of the medical service, both in his evidence to the Commissioners and in his letters home. After the war Longmore served in the Indian Mutiny and received rapid promotion to Deputy Inspector-General in 1858. Having gained a considerable reputation as a surgeon, on his return from India in 1860 he was appointed Professor of Surgery in the Army Medical School, being strongly recommended for this post by his friend Alexander. Longmore proved an able teacher of surgery and was an authority also on field organisation, transport and equipment. He published many useful texts, including studies relating to his experiences in the Crimean War. He relinquished his Chair in 1893. Longmore was outstanding as a regimental surgeon, as one who learned from his experience in the field, and as one who made it his life-work to transmit his knowledge to the future generations of army surgeons. It was said of him on his retiral, "the progress of military surgery for the last thirty years was more intimately associated with the name of Longmore than with any other".

THE NAVAL MEDICAL SERVICE AFTER THE WAR

The losses in the Navy during the war have been given in Chapter XV. Of the estimated 2,029 deaths of officers and men 77 per cent were due to disease, 12 per cent to accidents, and 11 per cent to wounds in action. The total of officers and men serving throughout the campaign in the two fleets and in the forces ashore is uncertain, but the losses do not seem excessive considering the climatic conditions and the hardships afloat and ashore. The number of medical officers who died during the war was only five, all of disease.[88] This was a small proportion considering the risk on board ship of contracting infective conditions such as cholera.

Unlike the Army Department, the Naval Medical Department escaped severe criticism, either of its pre-war planning or of its conduct during the campaign. At no time during or immediately after the war was any Commission or Committee appointed to enquire into alleged deficiencies. The low pay and poor conditions of service were only partially corrected during the war, when in 1855 the assistant-surgeons were granted ward-room status and allowed a single cabin (always provided that the commanding officer would allocate this, which in practice he seldom did). Not until 1859 did the naval doctors reach a level of payment equivalent to that of the army doctors. In 1875 the rank of assistant-surgeon was abolished and new entries were immediately rated Surgeons, a change which should have encouraged recruitment. The limited reforms which were a consequence of the Crimean War experience can be related to the careers of successive Directors-General. Sir William Burnett resigned in April 1855.

Burnett's successor, John Liddel[89], served with distinction at the battle of Navarino. He did not serve in the East during the Crimean War but had held responsible home appointments before becoming Director-General in 1855. During his term of office some important reforms were introduced, for example, improvements in the ventilation of ships. Alexander Bryson[90] became Director-General in 1864. He did not see active service in the Crimean War. He had done important work on the statistical methods employed in the medical service, but had never served in a naval hospital. As a result he was not a success as Director-General. He was succeeded in 1869 by Alexander Armstrong[91], who had served in the Baltic Fleet during the Crimean War as a surgeon, after making a name for himself in Polar exploration. Armstrong ensured that the medical service kept pace with the rapid advances in medicine and surgery at this time. In 1880 he was followed by John Watt Reid[92], who had served in the Black Sea Fleet in 1854 as an assistant-surgeon and been commended for his work during the cholera epidemic. During his eight years of office a Naval Medical School was established at Haslar Hospital, a Sick Berth Staff was introduced on a firm foundation, and female nurses were admitted to the naval hospitals.

Burnett and the four Directors-General who followed him were Scottish graduates. Two of the four had seen active service in the Crimean War. But the medical officer who distinguished himself most in the Crimean War was David Deas.[93] He rose rapidly in rank on account of his notable success in charge of naval personnel, afloat and ashore, in the Black Sea Fleet. By many it was considered that Deas rather than Bryson should have succeeded Liddel. In the event, however, he was himself retired, in 1867, at the age of 50, and was not subsequently recalled. Deas had contributed greatly to the good record of the Naval Medical Service during the Crimean War and was the most outstanding naval doctor on active service throughout the campaign. It is unfortunate that he is dismissed in the standard history of the naval medical service in only one line - "Much of the credit for the better record of the Navy must go to Inspector of the Fleet, Dr. David Deas".

The commitments of the Navy after the Crimean War did not often extend beyond the routine maintenance of 'Pax Britannica'. There was some involvement in the China War of 1858-1860, with 35 deaths in action, 110 deaths from cholera, and 239 deaths from dysentery.[94] The participation of a Naval Brigade in the Indian Mutiny has already been described. Between the Crimean War and the Great War of 1914-1918 there were no wars during which any major action was fought at sea. In consequence naval medical officers had little experience of war surgery. But in peace time it was necessary to make a constant effort to improve the general hygiene of fleets and of shore establishments, to control infective conditions more effectively, and to prevent disease.

An indirect result of the Crimean War was a vast improvement in the system of returns of the sick and wounded, instigated by Bryson.[95] In addition to a slow improvement in the ventilation systems of ships, the experience in the Crimea may be held to have influenced the introduction of safer water supplies on board ships, particularly by the use of distillation plants. But the most important gain was the gradual reform of the pay and promotion system, and of the general conditions of service of the naval doctor, the previous indifference to which had greatly discouraged recruitment to the medical service.

MISS NIGHTINGALE

On her return to England, Miss Nightingale threw herself into the immense labour involved in the preparations for the Royal Commission, in its procedure and report, and, not least, in the implementation of its recommendations. In 1858, as part of her determination to improve the lot of the British soldier, she pressed for the appointment of a Sanitary Commission for India.[96] Herbert was elected President of this Commission in May 1859 but was to die before the work was completed, and he was replaced by Lord Stanley. Four of the Commissioners were firm allies of Miss Nightingale: Alexander, Farr, Martin and Sutherland (of whom three had served on the Royal Commission). A lengthy report was published in 1863, written by Miss Nightingale and Dr. Sutherland. Appended to the second and third editions was a separate paper incorporating the personal observations of Miss Nightingale on the evidence.[97] For another twenty years Miss Nightingale was to exert a continuous influence on health affairs in India, not only those of the army but also those of the civilian population.

In 1859 Miss Nightingale turned her attention to the reform of the civil hospitals in Great Britain.[98] It was not until after the Crimean War that she became fully aware of the unsatisfactory state of these hospitals, even of some of the prestigious teaching institutions in London. In her **Notes on Hospitals,** published in the same year, she outlined the defects which required correction and stated her criteria for adequate ventilation, drainage, bed spacing, washing and toilet accommodation. Soon she was being consulted by doctors and administrators from all over the country, about either

EPILOGUE

the improvement of existing hospitals or the planning of new ones.

In November 1855 a public meeting had been called in London to discuss how Miss Nightingale's great work in the Crimean War could best be recognised. It was agreed to raise a 'Nightingale Fund' in her honour, by means of which there would be established, "an Institution for the training, sustenance, and protection of Nurses and Hospital Attendants".[99] A sum of £44,000 was soon collected, part of it from small contributions from the soldiers in the Crimea. She decided to found a Training School in St. Thomas's Hospital. Within a year fifteen probationer nurses had completed their training and been placed in other hospitals, to spread teaching methods, discipline, and the high moral standards of the St. Thomas course. The Training School gained a considerable reputation and became the pattern for other schools. Through these the nursing system in Britain was reformed and the status of the hospital nurse greatly improved.

Miss Nightingale also had had great influence, between 1861 and 1866, on the reform of Poor Law Administration and on the improvement of the conditions in workhouse hospitals. For instance, she collaborated with the philanthropist, William Rathbone, in the introduction of fully trained nurses to the Liverpool Workhouse Infirmary. A small group of nurses was sent by Miss Nightingale, to serve there under Miss Agnes Jones, one of Miss Nightingale's best pupils in the St. Thomas's School, and, in less than three years the conditions in the Workhouse Infirmary were transformed.[100] Miss Nightingale undertook many other humanitarian activities. She was consulted about the Census Bill of 1860, but her useful recommendation that details of the chronic sick and disabled should be included in the return was not accepted.[101] Again, prior to the Geneva Convention of 1864, as a result of which the Red Cross Society was founded, she was asked to advise the War Office on this innovation. When M. Henri Dunant read a paper in London in 1872 his opening words were as follows. "Though I am known as the founder of the Red Cross and the originator of the Convention of Geneva, it is to an

English woman that all the honour of that Convention is due. What inspired me ... was the work of Miss Florence Nightingale in the Crimea."[102] Again, during the Franco-Prussian War she gave advice to the various charitable organisations which carried help to the wounded of both sides.[103]

To some the reputation of Florence Nightingale rests almost entirely on her work at Scutari and her introduction of female nurses, thus initiating the reform of nursing in Great Britain. However it was not her activity at Scutari which in the end gained for her so much worldwide appreciation, rather it was her later activities which were most influential. Sir John McNeill wrote to her in December 1857, when she was so deeply involved in the preparations for the Royal Commission - "The nation is grateful for what you did at Scutari, but all that it was possible for you to do there was a trifle compared with the good you are doing now".[104]

A small group of doctors assisted Miss Nightingale in her work. Dr. John Sutherland first met Miss Nightingale when he came out to Scutari at the head of the Sanitary Commission early in 1855. Thereafter, for thirty-six years he acted as her adviser. To him, she admitted, she owed all her knowledge of Sanitary Science. He collaborated in collecting material for the Commissions and enquiries in which she was involved, and in writing the final reports. If Miss Nightingale was at times carried away by her ideas and impetuous in her criticisms, Sutherland provided cautious advice and urged her to "soften down her doctrines". Sir John McNeill was another favourite of Miss Nightingale. He first met her in the East when he came out with the Supplies Commission, and he then worked closely with her for some thirty years. He was of particular help in the preparations for the Royal Commission, providing her with details or army organisation which otherwise would have been inaccessible to her, but he also played a large part in the organisation of the Training School for Nurses. Among other doctors first met by Miss Nightingale at Scutari was Henry Parkes. He was appointed Professor of Hygiene at the Army Medical School, and until he died in 1876 he remained closely in touch with Miss Nightingale and kept her informed of all developments in the School. Dr. William Aitken who had come out with Dr. Lyons as a pathologist and who subsequently became Professor of Pathology at the Army Medical School, also kept in close touch with Miss Nightingale over the progress of the School.

After the war Dr. William Farr collaborated with Miss Nightingale for many years. He was of great assistance to her in the preparation of statistical tables for the Commissions. There were many other civilian doctors who corresponded with Miss Nightingale or collaborated with her on specific problems. Sir James Paget of St. Bartholomew's Hospital supported Miss Nightingale in her attempts to introduce better records in the civilian hospitals - she admired Paget more than any other contemporary surgeon. Even before the war Miss Nightingale had known Sir James Clark, and she was frequently given good advice by him. He supported her in all her causes, and was in a position to enlist the help of Queen Victoria in the furtherance of medical reform.

The course of events which allowed Miss Nightingale to enter the field of nursing, and the friendship with Herbert, through which he selected her to take a band of nurses to Scutari, triggered off a remarkable sequence of major reforms of the Army Medical Service, of civil nursing, of hospital design, and of many other fields of medicine, sanitary science, and social science. Of the many humanitarian pioneers of the Victorian era she stands out as one of the greatest.

It is relevant to refer at this point to the complex character of Florence Nightingale to remind the reader how it was she achieved so much during the Crimean War (and afterwards), but also how it was that she failed to be easily understood, indeed was frequently misunderstood, by many of those with whom she came in contact, particularly by regular army doctors hidebound by tradition. Of the many assessments of Florence Nightingale's character that by her early biographer, Cook, remains the most convincing, since it was made by one who was brought up in the Victorian age and was in a position to talk with many individuals who had known his subject. Later assessments have been slighter and tending to caricature, either because of the fashion set by Strachey of debunking eminent Victorians, or because writers have been more concerned to produce readable and popular works, often by over-dramatisation. In 1913 Cook wrote as follows.

> She was a woman of strong passions - not over-given to praise, not quick to forgive; somewhat prone to be censorious, not apt to forget. She was not only a gentle angel of compassion; she was more of a logician than a sentimentalist. She knew that to do good work requires a hard head as well as a soft heart ... Miss Nightingale knew hardly any fault which seemed worse to her in a man than to be unbusiness-like; in a woman, than to be 'only enthusiastic'. She found no use for angels without hands ... She had an equal contempt for those who act without knowledge, and for those whose knowledge leads to no useful action. She was herself laborious of detail and scrupulously careful of her premises ... When once her decision was taken, she was resolute and masterful - not lightly turned from her course, impatient of delay, not very tolerant of opposition ... The greatness of Miss Nightingale's character, and the secret of her life's work, consist in the union of qualities not often found in the same man or woman ... She was possessed by infinite compassion. Pity for the sick and sorrowful - a passionate desire to serve them - devotion to her 'children', the common soldiers - sympathy with the voiceless peasants of India: these were the ruling motives of her life ... Miss Nightingale's own peculiar genius was for administration and order; and she had to employ her genius within the fields of opportunity which her sex and her circumstances offered ... She was intensely conscious of a special destiny, and the tenacity with which in the face of many obstacles she clung to her sense of vocation enabled her to fulfil it.[105]

CONCLUSION

While it is appropriate to end this account with a recognition of the heroic and progressive role of Florence Nightingale, initiated by her involvement in the Crimean War, the opportunity may be taken to pay belated tribute to the doctors - military, naval and civilian - who played a no less worthy part in the campaign. Their devotion to duty, their courage, and their skills were not widely or substantially appreciated in the immediate post-war period. Army doctors who served in the Crimean Peninsula were awarded the Crimea War Medal, with bars for involvement in the actions of the Alma, Inkerman, Balaclava, and the siege of Sebastopol.[106] But army doctors who served only in the base hospitals were awarded no campaign medal, despite their greater risk of disease or even death. Naval doctors who served in the Baltic Fleet in 1854 or 1855 were entitled to the Baltic Medal, while those serving in the Naval Division or in the Marines ashore, together with some of those in designated warships in the Black Sea Fleet, were eligible for the Crimean War Medal, with appropriate bars (for instance, for the expedition to the Sea of Azov). A few of the civilian doctors who were transferred to the Crimea received the campaign medal, but those who worked only in the base hospitals had no such award. With the exception of the three doctors who were in retrospect awarded the Victoria Cross, the regimental surgeons and assistant-surgeons had no special recognition. French and Turkish campaign medals were awarded to selected medical officers, usually those of some seniority or those who had at some time assisted the Turkish Medical Service. After the war there occurred a moderately generous hand-out of orders of various grades, of which some were well deserved but many were only in virtue of seniority, as well as a reciprocal exchange of such decorations between the three allied governments.[107] Only the Turks awarded decorations to the medical officers of the Turkish Contingent.

Those medical officers who died in the Crimea were buried in the Divisional or Regimental Cemeteries scattered along the valleys and over the bleak uplands of the peninsula.[108] In the well-tended British Military Cemetery at Scutari, the grave-stones of most of the doctors who died in the base hospitals can still be seen.[109] At home a handsome memorial to the army doctors was erected in 1864 in the grounds of Netley Hospital, although regrettably the list of inscribed names was incomplete and inaccurate in other respects. But in 1973, a few years after the demolition of the main part of the hospital, the memorial was destroyed.

Scattered throughout the British Isles, in cathedrals and churches, are the names of some of the doctors who died, names inscribed either on regimental tablets or, more rarely, on individual memorials. The hero Thompson, who cared for Russian prisoners after the Alma, is commemorated by an obelisk on a hill near Forres, his birthplace. Alexander, dying while serving as the first post-war Director-General, has a statue at his birthplace, Prestonpans.

The political and international gains of the Crimean War may have been negligible but the sacrifices were not entirely in vain. Many factors, such as the public exposure of the appalling conditions of the campaign and the findings of numerous commissions, led to a general reform of the army, producing not least a more humane attitude to the common soldier. As far as the medical services were concerned, despite the strong recommendations of the Royal Commission reform was slow. Sadly it must be said that, in subsequent campaigns, even up to the two World Wars, some of the old errors were repeated. The dictum **si vis pace pare bellum** is never readily acted upon. In times of peace, expenditure is inevitably cut and the medical services suffer perhaps more than most. At the end of a war, many medical officers are retired and their experience is lost to the services. Hence, at the start of both the First and Second World Wars, the hard earned experience of previous campaigns was often forgotten and lessons had to be painfully re-learned. This applied particularly to the techniques of dealing with tissue-destructive wounds. A less pessimistic view is tenable following the Falkland War of the early 1980s, admittedly a small-scale campaign. Here it was possible to deploy at short notice a highly trained medical staff skilled in the most up-to-date techniques. The high standard of medical and surgical work owed much to the close co-operation of three services, and perhaps to the fact that, since the Second World War, service doctors on promotion to higher ranks are now often allowed to continue in clinical work, rather than being lost to this by the burden of purely administrative duties.

The medical departments of the armed services have evolved over many centuries. It is proper to conclude by suggesting that the high traditions of service doctors in more recent times owe something to the devotion and dedication of those of their predecessors who served in the face of exceptional hardships, constant problems, and often great peril, on several fronts during the Crimean War.

NOTES

1. **Med. Surg. Hist.**, 2:251, "Return showing primary admissions into hospitals of the Army in the East from 10th April 1854, to 30th June 1856, also deaths in Regimental and General Hospitals, in Hospital Ships, or suddenly from violence with the exception of those which occurred in action with the enemy".
2. F.H. Garrison, **Notes on the history of military medicine** (Washington, U.S.A., 1922), 171-172. See also R.L. Reid, 'The British Crimean disaster - ineptness or inevitability?', **Military Medicine** (1955), 420-426; also Cantlie, 2:185.
3. Garrison, **Notes**, 171.
4. Garrison, **Notes**, 172.
5. A. Seaton, **The Crimean War: a Russian chronicle** (London, 1977), 15.
6. **Royal Commission**, 405.
7. **M.T.G.** (1856), 1:645.
8. For accounts of the American doctors, see A. Parry, 'American doctors in the Crimean War', **South Atlantic Quarterly**, 54 (1955), 478-490; J.I. Waring, 'The journal of Dr. William Joseph Holt in the Crimean War', **South Carolina Med.J.**, 62 (1966), 24-28.
9. **Report from the Select Committee on Medical Department Army** (London, 1856). For the findings of this Committee, see **Cantlie**, 2:196-200; P.R. Kirby, **Sir Andrew Smith** (Cape Town, 1965), 323-324.
10. Thomas Balfour (1813-1891); L.R.C.S.Ed. 1833; M.D. Edinburgh 1834; joined as assistant-surgeon 1836; surgeon 1848; D.I.G. 1859; Head of Statistical Branch of the Army Medical Department 1859-1873; F.R.C.P. 1860 (obituary **B.M.J.** (1891), 1:204-2205; **Munk**; **Drew**; **DNB**).
11. **Report of the Commissioners appointed to enquire into the regulations affecting the sanitary condition of the army, of the organisation of military hospitals and the treatment of the sick and wounded, with evidence and appendix** (London, 1858).
12. George Beatson (1814-1874); L.R.C.S., M.D. Glasgow 1836; joined as assistant-surgeon 1838; staff-surgeon December 1854; served in the East September 1854 - June 1856; P.M.O. India 1863 - 1868, 1873 until death on service, in rank of S.G. (obituary **B.M.J.** (1874), 1:822; **Drew**; **DNB**).
13. John Taylor (1810-1892); joined as assistant-surgeon 1833; staff-surgeon March 1854; served in the East March 1855 - May 1856; retired 1863 as I.G. (obituary **Lancet** (1893), 1:65; **Plarr**; **Drew**).
14. **Royal Commission**, 1-8, 249-263, 327-333.
15. Ibid., 361-389.
16. Lord Stanmore, **Sydney Herbert. Lord Herbert of Lea: A memoir** (2 vols., London, 1906), 2:133-134.
17. For general accounts of the planning and building of Netley Hospital, see **Cantlie**, 2:211-214; **B.M.J.** (1966), 1:412-413.
18. E. Cook, **The Life of Florence Nightingale** (2 vols., London, 1913), 1:340-342. See also **B.M.J.** (1857), 1:450-451, 502-503, 528; **Royal Commssion**, 235-238, 316.
19. **Cantlie**, 2:217-233. Miss Nightingale failed at this stage to persuade the Army to establish a female nursing service - for the excessive delay in achieving this, see A. Summers, **Angels and Citizens** (London, 1988).
20. **Medical and Surgical History of the British Army which served in Turkey and the Crimea during the War against Russia in the years 1854-1855-1856**, vol. I, 'Military Medical History of individual Corps'; vol. II, 'Part I, History of disease: Part II, History of wounds and injury', 'Presented to both Houses of Parliament' (London, 1858). The copy I have used has bound with it a 21-page supplement and numerous statistical tables entitled, 'Mortality of the British Army, at home, at home and abroad and during the Russian War, as compared with the civilian population in England' (London,

1858). Although there is no acknowledgement, the statistics in this supplement undoubtedly originated from Dr. William Farr and Miss Nightingale.
21. William Hanbury (1823-1865); L.R.C.S.I. 1845; joined as assistant-surgeon 1846; staff-surgeon November 1854; served in the East November 1854 - June 1856 (**Drew**).
22. **Med. Surg. Hist.**, 1:469-496.
23. Ibid., 1:512-522.
24. Ibid., 522-524.
25. Ibid., 524-525.
26. Ibid., 526-530.
27. Ibid., 531-554.
28. Ibid., 555-558.
29. Ibid., 2:1-35.
30. Ibid., 34-201.
31. Ibid., 202-226.
32. Ibid., 227-245.
33. Ibid., 253-396.
34. Ibid., 465-480.
35. These tables were printed, without pagination, after p.480.
36. J.N. Radcliffe, **The hygiene of the Turkish Army** (London, 1858) - reviewed in **M.T.G.** (1858), 1:123.
37. E.A. Parkes, **A manual of practical hygiene prepared especially for use in the medical service of the army** (London, 1864).
38. T. Burgess, 'Studies of the surgery of the war from the Military Hospital, Portsmouth', **Lancet** (1856), 1:650-652.
39. G. Milroy, 'The sickness and mortality in the French Army in the Crimea from 1854-56', **M.T.G.** (1858), 1:466-467.
40. - Perrin, 'Scorbutus as observed in the French Army in the Crimea', **M.T.G.** (1858), 1:145-146.
41. T. Longmore, **Gunshot injuries: their history, characteristic features, complications, and general treatment: with statistics concerning them as they are met with in warfare** (London, 1877).
42. **Ed.Med.J.**, 1 (1855), 984.
43. G.H.B. Macleod, 'Notes on surgery of the war', **Ed.Med.J.**, 1 (1855), 984-1001, 1063-1087; 2 (1856), 37-55, 193-207.
44. G.H.B. Macleod, **Notes on the surgery of the war in the Crimea** (London, 1858).
45. W.H. Flower, 'Primary amputation in the Crimea', **M.T.G.** (18??), 1:308-309.
46. P. Fraser, **A treatise upon penetrating wounds of the chest** (London, 1859).
47. C. Kidd, 'On osteomyelitis after amputation', **Ass.Med.J.**, 7 (1856), 559-567.
48. G. Lawson, **On gunshot wounds of the thorax** (London, 1858).
49. Jeffrey Marston (1831-1911); L.S.A., M.R.C.S., M.D. St. Andrews 1854; joined as assistant-surgeon November 1854; served in the East March 1856 - June 1856; F.R.C.S. 1858; head of Statistical and Sanitary Department of Army 1882-1888; retired as S.G. 1889 (obituary **Lancet** (1911), 1:974-975; **Plarr; Drew**).
50. J. Marston, 'On the secondary affections resulting from gunshot wounds', **M.T.G.** (1857), 2:83-85, 243-245.
51. For a general account of the Mutiny, see C. Hibbert, **The Great Mutiny: India 1857** (London, 1978); for medical accounts, see **Cantlie**, 2:238-250; G.A. Kempthorne, 'Events in India 1857-1858', **J.R.A.M.C.**, (1931), 134-147, 223-229.
52. Detailed statistics are not readily found, but see **Cantlie**, 2:248.
53. Munro, **Records of Services and Campaigns in many lands** (London, 1887), 234-235.

54. This figure is derived from **Drew**, by extracting the names of medical officers awarded the service medal for the campaign. There may have been some acting assistant-surgeons.
55. For Home's citation, see [Anon.], **The medical Victoria Crosses** (Aldershot, n.d.).
56. William Bradshaw (1830-1861); L.R.C.S.I. 1854; joined as assistant-surgeon 1854; served in the East November 1854 - December 1855, April - July 1856; retired 1860 (obituary **M.T.G.** (1861), 1:310; **Drew**). For Bradshaw's citation, see [Anon.], **The medical Victoria Crosses**.
57. Stuart Moore (1828-1857); joined as assistant-surgeon 1851; served in the East April 1854 - May 1856 (**Drew**).
58. William Dumbreck (1834-1858); joined as assistant-surgeon April 1854; served in East April 1854 - May 1856 (**Drew**).
59. William Irwin (d. 1857); joined as assistant-surgeon February 1855; served in the East May 1855 - October 1855 (**Drew**).
60. Charles Nelson (d. 1857); joined as assistant-surgeon November 1854; served in the East for the duration (**Drew**).
61. W.B. Rowbotham, **The Naval Brigade in the Indian Mutiny** (Navy Records Society, London, 1947).
62. Cook, **Nightingale**, 1:371.
63. C. Woodham-Smith, **Florence Nightingale 1820-1910** (London, 1950), 316.
64. **Lancet** (1858), 1:175.
65. For a medical account of the China Wars, see **Cantlie**, 2:251-154; G.A. Kempthorne, 'The Army Medical Services (1857-69)', **J.R.A.M.C.**, 58 (1931), 54-69.
66. For Muir, see note 84.
67. William Rutherford (1816-1887); L.R.C.S.I. 1835; joined as assistant-surgeon 1841; M.D. Glasgow 1845; surgeon 1852; served in the East November 1854 - December 1855, October 1855 - June 1856; retired 1876 as S.G. (obituary **Lancet** (1887), 1:696; **Drew**).
68. Cantlie, 2:253.
69. Cook, **Nightingale**, 1:398.
70. **The Times**, 14.7.1858.
71. **B.M.J.** (1872, 2:230; **Lancet** (1872), 2:245; **M.T.G.** (1872), 2:244-245.
72. I.B. O'Malley, **Florence Nightingale 1820-1856** (London, 1931), 379.
73. S.N. Mitra, **Life and Letters of Sir John Hall** (London, 1911), 480-503.
74. The entries in the last years of 'Hall's Diary' are full of details of his search for a climate and diet which might improve his health.
75. **B.M.J.** (1866), 1:109.
76. W.H. Greenleaf, 'Biography and the amateur historian: Mrs. Woodham-Smith's Florence Nightingale', **Victorian Studies** (1959), 190-192.
77. 'Hall Diary', 11.11.1854
78. Cook, **Nightingale**, 1:288
79. **Cantlie**, 2:406.
80. R.E. Barnsley, 'Sir John Hall', **Transactions of the Cumberland and Westmorland Antiquarian and Archaeological Society**, 46 (1966), 418.
81. For Alexander, see note 16 to Chapter V; and for his period as D.G., see **Cantlie**, 2:215-217.
82. James Gibson (1805-1867); M.D. Edinburgh; joined as hospital assistant 1826; assistant-surgeon 1829; served in the East May 1854 - January 1856; D.I.G. May 1855; D.G. 1860; K.C.B. 1865; retired 1867 (obituaries **B.M.J.** (1868), 1:235; **Lancet** (1868), 1:331-332; **M.T.G.** (1868), 1:277 **Drew**; **DNB**). For Gibson's period as D.G., see **Cantlie**, 2:267-272.
83. Thomas Logan (1818-1896); M.D. Glasgow 1828; joined as hospital assistant 1828; assistant-surgeon 1830; D.I.G. December 1855; served in the East June 1855 - June 1856; F.R.C.P. 1867; D.G. 1867; K.C.B. 1869; retired 1874 (obituary **Lancet** (1896), 1:1764; **Munk**; **Drew**). For Logan's period as D.G., see **Cantlie**, 2:272-278.

84. William Muir (1818-1885); M.D. Edinburgh 1840; joined as assistant-surgeon 1842; surgeon February 1854; served in the East for the duration of the war; K.C.B. 1873; D.G. 1874; retired 1882 (obituary **B.M.J.** (1885), 1:1271; **Drew**). For Muir's period as D.G., see **Cantlie**, 2:278-282.
85. Thomas Crawford (1824-1895); L.R.C.S.Ed., M.D. Edinburgh, 1845; joined as assistant-surgeon 1848; surgeon February 1855; served in the East January 1855 - June 1856; D.G. 1882; K.C.B. 1885; retired 1889 (obituary **B.M.J.** (1895), 2:1005; **Drew**). For Crawford's period as D.G., see **Cantlie**, 2:282-287.
86. William Mackinnon (1830-1897); L.R.C.S.Ed., 1851; joined as assistant-surgeon 1853; served in the East April 1854 - June 1856; D.G. 1889; K.C.B. 1891; retired 1896 (obituary **B.M.J.** (1897), 2:1376, 1458-1459; **Drew**). For MacKinnon's period as D.G., see **Cantlie**, 2:287-289.
87. Thomas Longmore (1816-1895); M.R.C.S. 1841; joined as assistant-surgeon 1843; surgeon March 1854; served in the East for the duration of the war; F.R.C.S. 1856; retired 1876 as S.G; knighted 1886 (obituaries **B.M.J.** (1895), 2:956; **Lancet** (1895), 2:952-954, **Plarr**; **Drew**; **Cantlie**, 2:406-410).
88. This total includes Elliott who died during the war after his court-martial (as mentioned in Chapter XIII).
89. John Liddell (1794-1863); L.R.C.S.Ed. 1821, M.D. Edinburgh 1822; joined the Navy 1822 (**M.T.G.** (1855), obituary **B.M.J.** (1863), 1:574; **DNB**; **Keevil**, 4:67).
90. Alexander Bryson (1802-1868); M.D. Glasgow; joined the Navy 1827; D.I. 1854; F.R.C.P. 1860; D.G. 1864 (obituary **B.M.J.** (1869), 2:670; **Keevil**, 4:7-9; **DNB**).
91. Alexander Armstrong (1818-1899); L.R.C.S.Ed., M.D. Edinburgh 1841; joined the Navy 1842; F.R.C.P. 1860 (obituary **B.M.J.** (1899), 2:181; **Munk**; **DNB**; Anon., 'Sir Alexander Armstrong', **J.R.N.M.S.**, 22 (1936), 275-284; **Keevil**, 4:9-10.
92. John Watt Reid (1825-1909); L.R.C.S.Ed. 1844; M.D. Aberdeen 1856; joined as assistant-surgeon 1845 (**Keevil**, 4:10).
93. David Deas (1817-1876); L.R.C.S.Ed. 1827 (obituaries **B.M.J.** (1876), 1:145; **Lancet** (1876), 1:193).
94. Keevil, 4:210.
95. Ibid., 4:268.
96. Cook, **Nightingale**, 2:18-38.
97. **Report of the Royal Commission on the Sanitary State of the Army in India** (London, 1863).
98. Cook, **Nightingale**, I:415-427.
99. Ibid., 456-467. See also M.E. Baly, **Florence Nightingale and the nursing legacy**, London, 1986, chap.1.
100. Cook, **Nightingale**, 2:124-130; J.C. and J. Ross, **A gifted touch: a biography of Agnes Jones** (Worthing, 1989).
101. Ibid., 1:435-438.
102. Ibid., 2:205.
103. Ibid., 197-205.
104. Ibid., 1:362.
105. Ibid., 2:424-434.
106. L.L. Gordon, **British Battles and Medals**, 5th ed. (London, 1979).
107. For lists see **Ass.Med.J.** (1856), 1:119; **M.T.G.** (1856), 2:118.
108. I have regrettably been unable to discover whether or not these graveyards and memorials still survive.
109. The Scutari British Graveyard is cared for by the War Graves Commission, and most of the known memorial stones appear to have survived.

SOURCES

PRINTED MATERIAL

GENERAL HISTORY

Many texts concerning the Crimean War (general histories, descriptions of particular actions, biographies, etc.) have been consulted. Those of value in giving the background of the campaign or dealing with medical affairs are cited in the notes to relevant chapters. Kinglake's remarkable eye-witness account up to the death of Lord Raglan, which first appeared in 1863, is frequently quoted. I have used A.W. Kinglake, **The invasion of the Crimea. Its origin, and an account of its progress to the death of Lord Raglan** (9 vols., Edinburgh, 1901, reprint of 6th. (1876) ed.) - cited in the notes as **Kinglake**.

MEDICAL HISTORY

For the Army Medical Service, the first three chapters of Volume II of N. Cantlie, **A history of the Army Medical Department** (2 vols., Edinburgh, 1974), provide a concise review of the campaign. This work is cited in the notes as **Cantlie**.

For the Naval Medical Service, the history of its development and a brief account of the Crimean campaign are provided in J. Keevil, **Medicine and the Navy : Volume 1 1200-1649**; J. Keevil, **Medicine and the Navy: Volume 2 1649-1714**; C. Lloyd and J. Coulter, **Medicine and the Navy: Volume 3 1714-1815**; C. Lloyd and J. Coulter, **Medicine and the Navy: Volume 4 1815-1900** (Edinburgh, 1957-1963). Surgeon-Commander Keevil planned the whole work but died before its completion: it is cited in the notes as **Keevil**.

> There are innumerable papers on medical aspects of the Crimean War, and I have recently had the opportunity of reading J.W. Warburton, 'A Medical History of the British Expeditionary Force in the East, 1854-1856' (Ph.D. thesis, University of Keele, 1982). This is an able analysis of the administrative blunders of the campaign, exonerating the doctors from responsibility for the major health disasters and set-backs.

OFFICIAL REPORTS

For the Army, the indispensable text is **A Medical and Surgical History of the British Army which served in Turkey and the Crimea during the war against Russia in the years 1854-55-56. Presented to both Houses of Parliament** (2 vols., London, 1858). The scope of these volumes is indicated in Chapter XVIII. It is cited in the notes as **Med. Surg. Hist.**

> Page references to regimental reports included in volume 1 of this history, which in this respect is adequately indexed, are not supplied; but page references to the other volume, which is without an index, are supplied.

For the Navy a much shorter report is available: **Medical Statistical Returns of the Baltic and Black Sea Fleets during the years 1854-1855. Ordered by the House of Commons to be printed 27 February, 1857.** The scope of this report is indicated in Chapter XVIII.

The reports of the various Commissions and Committees appointed during the War are listed in Chapter XI. The important post-war Royal Commission has been widely quoted: **Report of the Commissioners appointed to inquire into the regulations affecting the sanitary condition of the army, the organisation of Military Hospitals, and the treatment of the sick and wounded, with evidence and appendix. Presented to both Houses of Parliament, 1858.** The scope of this very elaborate report is indicated in Chapter XVIII. It is cited in the notes as **Royal Commission**.

BIOGRAPHICAL SOURCES: (a) ARMY

Commissioned medical officers can all be traced in R. Drew, ed., **Medical Officers in the British Army 1660-1960** (2 vols., London, 1968), cited in the notes as **Drew.**

> The first volume, which includes those officers who served in the Crimea, has a useful introduction sketching the evolution of the Army Medical Service. For most entries it is usual to find dates and places of birth and death, medical qualifications, and service record (including the regiments to which the individual was attached, promotions, and decorations). In a few instances information is also given about publications, post-service careers, and other matters. But there are defective entries, particularly with reference to qualifications. Moreover, the date of death is not always known for those who resigned or left the army before completing service up to the usual retiral date.

SOURCES

The basic information in Drew can often be augmented by tracing an obituary (particularly in the **British Medical Journal** or the **Lancet**). Not all commissioned medical officers appear in the medical directories. I have used issues of **London and Provincial Medical Directory** for the period 1847-1859, and from 1860 the **Medical Directory**, which from 1865 included a separate list of "Army and Naval Medical officers".

> These lists sometimes provide additional information concerning qualifications but are otherwise only confirmatory of Drew. Each directory has an obituary list for the previous year. These notes are usually very brief but sometimes give additional information.

The more distinguished commissioned officers may be found in the **Dictionary of National Biography**, cited in the notes as **DNB**. Those who were awarded the F.R.C.P. are to be found in G.H. Brown, ed., **Lives of the Fellows of the Royal College of Physicians of London 1826-1925** (London, 1925), which is Volume IV of Munk's original Roll of the Fellows, and hence is cited in the notes as **Munk**. Those awarded the F.R.C.S. of England are to be found in **Plarr's Lives of the Fellows of the Royal College of Surgeons of England** (revised by D'Arcy Power, 2 vols., Bristol, 1930), which is cited in the notes as **Plarr**.

Commissioned medical officers in staff appointments during the war are listed in **Med. Surg. Hist.**, 1:512-524; but only initials, surnames and dates and places of service are given. There is a list of all medical officers who served in the East from April 1854 to 14 March, 1855, in **Military Medical Officers (Turkey) Return of the Medical Officers serving in Turkey**. This was published by the War Department under the signature of the Director-General.

> Indications are given of age, rank, regimental or staff appointment, and as to whether the officer was still serving in the East on March 14th 1855, or had died, or had gone home by that date. Unfortunately no similar list has been traced for the later part of the War.

Non-commissioned medical officers serving in the army are not so easily traced. Those serving in staff appointments appear in **Med. Surg. Hist.**, 1:512-524.

> By recognising the commissioned officers in this list (checked against Drew) it can be assumed that the remaining names are those of acting

assistant-surgeons who served in staff appointments. All the non-commissioned officers serving up to 14 March 1855, are found in the Director-General's list noted above. Some of those who joined after that date have been traced from reports in the medical journals, from chance discovery in the directories, or in various texts. It is likely that I have failed to trace a number of these doctors and, my total of army medical officers serving in the campaign, although higher than any quoted previously, is probably a slight underestimate.

BIOGRAPHICAL SOURCES: (b) NAVY

There is no source for the Naval Medical Service similar to Drew.

If names crop up in the medical journals, official reports, biographies or other sources these can be cross-checked with the contemporary Navy Lists, from which full name, date of promotion to current rank and, occasionally, qualifications can be obtained. A proportion of these doctors can be traced in the Directories or their obituaries located. A few names are to be found in Munk or Plarr. Probably the names of all the medical officers who served throughout the war could be traced in the various official Navy records held in the Public Record Office, but this extensive research I have not been able to achieve. There are some lists of appointments to ships in the contemporary medical journals, but these lists are incomplete.

BIOGRAPHICAL SOURCES: (c) CIVILIAN DOCTORS AND THE TURKISH CONTINGENT

In Chapter XII the sources of information concerning the civilian doctors who served in the East are given.

The lists in the medical journals are fairly accurate and most names can be found in the directories. A large proportion of obituaries have been found. Additional biographical details of Civilian doctors are supplied in Appendix I.

In Chapter XVI the sources of information concerning the doctors who served with the Turkish Contingent are given.

The lists in the medical journals are incomplete, but some additional names have been traced in biographies, in Medical Directories etc. Those who served before or after the War in the Indian Medical Service are to be found in D.G. Crawford, **Roll of the Indian Medical Service, 1615-1930** (London, 1930), cited in the notes as **Crawford**. Additional biographical details of selected doctors in the Turkish Contingent are supplied in Appendix II.

DEATHS OF MEDICAL OFFICERS

It has been shown that the calculations of the total number of deaths of Army medical officers published previously are inaccurate. I have traced additional deaths from a variety of sources noted for individuals. In addition I have made use of a minor and rare contemporary source, J. Colborne and H. Brine, **The Last of the Brave or Resting Places of our fallen heroes in the Crimea and at Scutari** (London, 1857).

> This work records all the officers and men who were buried in the Crimea, Scutari, or elsewhere in the theatre of war, and those commemorated on regimental or other memorials in the graveyards. The inscriptions on all memorials are given in full. The book is profusely illustrated with lithographs by E. Walker depicting all the regimental, divisional, and general graveyards.

NEWSPAPERS

Of the contemporary newspapers I have made most use of **The Times**. Quotations from this and other newspapers are to be found frequently in the contemporary medical journals. The **Illustrated London News** of the period is an invaluable source of information, not only because of the lavish illustrations of the campaign but also because of scattered items of news not recorded elsewhere. With some exceptions, such as the **Edinburgh Courant**, I have not been able to tap the provincial newspapers. I believe that further information might be found in these, either in letters from doctors who served in the East, or in obituaries in later years.

MEDICAL JOURNALS

The medical journals prior to 1854, particularly the **Lancet** and the **Medical Times and Gazette** have been consulted frequently in the preparation of Chapters I-II. The campaign of 1854-1856 is well covered in the **Association Medical Journal, Lancet,** and **Medical Times and Gazette.** Many other later journals have also been consulted.

Abbreviated references to journals cited in the notes are as follows.

Annals of Medical History	Ann.Med.Hist.
Annals Royal College of Surgeons England	Ann.R.C.S.Eng.
Association Medical Journal	Ass.Med.J.
British and Foreign Medico-Chirurgical Review	Brit.For.Med.Chir.Rev.
British Journal of Accident Surgery	Brit.J.Accident.Surg.
British Journal of Surgery	B.J.S.
British Medical Bulletin	Brit.Med.Bull.
British Medical Journal	B.M.J.
Bulletin of the History of Medicine	Bull.Hist.Med.
Caledonian Medical Journal	Cal.Med.J.
Edinburgh Medical Journal	Ed.Med.J.
Glasgow Medical Journal	Glas.Med.J.
Irish Journal of Medical Sciences	Irish J.Med.Sc.
Journal of the Royal Army Medical Corps	J.R.A.M.C.
Journal of the Royal College of Physicians of London	J.R.Coll.Phys.Lond.
Journal of the Royal College of Surgeons of Edinburgh	J.R.Coll.Surg.Edin.
Journal of the Royal Naval Medical Service	J.R.N.M.S.
London Medical Gazette	Lond.Med.Gaz.
London Medical Journal	Lond.Med.J.
Medico-Chirurgical Journal	Med.-Chir.J.
Medico-Chirurgical Transactions	Med.-Chir.Trans.
Medical History	Med.Hist.
Medical Press and Circular	Med.Press
Medical Times and Gazette	M.T.G.
Military Medicine	Military Medicine
Monthly Journal of Medical Science	Monthly J.Med.Sc.
Proceedings of the Royal Society of Medicine	Proc.Roy.Soc.Med.
South Carolina Medical Journal	S.Carolina Med.J.
Transactions of the Provincial Medical and Surgical Association	Trans.Prov.Med.Ass.

LIBRARIES

The official material and many of the rarer texts are of course available in the British Library. But I have been fortunate to have been able to consult, nearer home, many of the official reports in the Picton Library, Liverpool. And it has been a great advantage to have had easy access to the Library of the Liverpool Medical Institution, which has a remarkably complete collection of all the early medical journals and of many of the texts relating to the period of the war.

MANUSCRIPT SOURCES

ROYAL ARMY MEDICAL CORPS HISTORICAL MUSEUM, ALDERSHOT

A large collection of manuscript and other material relating to the Crimean War, formerly at Millbank, is easily accessible in the museum at Aldershot. The most important collection for our purpose is the Hall MSS - consisting of "medical registers, jotter books, reports, returns, correspondence, and diaries" (Historical Manuscripts Commission). Mitra, Hall's biographer, had access to the then unsorted trunk of papers bequeathed by Hall's descendants. Of some thirty small diaries, seven, travel-stained and worn, cover the Crimean period. The entries are brief but the depressions and exasperations suffered by Hall come through clearly. This source is cited in the notes as 'Hall Diary'. The vast collection of letters is of considerable interest, not least the communications between Hall and Smith, the Director-General; and of significance also are letters between Hall and his colleagues. These letters are cited in the notes as 'Hall/Smith Letters', 'Hall/Cumming Letters', etc. The many miscellaneous reports and returns mostly corroborate details in the official medical history of the war.

In addition, the R.A.M.C. archives contain the diaries, memoirs and letters of some of the junior medical officers who served in the Crimea. These eye-witness accounts give a vivid picture of the campaign and throw considerable light on the attitudes of the junior staff. Of these records the most useful are those of William Calder (cited as 'Calder Diary'), William Cattell ('Cattell Memoirs'), David Greig ('Greig Diary' and 'Greig Letters'), Henry Sylvester ('Sylvester Journals') and Arthur Taylor ('Taylor Letters'). None of these five items has been published in full. Major-General Barnsley published extracts from Cattell's Memoirs (see note 12 to Chapter III) and he prepared a full typescript of Taylor's Letters, but sadly was unable to find a publisher.

ROYAL COLLEGE OF SURGEONS OF EDINBURGH LIBRARY

In the College Library are the diary and letters of Patrick Heron Watson, and these are of special interest because he was more critical of the army medical service than others whose writings survive. They are cited in notes as 'Heron Watson Diary' and 'Heron Watson Letters'.

NATIONAL LIBRARY OF SCOTLAND

This library holds a collection of letters written by William Aitken which throw considerable light on the Pathological Commission. Cited as 'Aitken Letters'.

BOWMAN COLLECTION

The late Dr. K. Bryn Thomas very kindly provided me with photostats of letters in a private archive, the Bowman Collection, concerning the Struthers case (Chapter VIII) which he had brought to light while preparing his article, 'The manuscripts of Sir William Bowman', **Med.Hist.**, 10 (1966), 245-256. The relevant letters, mainly from Professor Simpson, are cited as 'Simpson/Christison Letters', 'Simpson/Herbert Letters', etc.

CANNING LETTERS

A collection of letters from Lady Charlotte Canning in London to Lady Stratford (wife of the Ambassador in Turkey) throws new light on the organisation for the selection of nurses for Scutari, and on Miss Nightingale.

These letters were seen by Sir Edward Cook only after he had published his biography of Florence Nightingale and he indicated that if he prepared a second edition he would include excerpts of importance, but there was no second edition. The collection was inherited by my wife through a Canning family connection and I am very grateful to her for allowing me to use the letters. Cited as 'Canning Letters'.

PUBLIC RECORD OFFICE, LONDON

The relevant material in the Public Record Office would take a life-time to study fully. Over the years I have examined a substantial proportion of those reports, returns, letters and other material which can be readily traced from the catalogues. This material is cited in the notes as **P.R.O.**

BIBLIOGRAPHY

A Lady Volunteer [F. Taylor], **Eastern Hospitals and English Nurses**, London, 1857

B. Abel-Smith, **The Hospitals 1800-1848**, London, 1964

J. Adye, **A Review of the Crimean War to the Winter of 1854-55**, London, 1860

M. Airlie, **With the Guards we shall go**, London, 1933

Z. Alexander and A. Dewjee, eds., **Wonderful Adventures of Mrs. Seacole in many lands**, Bristol, 1984

M. Aloysius, **A Sister of Mercy's Memoir of the Crimea**, London, 1862

Lord Anglesey, **Little Hodge, being extracts from the diaries and letters of Colonel Edward Cooper Hodge written during the Crimean War, 1854-1856**, London, 1971

S.T. Anning, **The General Infirmary at Leeds**, 2 vols., Edinburgh, 1963

Anon, **Two months in and about the camp before Sebastopol**, London, 1855

A. Armand, **Guerre de Crimée: Histoire Médicale-Chirurgicale**, Paris, 1858

B. Askwith, **Crimean Courtship**, Salisbury, 1985

E.T. Atkins, **The Moorfield Eye Hospital**, London, 1929

G.M. Ayres, **England's First State Hospitals**, London, 1859

M.E. Baly, **Florence Nightingale and the Nursing Legacy**, London, 1986

M.C. Baudens, **La Guerre de Crimée**, Paris, 1858

M.C. Baudens, **Souvenir d'une Mission Médicale a l'Armée D'Orient**, Paris, 1857

J. Beddoe, **Memories of Early Years**, Bristol, 1910

A. Benson, ed., **The Letters of Queen Victoria 1858-1861**, 3 vols., London, 1907-1908

N. Bentley, ed., **Russell's Despatches from the Crimea 1854-1856**, London, 1966

Lady Blackwood, **A Narrative of personal experiences and impressions during a residence on the Bosphorus during the Crimean War ...**, London, 1881

R.L.V.F. Blake, **The Crimean War**, London, 1971

J. Bland-Sutton, **The Story of a Surgeon**, London, 1930

V. Bonham-Carter ed., **Surgeon in the Crimea. The experiences of George Lawson recorded in letters to his family 1854-1855**, London, 1968

SOURCES

D. Bonner-Smith and A.C. Dewar, eds., **Russian War 1854. Baltic and Black Sea. Official Correspondence**, Navy Records Society, London, 1943

D. Bonner-Smith, **Russian War 1855. Baltic Official Correspondence**, Naval Records Society, London, 1944

A. Briggs, **Victorian People**, London 1958

C. Bruce, **England and France before Sebastopol looked at from the medical point of view**, London, 1857

A. Buchanan, **Camp Life as seen as a Civilian**, Glasgow, 1871

E.H. Burrows, **A History of Medicine in South Africa**, Capetown, 1958

T. Buzzard, **With the Turkish Army in the Crimea and Asia Minor**, London 1915

G. Cameron, **History of the Royal College of Surgeons in Ireland**, 2nd ed., Dublin, 1916

N. Cantlie, **A History of the Army Medical Department**, 2 vols., Edinburgh, 1974

P. Cassar, **A Medical History of Malta**, London, 1964

K. Chesney, **Crimean War Reader**, London, 1960

G. Clark and A.M. Cooke, **A History of the Royal College of Physicians of London**, 3 vols., Oxford, 1964-1972

P. Compton, **Colonel's Lady and Camp-Follower**, London, 1970

J. Colborne and F. Brine, **The Last of the Brave, or, Resting Places of our Heroes in the Crimea and at Scutari**, London, 1857

Z. Cope, **Florence Nightingale and the Doctors**, London, 1958

J.S. Curtiss, **Russia's Crimean War**, Durham N.C., 1979

A.C. Dewar, **Russian War, 1855. Black Sea Official Correspondence**, Navy Record Society, London, 1945

C.R. Dod, **The Parliamentary Companion**, London, 1854

R. Drew, ed., **Medical Officers in the British Army 1660-1960**, 2 vols., London, 1968

F. Duberly, **Journal kept during the Crimean War**, London, 1856

C. Falls, ed., **Diary of the Crimea: George Palmer Evelyn**, London, 1954

C. Fitzherbert, ed., **Henry Clifford V.C. His letters and sketches from the Crimea**, London, 1956

E.R. Frizelle and J.D. Martin, **The Leicester Royal Infirmary 1771--1971**, Leicester 1971

F.J. Gant, **Autobiography**, London, 1903

F.F. Garrison, **Notes on the History of Military Medicine**, Washington, 1922

M. Gelfand, **Livingstone the doctor. His life and travels**, Oxford, 1957

R. Gibbs, **The Battle of the Alma**, London, 1963

S. Goldie, 'I have done my duty.' **Florence Nightingale in the Crimean War 1854-1856**, Manchester, 1988

M. Goodman, **Experiences of an English Sister of Mercy**, London, 1862

L.C. Gordon, **British Battles and Medals**, London, 1979

T. Gowing, **A soldier's experience. A view from the ranks**, Nottingham, 1903

J. Harris, **The Gallant Six Hundred**, London, 1973

E. Hamley, **The War in the Crimea**, 10th ed., London, 1910

C. Hibbert, **The Destruction of Lord Raglan**, London, 1963

C. Hibbert, **The Great Mutiny. India 1857**, London, 1980

A.D. Home, **Service Memories**, London, 1912

Lady Hornby, **Constantinople during the Crimean War**, London, 1863

J. Hunter, **A Treatise on the blood, inflammation and gun shot wounds...**, 2 vols., London, 1794

L. James, **Crimea 1854-1856. The War with Russia from contemporary photographs**, New York, 1981

W. Jenner, **Lectures and Essays on Fevers and Diphtheria 1849-1879**, London, 1893

D. Judd, **The Crimean War**, London, 1975

J. Keevil, C. Lloyd, and J. Coulter, **Medicine and the Navy**, 4 vols., Edinburgh, 1957-1963

H. Keppel, **A Sailor's Life under four Sovereigns: Sir Henry Keppel**, 3 vols., London, 1899

A.W. Kinglake, **The Invasion of the Crimea. Its origin, and an account of its progress to the death of Lord Raglan**, 9 vols., Edinburgh, 1901 (reprint of 6th. ed., 1876).

P.R. Kirby, **Andrew Smith and Natal**, 2 vols., Van Riebeck Society, Cape Town, 1955

P.R. Kirby, **Sir Andrew Smith KCB. His life, letters and works**, Cape Town, 1965

G. Lawson, **On gunshot wounds of the thorax**, London, 1858

J.H. Lefroy, **Autobiography of John Henry Lefroy**, [privately printed, n.d., c.1895]

M. Levien, ed., **The Cree Journals. The voyages of Edward H. Cree, Surgeon R.N., as related in his private journals 1837-1856**, Exeter, 1981

G.A. Lindebloom, **Dutch Medical Biography**, Eindhoven, 1984

T. Longmore, **Gunshot Injuries. Their history, characteristic features, complications and general treatment: with statistics concerning them as they are met with in warfare**, London, 1877

H.W. Lyle, **Kings and Kings' Men**, Oxford, 1935

G.H.B. Macleod, **Notes on the Surgery of the War in the Crimea**, London, 1858

G. Macnamara, **A History of Asiatic Cholera**, London, 1876

- McNamara, **A trip to the Trenches**, London, 1855

W.R. Merrington, **University College Hospital and its Medical School. A History**, London, 1976

S.M. Mitra, **The life and letters of Sir John Hall, M.D., F.R.C.S., K.C.B.**, London, 1911

H. Morris, **Portrait of a Chef. The Life of Alexis Soyer**, Cambridge, 1932

H. Moyse-Bartlett, **Louis Nolan and his influence on the British Cavalry**, London, 1971

W. Munro, **Records of Service and Campaigning in many lands**, London, 1867

W. Munro, **Reminiscences of military service with the 93rd. Sutherland Highlanders**, London, 1873

F. Nightingale, **Notes on matters affecting the health, efficiency and hospital administration of the army ...** London, 1858

F. Nightingale, **Notes on Hospitals**, 3rd ed., London, 1863

E.M. Nolan, **Illustrated History of the War against Russia**, 2 vols., London, 1855

I.B. O'Malley, **Florence Nightingale 1820-1856**, London, 1931

S.G.O. Osborne, **Scutari and its Hospitals**, London, 1855

E.A. Parkes, **A Manual of Practical Hygiene prepared especially for use in the medical service of the army**, London, 1864

W.B. Pemberton, **Battles of the Crimean War**, London, 1962

P. Pincoffs, **Experience of a Civilian in Eastern Military Hospitals**, London, 1857

E.S. Pollard, **Florence Nightingale: the wounded soldier's friend**, London [n.d., c.1900]

F.N.L. Poynter, **The Evolution of hospitals in Britain**, London, 1964

J. Pudney, **Brunel and his world**, London, 1974

J. Radcliffe, **The Hygiene of the Turkish Army**, London, 1858

I. Rae, **The strange story of Dr. James Barry**, London, 1958

F. Robinson, **Diary of the Crimean War**, London, 1856

G. Rolleston, **Scientific Papers and Addresses by George Rolleston**, Oxford, 1884

L.T.C. Rolt, **Brunel and his World**, London, 1974

J.C. Ross and J. Ross, **A gifted Touch. A Biography of Agnes Jones**, Worthing, 1989

W.B. Rowbotham, **The Naval Brigade in the Indian Mutiny**, Navy Records Society, London, 1947

W. Russell, **The British Expedition to the Crimea**, London, 1858

H. Sandwith, **A narrative of the siege of Kars**, London, 1856

A. Seaton, **The Crimean War. A Russian Chronicle**, London, 1977

J. Selby, **The Thin Red Line**, London, 1970

J.A. Shepherd, **Spencer Wells. The Life and Work of a Victorian Surgeon**, Edinburgh, 1965

J.A. Shepherd, **Simpson and Syme of Edinburgh**, Edinburgh, 1969

J. Smyth, **The Story of the Victoria Cross**, London, 1963

A. Soyer, **Soyer's culinary campaign - with the plan of the art of cooking**, London, 1857

Lord Stanmore, **Sidney Herbert. Lord Herbert of Lea. A Memoir**, 2 vols., London, 1906

H.F. Stapylton, **The Eton School List. 1791-1877**, Eton, 1884

G. St. Aubyn, **The Royal George**, London, 1963

C.W. Strachan, **Wellington's legacy. The Reform of the British Army**, Manchester, 1984

A. Summers, **Angels and Citizens**, London, 1988

V. Surtees, **Charlotte Canning**, London, 1975

S. Terrot, **Reminiscences of the Scutari Hospitals**, privately printed, 1898

E.C.P. Tisdale, ed., **Mrs Duberly's Diary**, London, 1963

A. Tulloch, **The Crimea Commission and the Chelsea Board**, London, 1857

T.H. Ward, **Humphry Sandwith. Memoir**, London, 1884

S.G.P. Ward, ed., **The Hawley Letters. The Letters of Captain R.B. Hawley, 89th [Regiment] from the Crimea, December 1854 to August 1856**, Society for Army Historical Research, London, 1970

P. Warner, **The Crimean War. A Reappraisal**, Newton Abbot, 1972

E. Williams, ed., **The Autobiography of Elizabeth Davies, a Balaclava Nurse**, 2 vols., London, 1857

I.C. Willis, **Florence Nightingale. A Biography**, London, 1931

C. Woodham-Smith, **Florence Nightingale 1820-1910**, London, 1950

C. Woodham-Smith, **The reason why**, London, 1953

APPENDIX I

ADDITIONAL BIOGRAPHICAL NOTES ON CIVILIAN DOCTORS SERVING AT SCUTARI, SMYRNA AND RENKIOI

Edward Atkinson (1830-1905) qualified in 1852 from King's College Hospital. After the war he was surgeon to the British Hospital in Jerusalem for four years. He returned to Leeds, his family being closely associated with the famous line of the Heys who dominated surgery in Leeds for three generations. Appointed Surgeon in the Leeds Infirmary in 1874, he had a considerable reputation as a teacher as well as an operator.

Carl (or Charles) Bader (d. 1891) qualified in 1855 from Guy's Hospital. Of German origin, he developed an early interest in ophthalmology. After his service in Renkioi he returned to London to practise this speciality, and became Lecturer in Diseases of the Eye at Guy's Hospital and Curator of the Museum at Moorfields Hospital. He was a pioneer in the use of the ophthalmoscope and was noted for the remarkable series of pathological specimens which he prepared for Moorfields Hospital.

John Barclay (1820-1901) qualified in Edinburgh in 1842 and became a physician to the Leicester Infirmary. He resigned from this post to go to Smyrna but was re-elected, to serve the hospital with distinction. From his experience in Smyrna he became a strong advocate of nursing reform.

John Beddoe (1826-1911) qualified in Edinburgh in 1853. He was a house-surgeon in the Royal Infirmary at the same time as Joseph Lister. After his service at Renkioi he settled in Bristol and was Physician to the Bristol Infirmary. Beddoe became widely known for his works on anthropology, for which he was awarded the F.R.S.

Hugh Birt (d. 1875) qualified from U.C.H. in 1836 and obtained the F.R.C.S. in 1844 (by examination). Before the war he had worked in Brazil as a surgeon, and then for some time was attached to the Naval Hospital in Valparaiso. At Scutari (perhaps as the most senior and best qualified doctor) he is said to have been rated as "1st Class Civil Surgeon". After the war he practised in London but had no hospital attachment.

Anthony Brabazon (1821-1896) qualified in 1846 in Dublin. Before the war he lectured in Anatomy in the Dublin Schools of Medicine. After his service at Scutari he eventually settled in Bath where he became Medical Officer of Health and Physician to the Royal Mineral Water Hospital. In 1855 he sent a short account of his clinical experiences at Scutari to the **Lancet.**

Charles Bryce (d. 1875) qualified in 1825, his M.D. thesis being on his observations of the 1832 cholera epidemic in Glasgow. Before the war he must have acquired some reputation, but where he practised is uncertain. At the request of the Army Medical Department he produced a paper on fever. His appointment at Scutari was for a particular purpose. In Chapter X reference has been made to the controversy concerning the treatment of dysentery and fever cases and to the suggestion that the methods of the practitioners in Constantinople were superior to those employed by the army doctors. Dr. Bryce was sent out to investigate this question. He was given charge of 100 beds in Koulali Hospital and treated as having the rank of Staff-Surgeon. The Director-General requested him to carry out a comparative trial of the two methods of treatment. This investigation was done between April and September 1855 and the results, according to Cantlie, proved conclusively that there was no truth in the allegation that the treatment given by the army doctors was inferior. When Bryce returned home in May 1856 he set up practice in Brighton but did not become eminent in any way.

George Buchanan (1827-1906) qualified in Edinburgh in 1849, and was in general practice in Glasgow before the war. Buchanan arrived at Scutari at the end of June 1855. Before taking up his appointment at Renkioi he visited the Crimea and served briefly in the lines before Sebastopol. Late in August he went to Renkioi, but finding little to do there he was glad to volunteer for further service in the Crimea, where he remained for several months. On his return to Glasgow he engaged exclusively in surgical practice. He became in 1860 Professor of Anatomy and in 1874 Professor of Clinical Surgery (a chair he held until 1900) in the University of Glasgow. A popular teacher, he also wrote prolifically but made no major surgical advance.

Edward Complin (1830-1855) qualified in 1852 and before the war was medical officer to the hospital hulk "Dreadnought", moored in the Thames. He reported a severe outbreak of cholera on the ship in 1854 and was unusual at the time in condemning castor oil as treatment. While at Smyrna he volunteered to serve in the Crimea but soon after his arrival he contracted fever and dysentery and he died at Scutari after a long illness.

Holmes Coote (1815-1872) qualified from the Westminster Hospital in 1832. He held junior posts at St. Bartholomew's Hospital, and in 1844 was elected F.R.C.S., in the first 300 to be nominated. In the same year he became a lecturer in anatomy at St. Bartholomew's Hospital and later an assistant surgeon. He was well established in a surgical career when he went to Smyrna. From Smyrna he was transferred to Renkioi Hospital. When he returned to England he became a full surgeon at St. Bartholomew's Hospital. He wrote several useful texts but made no original contributions to surgery, although having a high reputation as a teacher.

John Cowan (1829-1896) qualified in Glasgow, where he subsequently was in general practice and served on the editorial staff of the **Glasgow Medical Journal**. He spent some time in the Crimea before taking up his post at Renkioi. Returning later to the Crimea, he was invalided home after a severe bout of fever. Eventually he took up the post of Lecturer in Medical Jurisprudence in Anderson's College, Glasgow, and in 1865 became Professor of Materia Medica in the University. Dogged by ill-health he resigned the Chair in 1870, but continued to exert considerable influence on University affairs.

Patrick Fraser (d. 1881) qualified from King's College Hospital in 1836. Before the war it is uncertain where he practised but he served for a time as a physician in the "War of Restoration in Portugal". After the Crimean War he was in general practice in London and acquired some honorary appointments to minor European royalties, but he died in obscurity.

Frederick Gant (1825-1905) qualified in 1845. Before the war he lectured in physiology and anatomy at the Hunterian School of Medicine, and in 1853 was appointed an assistant surgeon at the Royal Free Hospital. He first served in the Crimea and then at Scutari. After the war he returned to England to surgical work at the Royal Free Hospital and remained on the staff for another 35 years. He wrote several useful text books of surgery and served a term as President of the Royal Medical Society. He became F.R.C.S. in 1861 but his relations with the College were somewhat strained when he published a "Guide to the Examinations", which in the opinion of his colleagues gave away too many details to the candidates! If an eccentric in some respects he stands out as one of this group who made a significant contribution in the post-war years. Not least he was a strong advocate for the admission of women to the profession.

APPENDICES

Henry Goodeve (1807-1884) qualified in Edinburgh in 1829. He joined the Indian Medical Service in 1831, and in 1835 became Professor of Anatomy and Obstetrics in the newly founded Calcutta Medical School. In 1844 he was elected F.R.C.S. He returned to England in 1845. Goodeve was attached to the Indian Medical Service for another three years, during which he supervised the training of Bengali medical students in London. His activities between 1848 and the outbreak of the war are uncertain, but he attained considerable prominence in medical circles. After the war he seems to have retired from active practice and lived in Bristol. His most important contribution had been in the development of the Calcutta Medical School.

John Hulke (1830-1895) qualified in 1852 from King's College Hospital. At first he assisted his father, William Hulke of Deal, in his practice. When the Duke of Wellington died at Walmer Castle in September 1852, father and son attended him on his death-bed, and the younger Hulke prepared an account of the last hours of their illustrious patient for the press, "to prevent the appearance of sensational reports". (**B.M.J.** 1895, 1:682-683). Before the war Hulke was house-surgeon to Sir William Fergusson. While at Smyrna he volunteered to serve in the Crimea and remained there through the following winter. When he came home in 1856 he was appointed an assistant surgeon at King's. In 1858, now interested in ophthalmology, be became an assistant surgeon at Moorfields Hospital, to become a full surgeon in 1867. He had transferred to the Middlesex Hospital as an assistant surgeon in 1862, to become a full surgeon there in 1870. In 1893 he was elected President of the College of Surgeons. Hulke was an able general surgeon and a pioneer in his speciality, being one of the first to introduce the technique of perimetry. He published many able papers in the journals. He had great versatility and was known as an expert geologist and palaeontologist. (For his work in these subjects he was awarded the F.R.S.). Hulke died in harness having been called out late on a winter night to operate on an emergency in the Middlesex Hospital and, as a result, contracted a fatal pneumonia. He ranks with Spencer Wells as one of the two most distinguished surgeons who served at Smyrna.

John Kirk (1836-1922) qualified in Edinburgh in 1854 at the age of 18. While a student he became greatly interested in Botany and was elected a Fellow of the Edinburgh Botanical Society. Among his many general interests was photography, and when he was at Renkioi he took many photographs of the hospital and staff. Kirk spent some time at Scutari before going to Renkioi. After his service there he visited the Crimea briefly. Returning home in 1858, Kirk was appointed to the staff of the explorer Dr. David Livingstone (1813-1873), prior to his exploration of the Zambezi River. It was stipulated that Kirk should be the botanist in the party but that he should also assist Livingstone as a medical officer. Kirk remained in Africa until October 1853, participating in all Livingstone's journeys for five years. He became second in command of the party and was a tower of strength to Livingstone, sharing all the hardships, and caring for his colleagues who suffered greatly from sickness. In 1866 Kirk was appointed Consul at Zanzibar and was in a position to assist Livingstone and other explorers in the planning of their expeditions. At a later date as Government Medical Officer in Zanzibar, Kirk exerted a powerful influence in the political field, in the face of German competition in East Africa. He did much for the welfare of the Africans. His most important achievement was his part in the suppression of the slave trade in Zanzibar, ratified by the important Brussels Agreement of 1890. When he returned from Zanzibar Kirk had a long and peaceful retirement, dying at the age of 90, the last survivor of the Renkioi medical staff. He received many honours for his work in Africa, including a knighthood and the F.R.S.

Arthur Leared (1822-1879) qualified in Dublin in 1847. Before the war he was a physician to the Metropolitan Dispensary in London. He returned to London

APPENDICES

after the war to become a senior physician in the Great Northern Hospital. Leared became an authority on cardiac diseases and invented the "double stethoscope", used for teaching. He contributed important texts and articles on cardiac disease and many other subjects. He was a great traveller and investigated the diseases of all the countries he visited.

Robert McDonnel (1828-1889) qualified in Dublin in 1850. He obtained F.R.C.S.I. in 1853. From Smyrna he went to the Crimea, serving in one of the general hospitals there, and he was awarded the Crimean medal. He returned to Dublin to hold a variety of teaching appointments. His scientific attainments were recognised in 1865 by the award of the F.R.S. In 1863 he was appointed surgeon to Steven's Hospital and Professor of Descriptive Anatomy at that hospital, and in 1877 he became President of the Royal College of Surgeons in Ireland. McDonnel served on many important Royal Commissions in Ireland. He was a prolific writer on a wide range of medical and surgical topics.

George Macleod (1828-1892) qualified in Glasgow in 1853. His early career and the circumstances of his appointment to Smyrna have been recounted (Chapter XII). Despite his youth and lack of experience he was appointed a senior surgeon at Smyrna and, in addition, was Deputy Superintendent. Finding little surgery to do, Macleod took two weeks leave at the end of May to visit the Crimea. He had a letter of introduction to Hall who asked him to remain at the front. He was given the status of a staff-surgeon and dealt with many of the wounded following the assaults on Sebastopol. He stayed on in the Crimea until April 1856. After the war he published a text on war surgery. He soon became well established in Glasgow and in 1859 was elected Professor of Surgery in Anderson's College. Ten years later he succeeded Lister as Professor of Surgery in Glasgow University. Macleod, an excellent clinical teacher, wrote widely but made no original contribution to surgical practice. He was however of great influence in the progress of the Glasgow School. Few of the younger civilian doctors who went out to the war made so much of their opportunities.

John Meyer (1814-1870) was born in England and was of German extraction. He had graduated in Heidelberg in 1836. His early medical career is unknown. He was from 1846-1854 in the Colonial Service in charge of a Lunatic Asylum for convicts in Tasmania, an appointment which was held in much derision by his critics. He visited Scutari briefly in December 1854. After Smyrna was abandoned, he returned to England in December 1855 and worked in mental hospitals, finally having charge of Broadmoor Criminal Asylum. When he died there were no obituaries in the medical press but he had been thought worthy of election as F.R.C.P. in 1863. Belatedly the President of the College in his Annual Address paid tribute to Meyer as a distinguished public servant.

Edmund Parkes (1819-1876) qualified in 1841 from University College Hospital. He joined the army as an assistant-surgeon in 1842 and served in India for three years. He resigned in 1845 and returned to London to become Professor of Clinical Medicine and a Physician in his hospital. He wrote authoritatively on cholera and dysentery from his experience in India. In 1855 at the request of the Government he went out to Turkey to find a site for the second Civil Hospital. When Renkioi was closed Parkes returned to his work in U.C.H. In 1860 the Army Medical School was founded at Fort Pitt and by the influence of Herbert and Miss Nightingale Parkes was elected Professor of Hygiene, a post which he held when the School was transferred to Netley and until his death. In the post-war years he remained a close friend and collaborator of Miss Nightingale. He contributed greatly to the development and success of the Army Medical School. His "Manual of Practical Hygiene" was of great influence and was reprinted in several languages. For his writings he was awarded the F.R.S.

Peter Pincoffs (1815-1872) qualified in Leyden in 1837, and then studied in Paris, London, and Berlin. He was in practice in Brussels in 1839, and in Dresden in 1842, but in 1847 settled in England. He worked in Manchester for about five years, and then returned to Dresden. How he was selected to serve at Scutari is unknown but he was there from April 1855 to April 1856. His experience and his opinions of the Army Medical Service are described in his personal account (Chapter XII). After the war Pincoffs practised in Dresden, Beirut, and Naples.

William Robertson (1818-1882) qualified in Edinburgh in 1839 and, elected F.R.C.P.E. in 1843, became a Physician to the Royal Infirmary. He was Editor of the **Edinburgh Monthly Journal of Medical Science.** Recommended by Professor Christison (and perhaps also by General Sir George Brown, to whom he was related) he went out to Renkioi as Senior Physician. When he returned to Edinburgh after the war he forsook clinical medicine, becoming Superintendent of Statistics in the Scottish Registry Office. Like Kirk, Robertson was an able photographer and took many plates of Renkioi.

George Rolleston (1829-1881), after taking a brilliant degree in classics at Oxford, qualified in 1854. When he was appointed to Smyrna he was advised by the Master of Pembroke College - "You have profit and employment in what otherwise would be the dead time in your career, possibly an avenue to something great and permanent ... You will now be under official trammels. Pray be discreet as to your words". Rolleston impressed his colleagues with his intellect. A lady nurse wrote of him - "I had constant opportunities for understanding his fine character, so full of talent and energy, so kind, and with so much earnestness in his playful manner. Looking back I see a tall fair young man moving up and down the long corridors ... attending to every case most carefully, always kind and cheerful in his manner." While at Smyrna he made the most of the clinical opportunities. "I have had Dr. Martin's wards as well as my own to take care of ... by a little management I contrived to get a very large share of what are called the 'good cases'." Rolleston volunteered to serve in the Crimea but Dr. Hall had no vacancy for him. Like Wells he paid a brief visit to the front which he described vividly in letters to his sister. It was a recognition of his ability that he was retained at Smyrna until December, with the approval of Panmure, to assist Meyer in the winding-up of the hospital. After the war Rolleston soon returned to Oxford, to become a physician to the Radcliffe Infirmary. His interests became more scientific than clinical and in 1861 he was appointed Linacre Professor of Anatomy. He proved an excellent teacher and researcher. He wrote widely on scientific subjects, his learning being "the rare blend of classical culture and enlightened science". He remained on the hospital staff but his influence was more in the organisation of teaching than in clinical science. Rolleston married a niece of Sir Humphrey Davy and their son, Sir Humphrey Rolleston, achieved a greater fame in medicine than his father.

John Streatfeild (1828-1886) qualified from the London Hospital in 1852. His activities before the war are unknown. After the war he became an ophthalmologist and was made an assistant surgeon at Moorfields Hospital in 1856 and full surgeon in 1867. He later became Professor of Clinical Ophthalmic Surgery at University College Hospital. Streatfeild was recognised as a deft operator and introduced several new techniques in eye surgery.

Thomas Spencer Wells (1818-1897) qualified in 1841. His early career in the Navy has already been recorded (Chapter I). He was well established professionally in London before the war and had considerable influence as editor of the **Medical Times and Gazette.** Although on half-pay as a naval surgeon he was not called up. The Medical-Director of the Navy, Burnett, despite being short of experienced surgeons, must have agreed to Wells' acceptance of the post of Surgeon at Smyrna. This produced some caustic comments. In the **Association Medical Journal** there was disapproval of the rival editor. "Mr. Spencer Wells, Editor of the Medical Times and Gazette is allowed to retain his half pay as surgeon in the Navy." He was to prove the most energetic member of the Smyrna staff, throwing himself into all aspects of the work, whether administrative, medical or surgical. In June he paid a visit of two weeks to the Crimea and recorded his opinions of the army medical service. He did not apparently volunteer to serve in the Crimea (probably because he had already been told of his imminent transfer to be chief surgeon at Renkioi). When he returned home from Renkioi he was quickly re-established in London. At the end of the war the new Director-General of the Navy, Liddel, was less charitable towards Wells' evasion of naval service, and appointed him to a warship. On the grounds of a chronic chest complaint Wells was however discharged from the Navy. He was to become a gynaecologist of great eminence, particularly in his establishment of the operation of ovariotomy as an acceptable and relatively safe procedure. He became President of the Royal College of Surgeons in 1882. In the College and in many other fields he exerted great influence. Wells made a considerable contribution by his service at Smyrna and Renkioi, and in his subsequent career stands out as the most distinguished of the civil surgeons.

APPENDIX II

ADDITIONAL BIOGRAPHICAL NOTES ON DOCTORS SERVING IN THE TURKISH CONTINGENT

Alexander Boggs (1823-1890) qualified in 1854 after an initial training in the Madras Medical School. He was appointed an assistant apothecary in the I.M.S. in 1853. He is recorded as having served in the Crimea in 1854 and later being appointed to the Turkish Contingent. He may have been an acting assistant-surgeon but he did not qualify medically until 1856. He was made an assistant-surgeon in the I.M.S. in 1856, but resigned in 1861 and spent the rest of his life in Paris, taking the M.D. in 1866. He was for long the Paris correspondent of the **British Medical Journal** and a respected practitioner in the British community.

Thomas Buzzard (1831-1919) qualified in 1855 from King's College. His service in the Turkish Contingent is indicated in his memoir. While in the East he was a correspondent to the **Daily News.** After the war Buzzard was in general practice in London for six years. In 1863 he became a consultant with a special interest in neurology and was appointed Physician to the National Hospital for the Paralysed and Epileptic. He wrote widely on his speciality and was elected F.R.C.P. in 1873. One of his sons, Sir Farquhar Buzzard, reached considerable distinction as a physician.

Brudenell Carter (1828-1918) qualified from the London Hospital in 1851 and was in general practice before he joined the Turkish Contingent. He served as a staff surgeon 1855-1856, mainly in the Crimea. He met Russell and through him became a war correspondent to **The Times.** After the war he was in London and then moved to Nottingham where he had a part in founding the Eye Hospital. In 1862 he went to Stroud and was involved in the establishment of the Gloucester Eye Infirmary. Two years later, now F.R.C.S., he returned to London and became ophthalmologist to St. George's Hospital, as well as serving on the editorial staff of **The Times.** Carter wrote widely on ophthalmology. By his journalistic activities he informed the public of the views of the medical profession on all the topics of the day. He was President of the Medical Society of London in 1886.

Archibald Cockburn (d. 1862) qualified in 1842 from St. Andrews. His appointment to a "high professional post in the Turkish Contingent" comes to light in a letter written by Dr. Tyler concerning the case of the naval surgeon Elliott. Cockburn practised in London before the war. He allegedly entered into partnership with an American cancer quack, and the Edinburgh College of Surgeons (of which he was a Fellow) suspended him. He was re-instated by the College and a short time later was appointed to the Turkish Contingent in the rank of Deputy-Inspector-General. In view of his past record Dr. Tyler thought the appointment was quite disgraceful. No details of Cockburn's activities in the Turkish Contingent have been found. After the war he became Deputy-Inspector for Lunacy in Scotland.

Alexander Farquhar (d. 1890) qualified in 1838, practised in Chelsea until about 1845, and then went to Egypt. He was in Alexandria for ten years, attached in some capacity to the "Marine Hospital". From there he joined the Turkish Contingent and served ably in the rank of Inspector-General in Eupatoria and Trebizond. He was elected F.R.C.S. in 1856 but little is known of his post-war career. In his last years he lived in Aberdeenshire but did not apparently practise there.

William Harris (1830-1914) qualified in 1851 from the London Hospital. He was commissioned in the I.M.S. as assistant-surgeon in 1853. Seconded to the Turkish Contingent in 1855 he served in the Crimea. After the war he returned to India and saw active service in the Mutiny. He was for some time Professor

APPENDICES 647

of Midwifery in the Madras Medical College. He retired with the rank of Deputy Inspector-General in 1875.

James Keeling (1832-1909) qualified in Edinburgh in 1852. He seems to have gone out late in 1854 to serve with the Turks as a volunteer and subsequently became officially attached to the Turkish Contingent. After the war he became a gynaecologist of distinction in Sheffield.

Robert Lewins (1817-1895) qualified in Edinburgh in 1832. He joined the army in 1842 and was appointed surgeon to the 63rd Regiment in March 1854. The regiment arrived in Varna just before the invasion fleet sailed, and was not landed in time to take part in the battle of the Alma, however it suffered heavy losses at Inkerman. Lewins went sick in January 1855 and was on half pay from June 1855. It is possible that for a short period in 1855 he was attached to the Turkish Contingent. He served in the army again from July 1858 until he retired in 1868. After his retiral Lewins gave up medical practice for philosophical studies; "he devoted himself obsessively to the propagation of irreligion". He found disciples for his philosophy (which he termed "hylozoism") particularly among the intellectual and militant young ladies of the late Victorian period.

Thomas Littleton (1824-1878) qualified in 1847 from University College Hospital, and is believed to have served in the navy as an assistant-surgeon for a few years. He became F.R.C.S. in 1849. In practice in Plymouth with his father before the war, he acted as medical officer to the firm constructing Saltash bridge, which led him to publish observations on the symptoms of "caisson disease" (diving bells were used in the construction of the bridge) (**Ass.Med.J.** 1855, 127-128). It is not clear whether Littleton went out to the Crimean War as a naval reservist or as a civilian doctor. His name appears in a short list of five medical officers appointed to the Turkish Contingent in the rank of staff surgeon, as well as in relation to his retirement from the Contingent in the November list of 1855. After the war he returned to Plymouth to become the first M.O.H. of that city.

William McEgan (1817-1857) qualified in 1840, and became an assistant-surgeon in the I.M.S. in 1847. He was listed as a civil surgeon in Scutari in 1855 and recorded as being attached to the Turkish Contingent from March 1855 to March 1856. There is evidence in various letters that when McEgan was in Scutari he was not popular with his seniors. His early use of anaesthesia for the wounded and his death during the Mutiny have already been described (Chapter II).

Duncan MacPherson (1812-1867) qualified in 1835 at Edinburgh, and was commissioned in the Indian Medical Service as assistant-surgeon in 1836. He saw active service in China in 1841 and was severely wounded. Promoted surgeon in 1852, he was probably on leave in England early in 1855 when he was placed in command of the Turkish Contingent in the temporary rank of Inspector-General. After spending several months in recruiting he went out about November 1855 to take charge of the Turkish Contingent, which he did with considerable efficiency. During his stay in Kertch he found time to make archaeological studies and publish papers on this subject, as well as sending specimens to the British Museum. He returned to India after the war and rapidly rose to the permanent rank of Inspector-General. He was appointed to the important post of President of the Sanitary Commission in Madras but died suddenly.

John Radcliffe (1830-1884) qualified about 1851 from the Hull Medical School. He served in the Turkish Contingent in Varna, Sinope, and the Crimea, and was attached for some months to the Turkish Hospital at Balaclava (on which he published a detailed report). When he returned home he became Superintendent of the National Hospital for the Paralysed and Epileptic. He was especially interested in epidemiology and was Secretary of the Epidemiological Society. Increasingly consulted by the Government on health matters, he conducted enquiries into the cholera outbreak of 1861 and many other epidemics. In 1869 he became an Inspector of Public Health. His help was sought by many other countries in the investigation of epidemics of plague and cholera.

Humphry Sandwith (1822-1881) qualified in 1846 from St. Bartholomew's Hospital, and in 1847 was a house surgeon at Hull Infirmary. Having set up in practice in London without success, he went out to Constantinople in 1849 with letters of introduction to the British Ambassador. He met Layard, the explorer and archaeologist, and accompanied him on expeditions to Mesopotamia. He established himself in practice by his contacts with the Embassy, to which he was unofficially physician, and in 1853 he became a correspondent to **The Times**. In July 1854 Sandwith was appointed to serve in Varna with a force of bashi-bazouks under General Beatson, in the capacity of both interpreter and medical officer. There he established a primitive hospital, and being short of medicines, he prepared these himself from herbs collected in the countryside. When Beatson's force was disbanded Sandwith went to Erzerum to serve under General Williams (H.M. Commissioner with the Turkish army in Asia). His experiences during the siege of Kars are described in his book. When he returned to London he was received as a hero and the publication of his narrative of the siege of Kars gained him considerable fame. In June 1856 he was in Russia as physician to the British Ambassador at the time of the coronation of Alexander II. In 1857 he went out to Mauritius as Colonial Secretary, but three years later had to resign this post because of ill-health. He now became deeply involved in politics, particularly the Eastern question. He visited Serbia and Turkey and in both countries was seen as a powerful supporter of national interests. Among the humanitarian causes in which he became involved were the National Aid Society (a charity to help the victims of the Franco-Prussian War), and the care of the sick and wounded in the Serbo-Turkish War. He stood for parliament in 1868 but was not elected. His influence on foreign affairs seems to have been appreciable although exerted from behind the scenes. He was elected F.R.C.P. in 1859 but did not practise medicine thereafter.

INDEX OF PERSONS

Aberdeen, Lord: 288,381
Acton, W.: 560
Adair, R.: 3,12
Adams, -: 377
Ainger, M.: 561
Airey, General: 510
Aitken, W.: 88,405-9,419,596,617
Albert, Prince: 242
Alexander T.: 117,131-2,231,235,
    376,510,593-4,602,610,614,
    619
Alibert, -: 362
Alkin, Elizabeth: 15
Aloysius, M.: 275-6
Ancell, M.: 491
Anderson A.: 138
Anderson, D.: 200-1
Anderson, G.: 223-4,231,235,312
Anderson, W.: 328-9
Armand, A.: 326
Armstrong, A.: 612
Arnott, J.: 584
Atherstone W.: 58
Atkins, J.: 17
Atkinson, E.: 426
Atkinson, J.: 420

Bader, C.: 440,443,640
Bakewell, H.: 344,348-9,359-60,
    490-1
Balding, C.: 562
Balfour, T.: 593
Ballingal, J.: 13-4,53
Banbury, R.: 561
Barclay, A.: 425-6
Barclay, J.: 425-6
Barnes, Miss: 526
Barry, D.: 580
Barry, J.: 580
Bartlett, Miss: 552-3
Bassano, C.: 578
Baudens, M.: 318,326,530
Baxter, T.: 77
Bayford, C.: 508
Beale, T.: 561
Beatson, G.: 427,434,594
Beatson, General: 559,648
Beckwith, H.: 245
Beddoe, J.: 440,443-4,640
Beith, R.: 541
Bell, C.: 6
Bell, J.: 13
Bellot, T.: 550
Bent, J.: 488
Bentinck, General: 384
Beveridge, -: 528
Bird, -: 560
Birnie, T.: 476
Birt, H.: 415,640

Blackwood, Lady: 267,507-8
Blake, E.: 471
Blakeley, -: 384
Blane, G.: 4,17-8,20
Blantyre, Lord: 281
Blenkins, G.: 582
Boggs, A.: 561,646
Boldero, -: 47
Bosquet, General: 124
Boustead, R.: 562
Bowen, R.: 582
Bowen-Thomson, J.: 420-1
Bowman, W.: 255,266,276,281
Boxall, R.: 560-8
Boxer, Admiral: 171
Boyle, E.: 328-9
Brabazon, A.: 415,640
Bracebridge, G.: 253,263,266,271,
    273-4,366,499,501,522-3,553,
    586
Bracebridge, Mrs.: 253,261,263-4,
    266,275,366,431,499,522-4
Bradshaw, W.: 603
Brady, M.: 488
Brett, F.: 37-38
Bridgeman, Mrs.: 271,276,532,586-7
Brokelsby, R.: 2
Brodie, B.: 13,436
Brown, General: 41,90,455,510
Brown, J.: 560
Browne, W.: 201
Brunel, I.: 436-9,446
Brunton, -: 431,438-439
Brush, J.: 208,219,225,297,308-9
Bryce, C.: 415-6,521,640-1
Bryson, A.: 52,612-3
Buchanan, J.: 440,443-5,641
Buller, General: 306
Burgesh, Lord: 510
Burgess, -: 600
Burgoyne, General: 384
Burnett, W.: 21,23,552,605
    early career: 44-5; planning
    in war: 45-6,48-52; views on
    chloroform: 60-1,98; views on
    cholera: 97,104-5; retiral:
    612,644
Burrell, W.: 38,51,66,68
Buzzard, T.: 560,562,564-5,646
Byron, Lord: 256,443

Calder, W.: 136
Calvert, -: 386,439,443-4
Campbell, C.: 217,274,503-5
Campbell, E.: 561
Campbell, G.: 413
Cambridge, Duke of: 23
Canning, Lady : 271,431,441,524-
    5,603-4

Canrobert, General: 124,454
Cardigan, Lord: 220-1,383
Carlaw, J.: 561-2
Carr, G.: 171
Carter, B.: 561,646
Casselas, -: 530
Cathcart, General: 217
Cattell, W.: 78,82-3,167
Cattle, W.: 561
Chapman, P.: 496
Chapple, R.: 225
Chenery, T.: 145-6
Christison, D.: 440,443
Christison, R.: 282
Clare, Rev. Mother: 523,526,532
Clarendon, Lord: 188,257
Clark, H.: 561
Clifford, H.: 239,291,306,324,
    462,510-1
Clough, Miss: 274-5,503-5,524
Clowes, W.: 1
Coates, -: 562,568
Cockburn, A.: 561,646
Cocking, J.: 333
Codrington, General: 486,508,572
Complin, E.: 426,443,641
Cooper, R.: 83,375
Coote, C.: 426
Coote, H.: 426,440-1,443
Coote, Mrs.H.: 431-2,443
Corbett, J.: 549
Cowan, James: 470-1
Cowan, John: 438,440,443-5,641
Cowper, J.: 561
Cranworth, Lady.: 532-3
Crawford, T.: 319,610-1
Cree, E.: 99-100,544,547-8
Cromwell, O.: 1,15
Crosse, J.: 223
Cruikshank, W.: 76,117,351,353
Cubitt, -: 560
Cullen, W.: 415,426
Cumming, A.: 185,272-4,278,350-3,
    357-8,374,406-7,431,521,524,
    530,580
Czadky, A.: 561

Dalby, W.: 550
Davidson, J.: 444,550,552
Davis, F.: 106
Davis, Mrs.: 274-5,500,502,505
Dawson, Sergeant: 382,384-5
Deas, D.: 107,333,538,613
De Chaumont, F.: 582-3
Dee, J.: 561
Delane, J.: 43,146,263
De Lisle, R.: 64
Derby, Lord: 425
Derriman, E.: 334,549
Dingan, -: 56
Dix, J.: 440

Dixon, T.: 440
Domville, H.: 106-7
Doyle, -: 406-7
Drake, Mrs.: 264,503,505
Drummond, H.: 288
Drummond, J.: 31
Duberly, Mrs.: 91,311,505
Duigan, D.: 99,333,494-5
Dumbreck, D.: 38-41,64,67,76-7,
    86,117,130,159-60,165,185,
    296,325,382,388,597
Dumbreck, W.: 603
Dunant, J.: 615-6
Duncan, W.: 395
Dundas, Admiral: 33,101-2,210,213,
    539,542
Dundas, G.: 188,191-2,382,390
Dyneley, -: 487

Easton, R.: 541
Eddowes, J.: 426,430
Edsall, -: 561,565,568
Edwards, -: 560
Elkington, A.: 232
Elkington, J.: 560
Ellice E.: 351
Elliot, Richard: 143,488
Elliot, Robert: 420
Elliott, James: 494-8
Elliott, John: 333
Elliott, R.: 420
Errol, Lady: 91
Erskine, Miss: 552-3
Esdaile, J.: 584
Estcourt, General: 162,308,312-3,
    455,509-10
Evans, General: 226,384
Evelyn, G.: 121
Evelyn, J.: 15

Fair, G.: 471
Falconer, J.: 426
Farley, N.: 578
Farquhar, A.: 560,646
Farr, W.: 614,617
Fauvel, -: 530
Fawcas, J.: 440
Fell, T.: 420
Field, -: 440
Filder, -: 404
Fitzgerald, -: 532,587
Fitzpatrick, J.: 4
Fitzroy, Lord: 201
Fleidner, T.: 252-3
Flewitt, J.: 420,529
Flower, W.: 235,382,388,
    601
Fogo, J.: 488
Foote, -: 560
Forbes, J.: 425-6
Forester, Lady: 256-7

Forrest, J.: 76,117,351,360, 382,388
Forteath, A.: 138
Foster, -: 148-9
Fowler, R.: 252
Fox, -: 440
Francis, J.: 440
Fraser, P.: 415,601,641
Fraser, T.: 466
Freeth, Rev.: 359
Fuller, J.: 559-60
Furlong, J.: 504

Gale, T.: 1
Gallaghar, J.: 97-8
Gant, F.: 415-6,641-2
Gaskell, Mrs.: 255-6
Gavin, H.: 395,398,492
Gibbon, S.: 426,429
Gibbons, J.: 488
Gibson, J.: 128,594,610
Gilborne, J.: 578
Gladstone, Mrs.: 271
Goodeve, H.: 440,443-5,642
Gordon, A.: 128,130
Gordon, T.: 5
Gordon, W.: 99
Gowing, T.: 122,134,237-8,510
Grabham, J.: 362
Graham, J.: 47
Grainger, R.: 426
Grant, -: 79
Grant, J.: 6
Gray, C.: 420
Greer, A.: 488
Greig, D.: 184,263,280-1,361, 490
Grey, Admiral: 396-8
Guthrie, G.: 5-9,12,14,42-3,52-4, 60,146,477,479

Hadaway, G.: 58,530
Hadley, J.: 500-1
Haire, -: 55
Hale, R.: 440,445
Hale, T.: 487
Hall, J.: 8,38,178,190,199,207, 215,235-6,241,259,279,302-4, 306-8,312-3,315,325-6,335-6, 350-3,357-8,391-3,406,463, 469-71,490,509-10,521,523, 525,534,566,577,580,582-7,594
  early career: 66-68; Bulgaria: 76-78; directive on cholera: 79-82; preparations for invasion: 112-4; the Alma: 127-32,154-5; criticisms of Hall: 161-7; visit to Scutari: 171-3; defence against critics: 400-1; civil surgeons: 421-2,444-5,447;

civil hospitals: 434-5,438; Miss Nightingale: 498-502; post-war criticism: 606-609; character: 609
Hamilton, -: 544
Hamilton, J.: 561
Hanbury, W.: 597,600
Harness, J.: 21
Harris, W.: 561,646-7
Harrison, -: 420
Hawes, B.: 434,436,524
Hearn, C.: 63-4,84,240
Heath, C.: 542
Hennen, J.: 7,12,33,53
Herbert, L.: 582
Herbert, Mrs.: 261-2,271,273,275, 524,532
Herbert, S.: 7,150,188,248,253, 277-9,289,301,308,352,355, 364-5,396,405,413,501,505, 529,534,552,587-9,604
  Miss Nightingale to Scutari: 257-261,265,268; Stanley affair: 271-3; Struthers affair: 281-3; First Commission: 389-90; Sanitary Commission: 593-7,604; Indian Commission: 614; death: 614
Hodge, E.: 155,299-300,305,307,329, 462
Holl, H.: 415
Holland, T.: 440
Holthouse, C.: 426
Home, A.: 603
Home, E.: 3
Hooker, J.: 23
Hooper, -: 440
Hope, W.: 487
Hornidge, T.: 426
Howard, E.: 415
Hughes, J.: 415
Hulke, J.: 426,430,444,642
Hume, J.: 10
Hume, T.: 582
Humfrey, W.: 423,427,429
Humphrey, J.: 440
Hunter, J.: 3,55
Hunter, T.: 423
Hutcheon, P.: 562
Huthwaite, F.: 141
Huxley, T.: 23

Irvine, Alexander: 561
Irvine, Archibald: 561
Irwin, William (Sen.): 58
Irwin, William (Jun.): 603

Jackson, R.: 3,7,12
Jameson, T.: 81,117
Jane, M.: 362
Jardine, J.: 426,430

Jeeves, W.: 488
Jenkin, E.: 89
Jenkins, -: 560
Jenkins, J.: 333
Jenner, W.: 439
Johnston, A.: 529
Jones, Agnes: 615

Keeling, J.: 561,647
Keith, T.: 181
Keppel, H.: 495-6,546-7
Ker, C.: 5
Kidd, C.: 601
Kinglake, A.: 73,110-1,144,205, 221,511
Kirk, J.: 440-1,443,642
Kirkland, J.: 258
Korniloff, Admiral: 205,214

Laennec, H.: 45
Laing, P.: 374,378
Lakin, J.: 426
Lamont, J.: 329
Langham, J.: 329
Langston, Miss: 502
Larkin, E.: 561
Larrey, D.: 53
Latta, T.: 56
Lawrence, J.: 582
Lawson, G.: 62-3,118,121,244-7, 290,300,302,360,462,488-9, 500,507,601
Lawson, R.: 161-2,166-7,351, 353,358,378,524
Layard, A.: 381-2,390
Leared, A.: 426,429,642-3
Le Blanc E.: 328
Lefroy, J.: 529-30
Le Mesurier F.: 560,564
Le Mesurier, Mrs.: 432
Leshley, W.: 330
Lewer, R.: 542
Lewins, R.: 561,647
Liddel, J.: 23,52,594,612-3,645
Lind, J.: 17-9,54,87,106
Lindsay, C.: 381
Linnaeus, C.: 53
Linton, W.: 38-9,76,80,117,128, 173,244,296,325,415,466,530-1, 534,597,603
Liprandi, General: 216
Lister, J.: 129,181,359,361,640
Liston, R.: 57-8
Littleton, T.: 561,647
Logan, T.: 610
Longmore, J.: 491-2
Longmore, T.: 491-2,596,601,611
Lovelace, Lady: 256
Lowe, P.: 1
Lucan, Lord: 220-1,383-4
Ludlow, H.: 522

Lushington, S.: 332,334,495
Lyons, Admiral: 101,110,143,332, 498,543
Lyons, R.: 405-9,415,444,582,617

Macalister, J.: 561
Macartney, C.: 491
Macartney, F.: 362
McCauley, -: 561,568
McCormack, J.: 394
McCormick, R.: 23,45
McCraith, J.: 430
Macdonald, J.: 188,192-3,263,265-6, 383,391
Macdonnel, A.: 224-5
McDonnel, R.: 426,430,643
McDowall, C.: 561
McEgan, W.: 59,415,561,647
Macfie, W.: 561
McGrigor, A.: 169,186,191,267,278-9,353,366,379,418,521,524,528
McGrigor, J.: 6-8,10-2,33-5,385, 394,412,605
McIlree, J.: 353
Mackay, G.: 60,215-6
McKechnie, A.: 100
Mackenzie, Mrs. J.: 551-4
Mackenzie, Rev.J.: 551-2
Mackenzie, R.: 88-89,129,131-4,141, 358,412-3,471
Mackey, P.: 142
McKinnon, D.: 247
McKinnon, W.: 611
McKutcheon, A.: 529
MacLaren, J.: 440
Macleod, G.: 412-3,415,426,430,444, 450,583-5,601,643
Macnamara, -: 357
McNeill, J.: 401-4,592,607,616
MacPherson, D.: 559,561,567,647
Macaulay, J.: 436
Manning, Cardinal: 254,270,275
Mapleton, H.: 382,388,594
Marks, Miss: 526
Marlow, B: 244
Marshall, H.: 7,12,402
Marshall, J.: 362
Marston, J.: 602
Martel, P.: 117
Martin, J.: 614
Martin, R.: 426
Mason, R.: 415
Massy H.: 244
Matthew, T.: 138,474,597
Maule, L.: 274,504
Maunder, C.: 440,443,477
Maxwell, -: 374,379,383,391
Mayne, J.: 528
Menshikov, Prince: 123-4,143,205

Menzies, D.: 66-7,147,168-172, 177-8,185-6,190,192-3,199,259, 277-9,348,351-2,355,382,386-8, 390,392
Menzies, E.: 583
Mercer, C.: 562
Meyer, J.: 273,421,425-8,430-3, 435,440,559,594,643
Millard, R.: 560,568
Milnes, M.: 253
Milroy, G.: 105,398-9,600
Milton, -: 355
Mitchell, J.: 38,40,76,141,173,597
Mitchell, T.: 529
Moore, S.: 603
Moore, Mrs: 526
Moorhead, T.: 423
Morgan, -: 106
Morris, C.: 389
Morton, Miss: 532
Mouat, J.: 209,222-3,247,477,530, 584,594
Moyle, J.: 16
Muir, W.: 610
Munro, W.: 118,128,131-2,210, 215,218,224,602

Napier, Admiral: 33,94,539
Napoleon, I.: 194
Napoleon III: 73,453-4
Nelson, C.: 603
Nelson, Lord: 20
Newcastle, Duke of: 73,352,374,389, 391,461
Newlands, -: 395
Newman, Mrs: 441
Newton, J.: 353,361
Nicholas, I.: 30
Nightingale, Florence: 7,12,91, 164,175,180,188,194,340-3,345, 347,369,38,390-1,393,398,401, 403-5,407,409,416-7,424,431, 436,438-9,441,444,503-6,511, 517,520-3,529,531-6,580,597, 599,603-4,606-10
  early life: 252-3; nursing experience: 255-6; call to the East: 256-68; religious problems: 269-70; Stanley affair: 270-6; relations with doctors: 276-81; Struthers affair: 281-4; account of Crimean winter: 289-90; evidence to First Commission: 379; opinion of Sanitary Commission: 399; visit to Crimea: 498-500; illness: 500-2; increasing problems at Scutari: 523-5; second visit: 586-7; third visit: 587-8; active in planning Sanitary Commission: 593-4; evidence to Commission: 595; Netley Hospital: 596; India Commission: 614; hospital reform: 615; Nightingale Fund: 615; poor-law reform: 615; medical advisors, 616-7: character, 617-8
Nightingale, Mrs.: 252-4,257
Nightingale, W.: 252,254-5
Nolan, L.: 220-1
Norris, J.: 245

O'Connor, N.: 350,353,578
Odevaine, F.: 561
Ogilvy, J.: 508
O'Leary, J.: 246
Omar, Pasha: 32,73,288,560,565,567
Ormerod, L.: 560,568
Osborne, Rev.: 164,188-91,198,200, 266,383,390-1,393
Owens, J.: 84

Pagan, -: 441
Paget, J.: 617
Paget, Lady: 505-6,510
Paget, Lord: 505,510
Pakington, J.: 381
Palmerston, Lord: 30,257,288-9,404, 488
Panmure, Lord: 289,365,368-9,393, 396,399,405,422,435,453,488-90, 529,586,593,606
Paré, A.: 1
Parker, Rev.: 393,390-1
Parkes, E.: 438-43,594,596,600, 616-7,643
Parry, -: 440
Patteson, -: 561
Paulet, Lord: 354,389,396-7,406-7, 444,524
Pauloff, General: 227
Pearse, J. : 15-6
Peele, General: 381
Pelissier, General: 454
Pennefather, General: 455
Pepys, S.: 15
Percy, J.: 273,382,390,393
Peters, J.: 138-9
Phelps, J.: 488
Philips, -: 560
Pincoffs, P.: 415-8,444,521,530,644
Pitcairn, G.: 89
Pine, C.: 329
Playne, A.: 440
Pont, -: 560
Prendergast, J.: 509-11
Pringle, J.: 2-3,12,53-4,335
Pusey, E.: 262

Quetelet, L.: 260

Radcliffe, J.: 560,563,600,647-8
Raglan, Lord: 3,32,41,73-4,77,101,
112-3,116,123,127,154-5,168,
191,210,217-8,220,222,226,233,
259,288,388,392,396,399,412,
453,455,487,498-503,505-6,523,
580,594
 gives no credit to doctors: 134-5; blamed for medical organisation: 147; blames doctors for transport: 160-7; sends wounded to Scutari: 237; supports Miss Nightingale: 266; requests nurses in Crimea: 274; ignorance of medical problems: 301-3; death: 510; character: 510-1
Ramsden, -: 230
Ranke, -: 426,430,477
Rathbone, W.: 615
Rawlinson, R.: 395-6,398,401
Reade, G.: 201,355
Reade, H.: 201
Reade, J.: 201
Reed, A.: 99
Rees, J.: 103-6
Regan, -: 333
Reid, A.: 142
Reid, J.: 612-3
Reid, W.: 401
Renwick, W.: 329
Reynolds, V.: 137
Richards, -: 225,486
Richards, -: 486
Richardson, J.: 23,45,60
Richardson, R.: 561
Ricketts, C.: 230
Risk, A.: 561
Riskillah, Habib: 561
Roberts, B.: 430,440,443
Roberts, Mrs.: 264,499-500,523,532
Robertson, W.: 440,644
Robinson, F.: 230
Roebuck, J.: 288,380-1,395
Rogers, -: 355
Rolleston, G.: 426,430,433,644
Rooke, H.: 415
Rooke, W.: 440,443,477,490
Rowdon, H.: 415,418,434,521,594
Russell, W.: 42-4,63,65,75,77,82,
110,145,217,232,297-8,308
Rutherford, W.: 604

Sabin, Rev. - : 188-9,356
Salisbury, Miss: 524,531
Salter, J.: 248
Sandwith, H.: 559,565-6,648
Schliemann, H.: 443
Sclaveroni, -: 583
Scarlett, General: 218
Scot, T.: 87,241

Scott, G.: 110
Seacole, Mrs.: 506-7
Sellon, Miss: 261-2,281
Shaftesbury, Lord: 399
Shegog, G.: 89
Shelton, G.: 466
Shorrock, J.: 141
Sibbald, -: 562,568
Sillery, -: 168,170,354,389-90,392
Sim, R.: 562
Simons, R.: 522
Simpson, General: 455,487,511
Simpson, J.: 53,58,181,199,281,354,
435
Simpson, W.: 491
Skelton, J.: 234
Skinner, -: 562
Smart, W.: 333-4
Smith, A.: 8-9,64,67-8,79,131,
168-9,171-2,177-8,185,190,248,
257,262,277-8,282,296,298,300,
303-4,316,326,348,351-2,609-10
 early life: 33-4; appointed M.D.G.: 35; prepares for war: 35-43; criticism: 145-50, 154, 159-60; views on nurses: 278-9; plan for First Commission: 373; evidence to Roebuck Committee: 382-3,385-7, 389; continued criticism: 393-5; Sanitary Commission: 593-4; evidence to Commission: 595-6; last years: 605; character: 605-6,609-10
Smith, F.: 329
Smith, G.: 171,186,198-200,357,383,
414
Smith, J.: 231
Smith, Mrs.: 7
Smith, S.: 257
Smollet, T.: 17
Smythe, Miss: 432
Snow, J.: 56,96,466-7,600
Soimonofff, General: 227
Soyer, A.: 366-70,499-500
Spence, T.: 190,245,248,263,374,385
St. Arnaud, General: 73,111-2,123,
125-6
Stafford, A.: 188,190-1,382,390,
393,593
Stanley, Lord: 614
Stanley, Mary: 259,261,270-4,276,
350,362,365,425,431,502-3,524,
526,531
Steele, G.: 60
Sterling, A.: 506
Stewart, G.: 362
Stewart, J.: 420
Stewart, Mrs.: 502-5,523,532,587
Stirling, R.: 562
Storks, General: 354,424,430-1,
524-5,531

Stratford de Redcliffe, Lady: 271,
    354,359,431,441,524,534-5
Stratford de Redcliffe, Lord: 170,
    190,266,381,386,391,504-6
Streatfeild, J.: 426,644
Stretton, S.: 440,443
Struthers, A.: 281-3,361-2
Summers, J.: 353
Sutherland, G.: 561
Sutherland, J.: 356,395-6,398-9,
    401,533,614,616
Swain, W.: 542
Sylvester, H.: 135,487
Syme, J.: 14,115,281,354,406

Tate, W.: 561
Taylor, A.: 185,280,338,488
Taylor, John: 594
Taylor, Joseph: 420
Taylor, Miss: 350,362-5
Teasdale, -: 566
Temple, W.: 351
Temple, W.R.: 561
Terrot, Miss: 345
Thomson, A.: 406-7
Thomson, John: 6,13
Thornton, R.: 582-3
Tice, J.: 138,160
Tindall, W.: 562
Todleben, General: 205
Trotter, T.: 17-20
Tufnell, T.: 14
Tuke, W.: 45
Tulloch, A.: 401-2,404,592,607
Turner, -: 561

Upton, - : 462

Van Millingen, - : 7
Vaughan, J.: 551
Vaux, J.: 382,389
Veale, T.: 440
Velpeau, A.: 58-9
Vesey, Miss: 552-3
Victoria, Queen: 288,403,500,
    544,572,617

Wakly, T.: 22,66
Walford, Mrs.: 526
Walker, -: 377
Wall, T.: 549
Walsh, J.: 333
Ward, -: 168-9,354-5,378
Ward, Lord: 501
Wason, E.: 361-2
Watson, -: 106
Watson, P.: 185,283,350-1,358-9,
    361,553
Weare, Miss: 505
Webb, S.: 31
Weir, J. (Army): 5-6

Weir, J. (Navy): 21
Wellington, Duke of: 6,8,10,32,
    192,220,316,463,553,642
Wells, Mrs.: 443
Wells, T.: 22-23,42,,58,394,
    422,426-30,440-1,443-4,469,
    474,484-5,644-5
West, -: 377
Whistler, D.: 15
White, C.: 375
White, J.: 491
Wigan, E.: 561
Wilkin, J.: 222
Wilkinson, R.: 426
Willet, -: 561
Williams, General: 565,648
Williams, J.: 581
Williams, St. G.: 561,566
Wilson, -: 395
Wilson, R.: 232-3
Wilson, W.: 99
Wise, J.: 106
Wishart, J.: 522
Woolaston, R.: 415
Wolseley, R.: 233
Wolseley, W.: 561
Wolsten, C.: 561
Wood, B.: 426
Wood, H.: 528
Woodal, J.: 1,15
Woodfull, S.: 420
Woodward, Miss: 500
Wordsworth J.: 415,426,430
Wreford, -: 169,334-5,378
Wrench, E.: 485-6,488,509
Wyatt, J.: 234-6,241,325

Yates, G.: 561
Yea, L.: 299
Yonge, J.: 16

INDEX OF SUBJECTS AND PLACES

Ambulance service: 37,43,79,116, 119,122,133,375,386,463
American doctors in Russian service : 592
Amputations: see 'War wounds'
Anaesthesia:
  use in Crimean War: 98,114-5, 131-2,199,215-6,234-6,435, 471-3,584-5; use in Services before Crimean War: 57-61
Army hospitals: (see also 'Field Hospitals' and 'Regimental Hospitals')
Army hospitals in Crimea:
  Balaclava General: 207,245,292,311,314,369,375, 499-500,502-3,532,577,586-7;
  Camp General: 469-470,503,577;
  Castle: 468-9,500,502-5,577, 587;
  Land Transport: 442,469,503, 587;
  Monastery: 469,503,577-8
Army hospitals in Bulgaria and Turkey:
  Abydos: 67,158,168,176,342, 420,435,599;
  Barrack: 64-5,67,168-9,174-8, 185-6,189,191-2,264-5,267,275, 278,280,340-343,347-9,362-4, 366,368-9,379-80,386-38,397, 407,418,517-22,526-30,534-6;
  General: 66-7,168-9,173-8,185, 264,340-3,347-9,351-4,386-91, 407,517-2,526-30,534-6;
  Haidar Pasha: 168,342,397,526, 335;
  Koulali: 67,168,175-6,274, 340-3,347,351,359,362,364-5, 387-8,415,421,526,534;
  Palace: 175-6,397,526;
  Varna: 76-9,598-9
Army hospitals (at home):
  Fort Pitt: 11,34,358,409,596;
  Netley: 596
Army medical officers: at the Alma: 127-31; at Balaclava: 219,222-6; briefing: 51-3; in Bulgaria: 76,83,89; conditions of service: 11,489,579-80; at Inkerman: 229-37; mobilisation in 1854: 38; national roots: 12-3; at Siege of Sebastopol: 214-5,245-6,456-7,470-1,484-9, 491-2; in Turkish Contingent: 560-1
Army Medical School: 13,409,596-7

Army Medical Service:
  seventeenth century: 1-2; eighteenth century: 2-4; nineteenth century: 4-14; state in 1854: 36-8

Bakewell case: 490-1
Balaclava, town and harbour: 65,310-3,399,542-3,573
Battles and sieges (Army) (see also 'Sebastopol'):
  Alma: 123-42,198,376;
  Balaclava: 216-6,264;
  Inkerman: 198,227-39;
  Kars: 565;
  Little Inkerman: 226-7;
  Tractir Bridge: 455
Battles and sieges (Army, earlier wars):
  Corunna: 5;
  Toulouse: 5;
  Waterloo: 5,8,42,412
Battles and sieges (Navy):
  Algiers: 23;
  Armada: 15;
  Navarino: 52;
  Trafalgar: 20
Bleeding (venesection): 54,57,475-7
Boards, Commissions and Committees - see 'Chelsea Board', 'First Commission (Newcastle)', 'Parliamentary Committee 1856', 'Pathology Commission', 'Roebuck Committee (Sebastopol Committee)', 'Sanitary Commission', 'Royal Sanitary Commission'
Bowel conditions: 84-5,96,103,196-7,243,317-8,344,463-4,518-9, 527,545-6,551,555,574-5

Campaigns:
  Afghan: (1838); 8
  Austrian Succession (1742): 2;
  Burma (1824): 8;
  China (1839): 8,22;
  China (1858): 604,613;
  Egypt (1801): 8;
  Egypt (1882): 611;
  French Wars (1793-1815); 3-7
  Indian Mutiny (1857); 602-4
  Ireland (1690): 2;
  Peninsula (1808): 5-6,278;
  Sikh (1845): 8;
  West Indies (1793): 3
Camps: 74-6,207-10,313
Chairs of military surgery: 6,13-4
Chelsea Board: 403-4,592

Chest diseases: 18,98,197,320-1, 346,467,519,528,541,547,551, 555,575
Chloroform - see 'Anaesthesia'
Cholera: 36,43,48,51,53,56-7,64,74-5,77-84,95-8,100,102-6,116-7, 119-21,129,132-3,135,137-8,140-2,144,197,243,245,255-6,316-8, 321-3,347,465-7,496-7,519-20, 526-9,540-1,546,565,574-5,577, 582,599-600
Civil hospitals:
assessment of value: 432-4,446-7; nursing staff: 424,428,431-2,441; planning: 421-7,435-9; Renkioi: 430-1,435-7; Smyrna: 273,390,394,413,421, 435,438,440,442,444,447,599
Civilian hospitals - comparison with Scutari Hospitals: 179-184
Civilian hospitals (at home):
Edinburgh Royal Infirmary: 129,181;
King's College: 62,255;
Leeds Infirmary: 180-1;
Middlesex: 255;
St. Thomas's: 264,615;
Salisbury Hospital: 252;
Shrewsbury Infirmary: 182
Civil surgeons:
in Crimea: 413,415,420-1,430, 443-5,447,484-5,492; at Renkioi: 440-1; in Scutari hospitals: 415; at Smyrna: 426-7
Civilian practice - comparison with Service practice: 55-6
Climate: 8,65,81,290,296-7,458-9, 576
Clothing (Army): 8,39-41,65-6,120, 241-2,290,298-304,387,450-9
Clothing (Navy): 330-1
Commissariat: 36-7,401-4
Commissions - see 'Boards' etc.
Committees - see 'Boards' etc.

Diet (Army): 74,81,208-9,240,289-0, 306-8,460
Diet (hospitals): 316,360,362-3, 366-9,379
Diet (Navy): 18,49,211,331,555
Diseases - see 'Bowel conditions', 'Chest conditions', 'Cholera', 'Eye conditions','Frost-bite', 'Heat-stroke', 'Malaria', 'Scurvy', 'Smallpox', 'Typhoid fever', 'Typhus', 'Venereal disease', 'Yellow Fever'
Dressers (Army): 419-0
Dressers (civil hospitals): 441
Dressers (Navy): 48,99,541-2

659

Dressers (Turkish Contingent): 560
Drunkenness: 7-12,17-8,63,74,79,82, 326-7,379,525

Edinburgh Medical School: 283,354, 359,441
Elliott case: 496-8
Eye conditions: 577-8

Fever: 85-7,95-6,102,195-6,243,318-20,344-5,429,464-5,519,527,540, 545,551,555,574,577,583,600
Field Hospitals: 470-1,494
First Commission: 315,352,373-80
Flank March: 142-5
Flogging: 12,66,327
French Army: 32,591
French medical service:140,193,415, 417-8,529,588,592,600
Frost-bite: 197,316,323-4,333,346, 428-9,528,551,575-6,582

Gallipoli: 62-4,80
Great Storm: 210,240,242,246-8,310, 374

Heat-stroke: 65,120,145,602
Honours and decorations (see also 'Victoria Cross'): 11,134-5, 487-9,606-7,618-9
Hospital orderlies: 37-8,79,363, 380,431,441-2,533-4
Hospitals: see 'Army hospitals in Crimea', 'Army hospitals in Bulgaria and Turkey', 'Army hospitals (at home)', 'Civil hospitals', 'Civilian hospitals (at home)', 'Field Hospitals', 'Naval hospitals (Crimea)', 'Naval hospitals (East - other than Crimea)', 'Naval hospitals (at home)', 'Poor-Law hospitals', 'Regimental Hospitals', 'Turkish hospitals'
Hospital ships:
'Belleisle': 50,100,541, Plate VII
'Diamond': 212,333-4';
'Mauritius': 604;
'Melbourne': 604;
'Minden': 22
Hospital transports:
'Andes': 116,139,148,201,362, 389,548;
'Arthur the Great': 136,157;
'Avon': 161,164,166,167,353, 608;
'Brandon': 522;
'Caduceus': 136,142;
'Cambria': 116,139,474;
'Cleopatra': 378;

'Colombo': 149,164,328;
'Cornwall': 142;
'Dunbar': 135;
'Echunga': 157;
'Emue': 330;
'Golden Fleece': 329;
'Gomelza': 156;
'Harbinger': 389;
'Kangaroo': 135,142,390,522;
'Medway': 361;
'Niagara': 378;
'Shooting Star': 341;
'Trent': 162,522;
'Victoria': 388
Hospital transports, organisation: 41-2,154,156-63,167,341,360, 458,599
Hounslow flogging case: 66-7,607
Hulks: 158,169,190,193,342,397-8
Huts: 210,241,295,305-6,461,578
Hygiene: 12,39,82-3,176-7,191, 308-9,312-3,459,600

Indian Medical Service: 559-61,567
India, Sanitary Commission: 614
Invasion of the Crimea: 110-9

Kaiserswerth Institution: 252-4, 259
Kamiesh: 143,543,573
Kars: 565,573
Kazatch: 143,543,546,548,573
Kertch: 543,546,573
Kilt: 240
Kinburn: 544,547-8,573

Malaria: 4,39,52,86,102,459
Marines: 101,218,330,496-8.549
Medical societies:
    Crimean Medical Society: 581-5;
    Medical Society of Constantinople: 530;
    Medico-Chirurgical Society of Smyrna: 428-429
Mortality of medical officers:
    British Army: 591-2; British Navy: 592,612; French Army: 592; Russian Army: 592
Mortality, total:
    British Army: 591-2; British Navy: 554; French Army: 592; other doctors: 592; Russian Army: 592; Turkish Contingent: 592

Naval Brigade: 101-2,210-3,330-5, 492-6,603
Naval hospitals (abroad):
    Bighi (Malta): 50;
    Naval Brigade Hospital (Crimea): 492;
    Therapia (Turkey): 50,107,192-3,212,216,274,333-4,444,492, 547,549-4;
Naval hospitals (at home):
    Chatham: 19;
    Greenwich: 16;
    Haslar: 19-20,49,51,179,541;
    Plymouth: 20,49,179;
    Yarmouth: 50,541
Naval Medical Officers:
    at Battle of the Alma: 127,137-9; in Baltic Sea (1854): 97-101; in Baltic Sea (1855-1856): 541-2; in Black Sea (1854): 103-7; in Black Sea (1855-1856): 544,548-9,550,552-3; briefing in 1854: 52-3; conditions of service before 1854: 21-2,44-8; Marines: 101-102,496-8,549; mobilisation in 1854: 47-9; surgeon naturalists: 23
Naval Brigade: 101-2,333-5,494-6
Naval Medical Service:
    seventeenth century: 14-5; eighteenth century: 16-20; nineteenth century (first half): 20-3; state in 1854: 45-51
Nightingale Fund: 615
Nurses: in Crimea: 247,498-500,502-5,532,586-8; at Regimental Hospitals: 274,503-6,532; at Renkioi Hospital: 438-9,441; at Scutari Hospitals: 261-4,283, 362-6,520-6,331-3; at Smyrna Hospital: 424,428,431-32; at Therapia Hospital: 550-4
Orderlies - see 'Hospital orderlies'

Parliamentary Committee (1856): 433,592-3
Pathology Commission: 383,405-9
Poor Law hospitals: 179,183-4,615
Purveyors: 265-7,354-5,363

Railroad: 462-3
Regimental Hospitals: 84-5,209-0, 213-4,219,222-3,234,244-7,292-5,314-28,375,391,458,470-1, 533,574-6
Respiratory tract diseases - see 'Chest diseases'
Rheumatic diseases: 18,197,346,519
Roebuck Committee: 288-9,351-2,373, 380-395
Royal College of Physicians: 1,3,19

661

Royal College of Surgeons, Edinburgh: 605
Royal College of Surgeons, England: 130,466
Royal Sanitary Commission: 259,401, 408,433-4,533-4,593-7
Russian Army: 32,591
Russian wounded: 133-4

Sanitary Commission: 356,380,395-401,404,433,499-500
Sardinian Army: 32,455,583
Scurvy: 16-8,54,87,95,106,197, 209,244,307,316,324-6,460, 472,541,547,551,600
Scutari harbour and town: 65
Sebastopol, siege of: First Bombardment: 213-216; Second Bombardment: 454-455; Third Bombardment: 455; Fourth Bombardment: 455; Fifth Bombardment: 455-456; naval bombardment: 215-6,543-4; capture: 455-6
Ships - see 'Hospital ships', 'Hospital transports', 'Ships (miscellaneous)', 'Warships'
Ships, miscellaneous:
  'Egyptus': 275;
  'Howard': 31;
  'John Masterman': 159;
  'Jura': 501-2;
  'Metropolitan': 299;
  'Pride of the Ocean': 334;
  'Prince': 139,246-8,298;
  'Vectis': 263
Shock: 473
Sinope: 30-1,434,438
Smallpox: 4,54,96,102,540,546-7
Stanley Affair: 270-6
Stethoscope: 45
Storm - see 'Great Storm'
Struthers Affair: 281-3
Supplies Commission: 373,401-4, 607
Tents: 63-4,240-1,304-5,375, 383,460
Tetanus: 45
The Times Fund: 263,267
Turkish Army medical service: 89,173,562-5
Turkish Contingent: 559-68
Turkish hospitals: 88,173,562-6
Typhoid fever: 53,86,102,243,317, 464,545
Typhus: 5,16-8,39,53-4,86,102,196, 318-9,345,350,427,442,465, 519,545,574

Varna: 74-82,84,86,88-9,168
Venereal disease: 98,327

Ventilation in warships: 18,612
Victoria Cross: 222,487,603

Walcheren Disaster: 4-5,336
War correspondents: 43-4,145-9, 155,163-4
Warships:
  'Agamemnon':103,139,215;
  'Ajax': 96;
  'Albion': 102-3,215,545,551;
  'Algiers': 545;
  'Amphion': 540;
  'Apollo': 141;
  'Arethusa': 48,60;
  'Arrogant': 540;
  'Bellerophon': 102;
  'Britannia': 103-4,497;
  'Cambria': 139;
  'Caradoc': 112;
  'Colossus': 541;
  'Conflict': 99;
  'Curacoa': 546;
  'Dauntless': 547;
  'Diamond': 103,333;
  'Duke of Wellington': 540;
  'Exmouth': 542;
  'Furious': 103;
  'Hannibal': 545;
  'Hecla': 98;
  'Imperieuse': 542;
  'James Watt': 96;
  'Jean d'Acre': 546, Plate IX;
  'London': 102,547;
  'Leopard': 549;
  'Neptune': 96;
  'Niger': 137;
  'Odin': 99-100,544;
  'Queen': 102,545;
  'Retribution': 31;
  'Rodney': 106,545,548;
  'Rosamond': 95;
  'Royal': 545;
  'Sanspareil': 215;
  'Sidon': 141;
  'Tiger': 106-7;
  'Trafalgar': 103,106;
  'Tribune': 545;
  'Vulcan': 138-9
War wounds, specific:
  abdominal wounds: 98,478-9;
  amputations:54-5,106-7,128-32, 137,140,198-200,214-6,219, 223-5,300,323,328,333,347,471, 479-84,493-4,520,528,541,551, 583;
  chest wounds: 477-8;
  facial wounds: 477;
  gangrene: 474-5;
  genito-urinary tract wounds: 479;
  head wounds: 476-7,493;

    joint resection: 483-4,583;
lower limb wounds: 479-82,493;
nerve injuries: 480;
surgical techniques: 473-474, 482;
upper limb wounds: 480-481,493;
vascular wounds: 479-480
War wounds, general: evolution of treatment: 1-3,5-6,9,17,23,54-5,57; hospital policy: 469-70, 520; infection: 474-5,494-5; various missiles: 473,601
Women in Crimea (other than nurses): 89-92,267,505-9

Yellow fever: 3,22,52

ILLUSTRATIONS

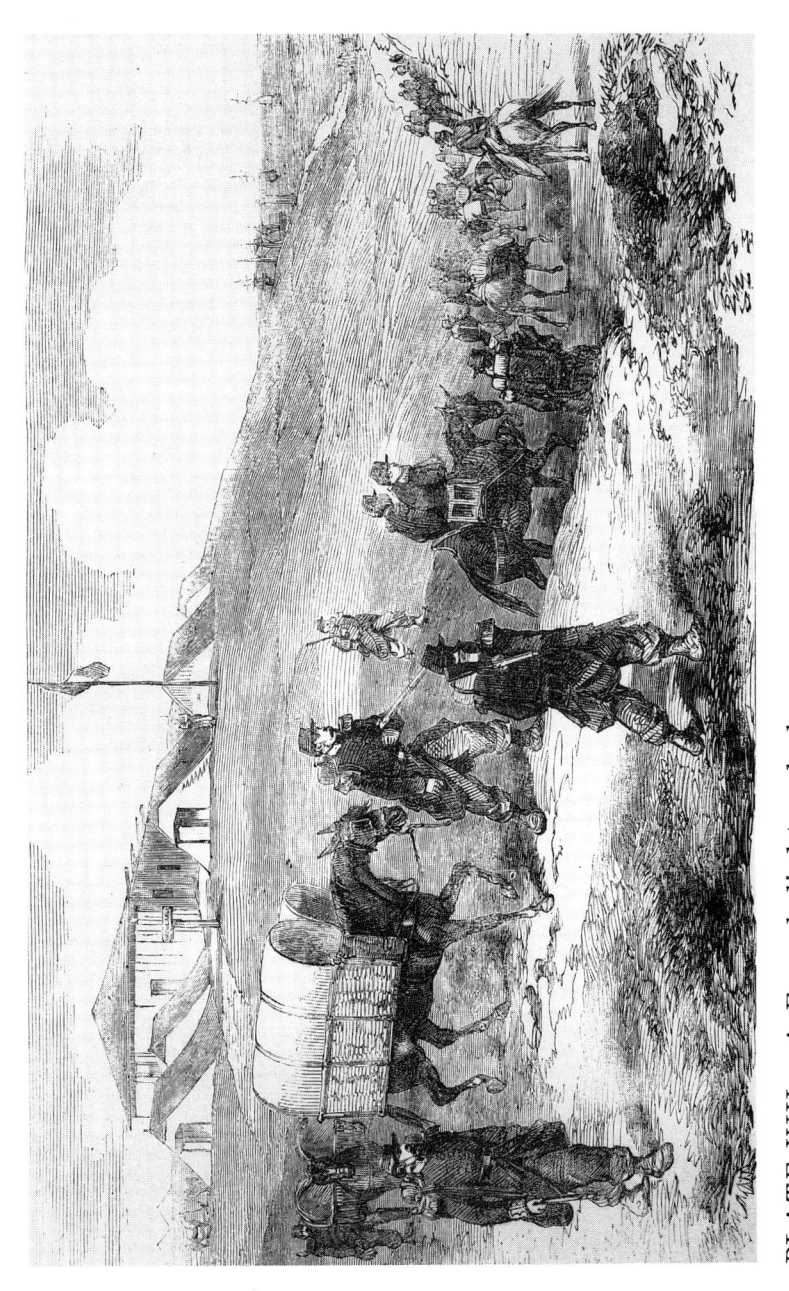

PLATE XIII: A French light ambulance.

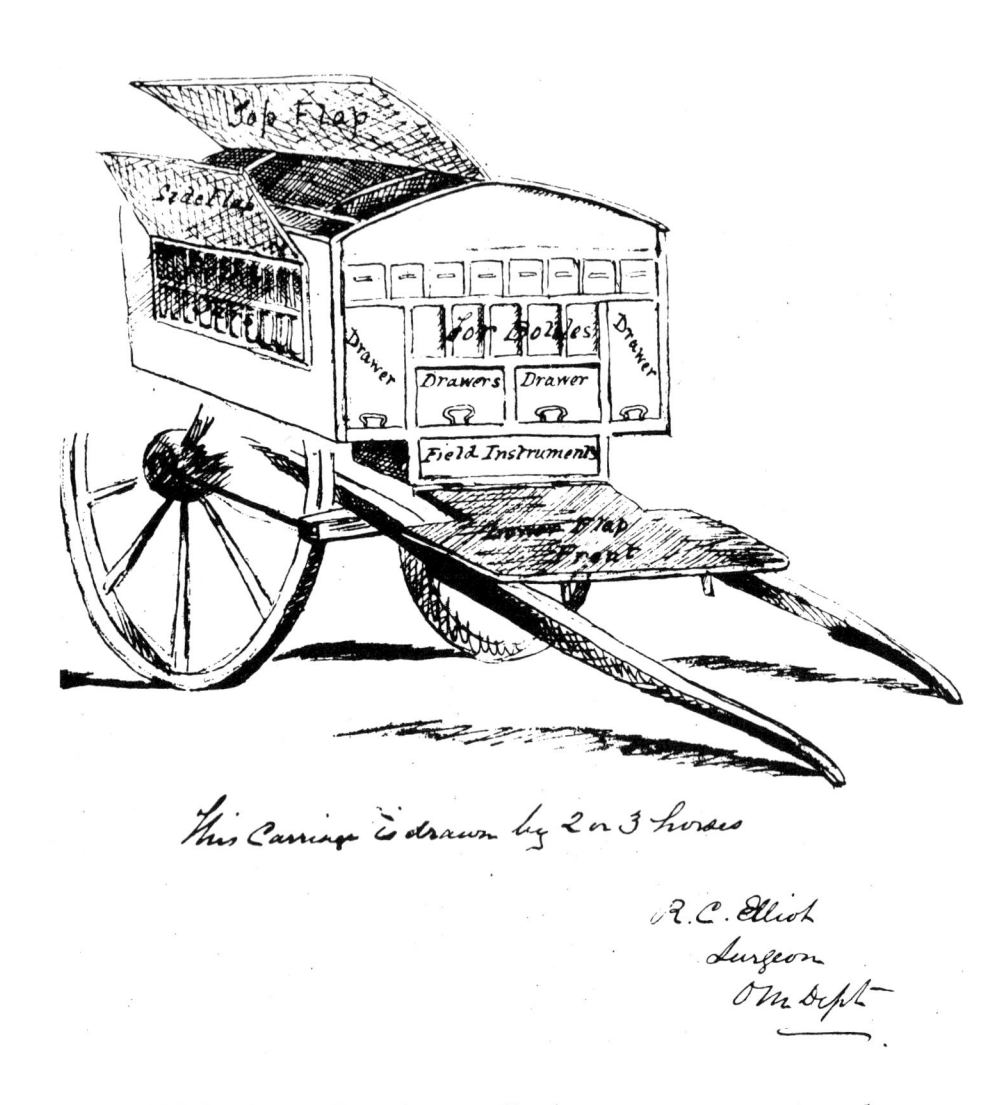

PLATE XIV: A Russian medical stores cart captured on the Flank March. Sketched by Surgeon Elliot.

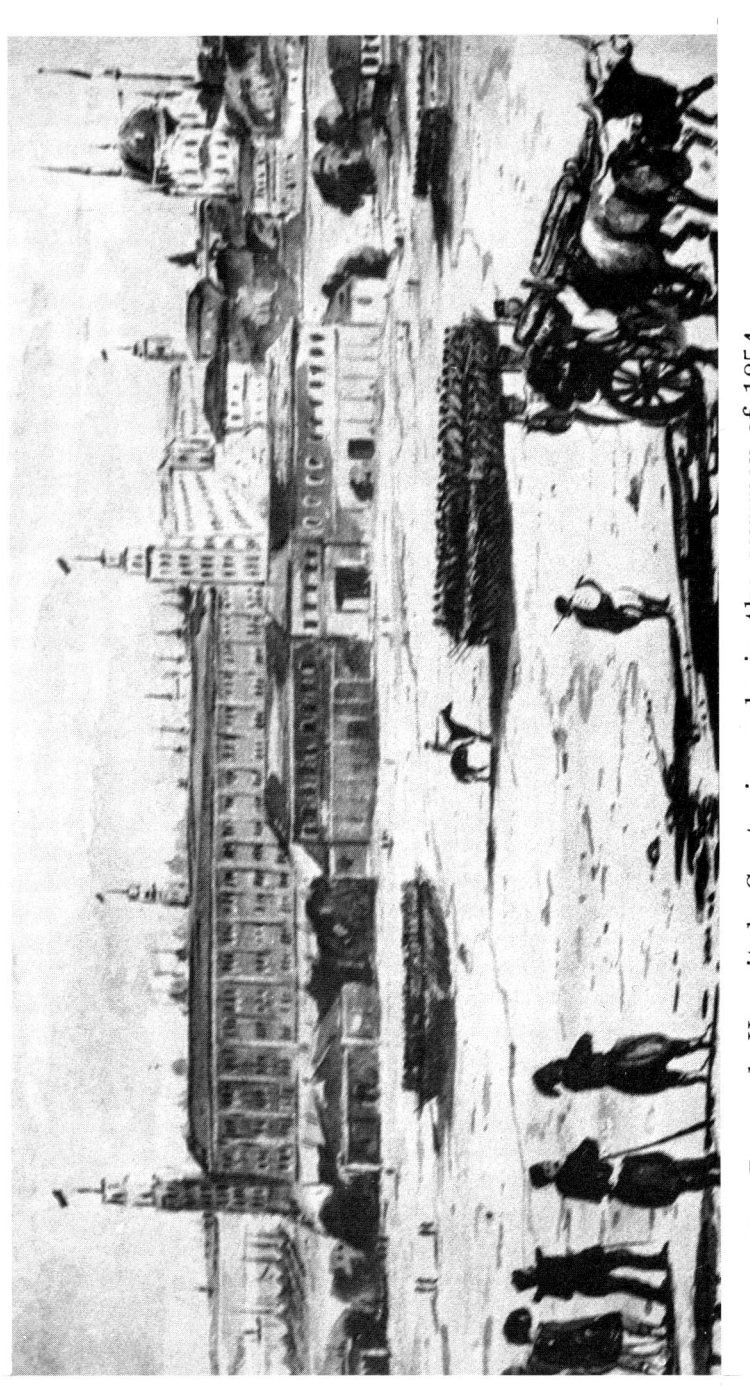

PLATE XV: Barrack Hospital, Scutari, early in the summer of 1854. Note the Turkish 'araba' in the right foreground.

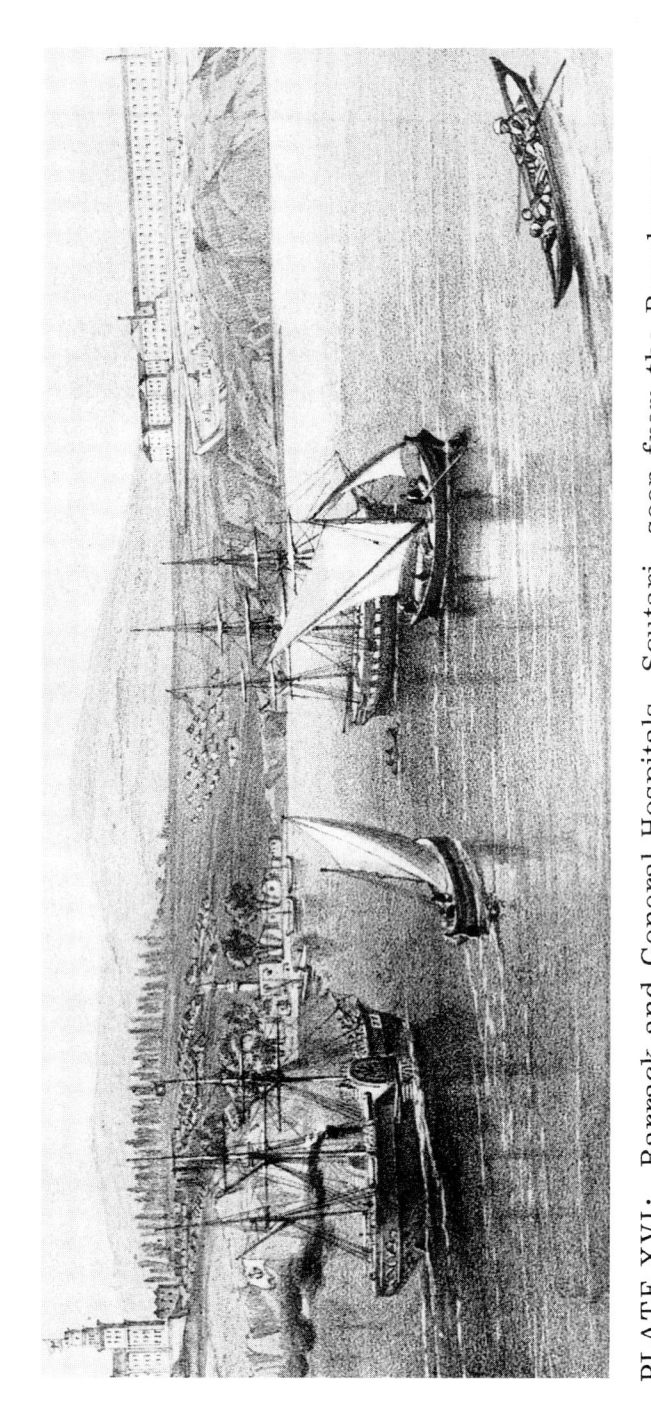

PLATE XVI: Barrack and General Hospitals, Scutari, seen from the Bosphorus.

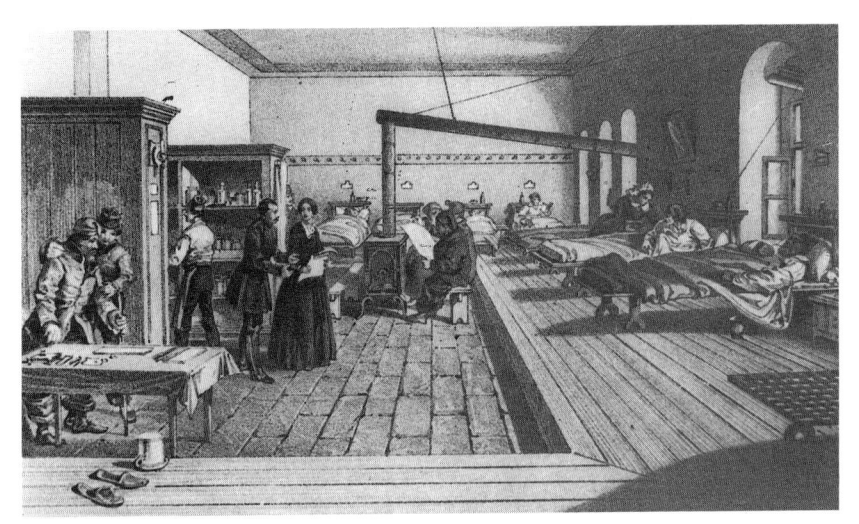

PLATE XVII: A ward in Barrack Hospital. Florence Nightingale with medical officers. Note the raised platform for the beds.

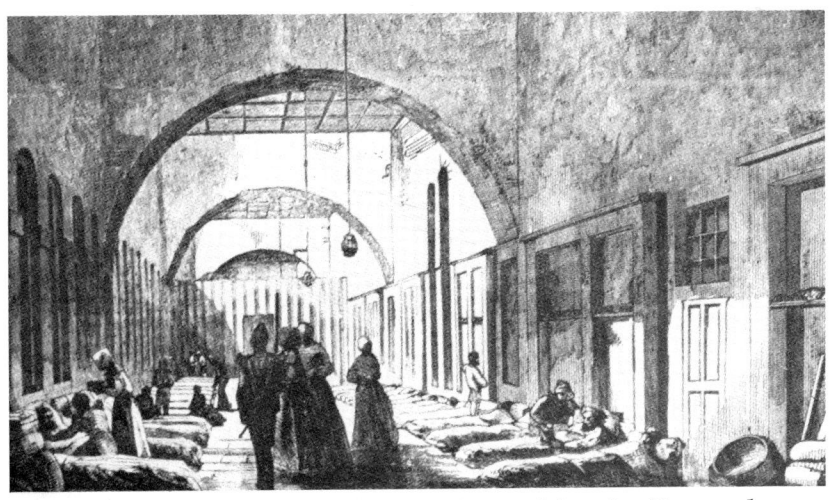

PLATE XVIII: An overcrowded corridor in Barrack Hospital, in the winter of 1854-55.

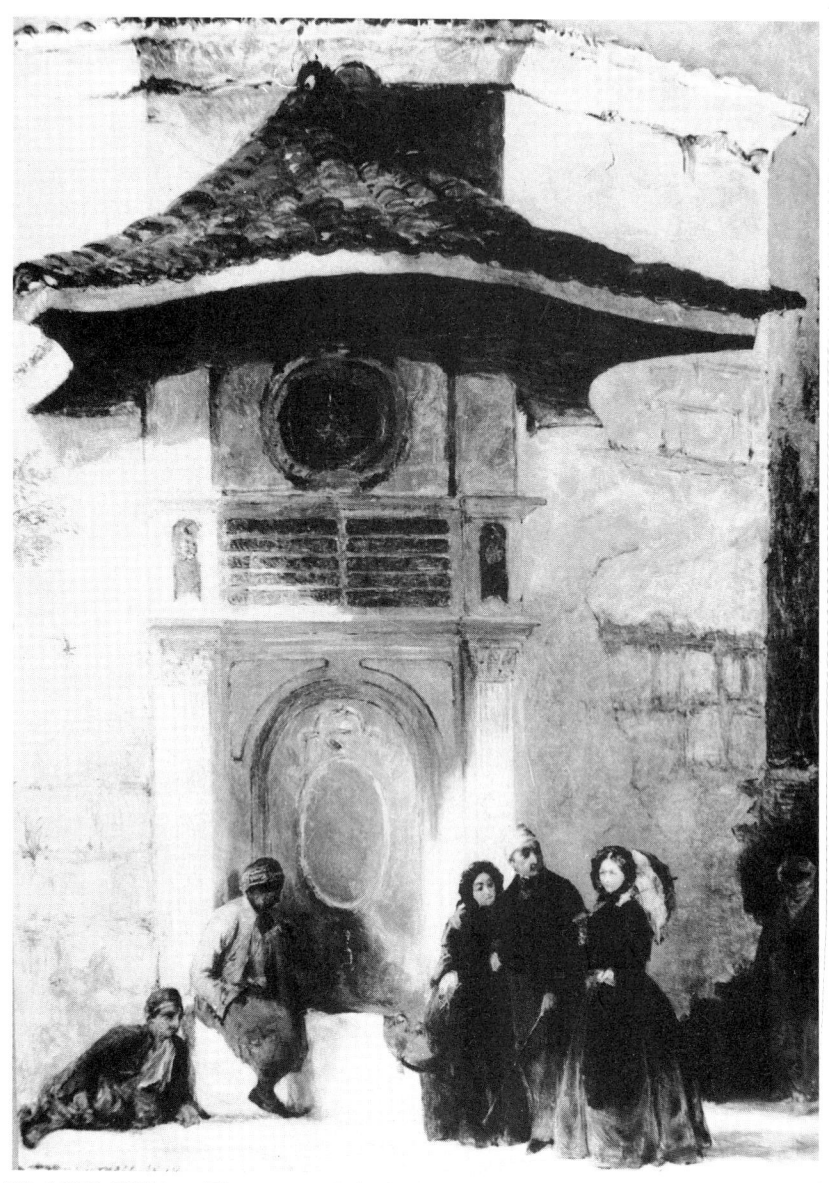

PLATE XIX: Florence Nightingale with the Bracebridges, on one of her rare expeditions to Constantinople.

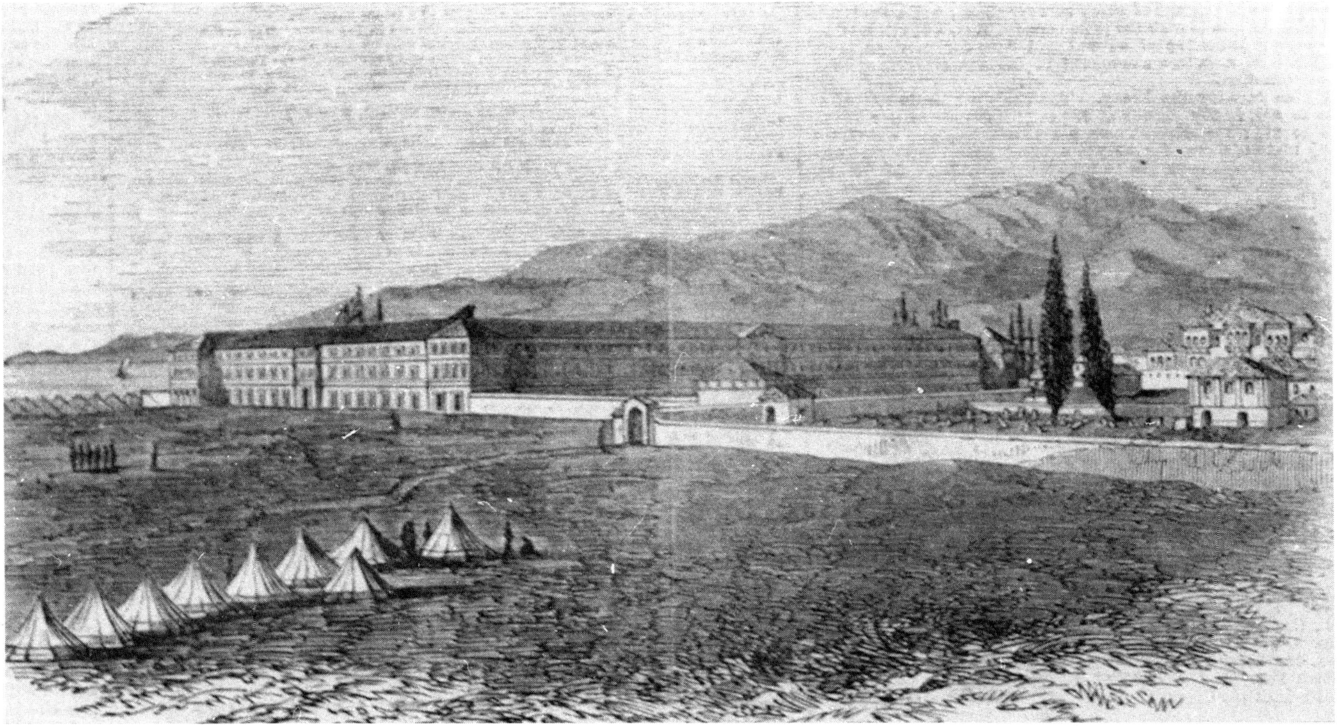

PLATE XX: Smyrna Hospital.

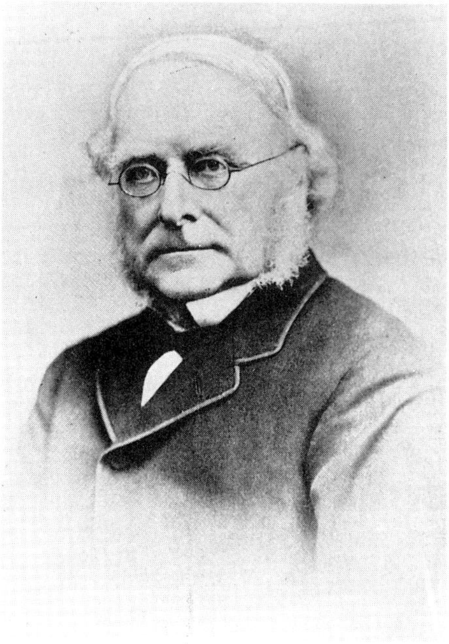

PLATE XXI:
Thomas Spencer Wells
(1817-1897),
naval surgeon prior to
the war, civil surgeon
in the East (1855-1856).

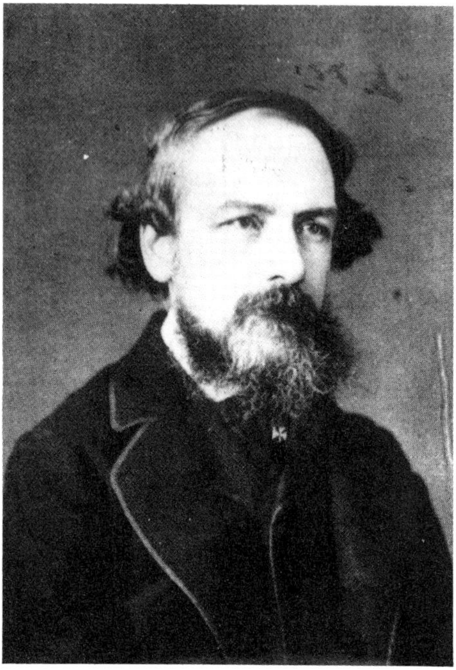

PLATE XXII:
John Hulke
(1830-1885),
civil surgeon in
the East (1855-1856).

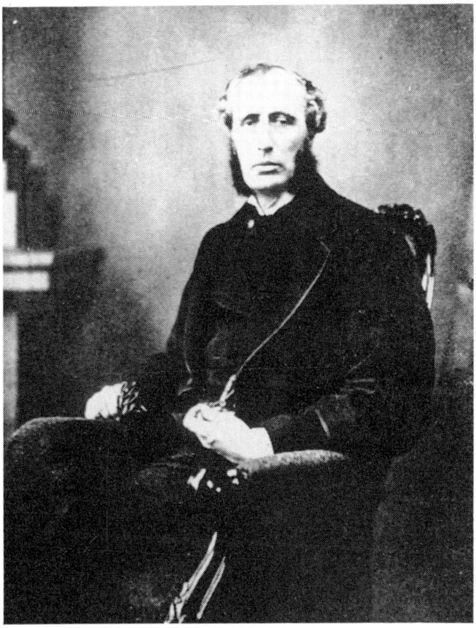

PLATE XXIII:
George Macleod
(1828-1892),
civil surgeon in
the East (1855-1856).

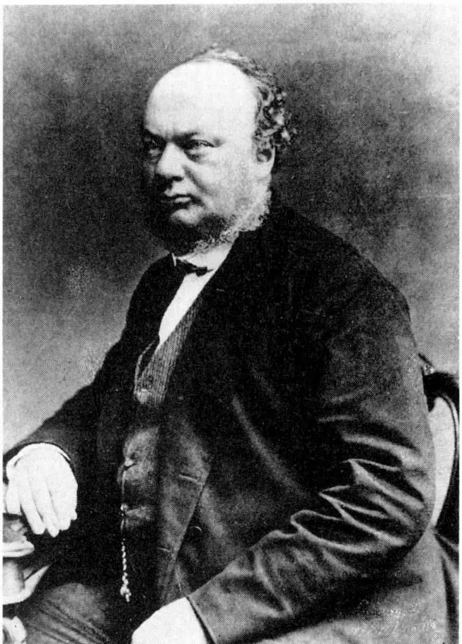

PLATE XXIV:
Holmes Coote
(1815-1872),
civil surgeon in
the East (1855).

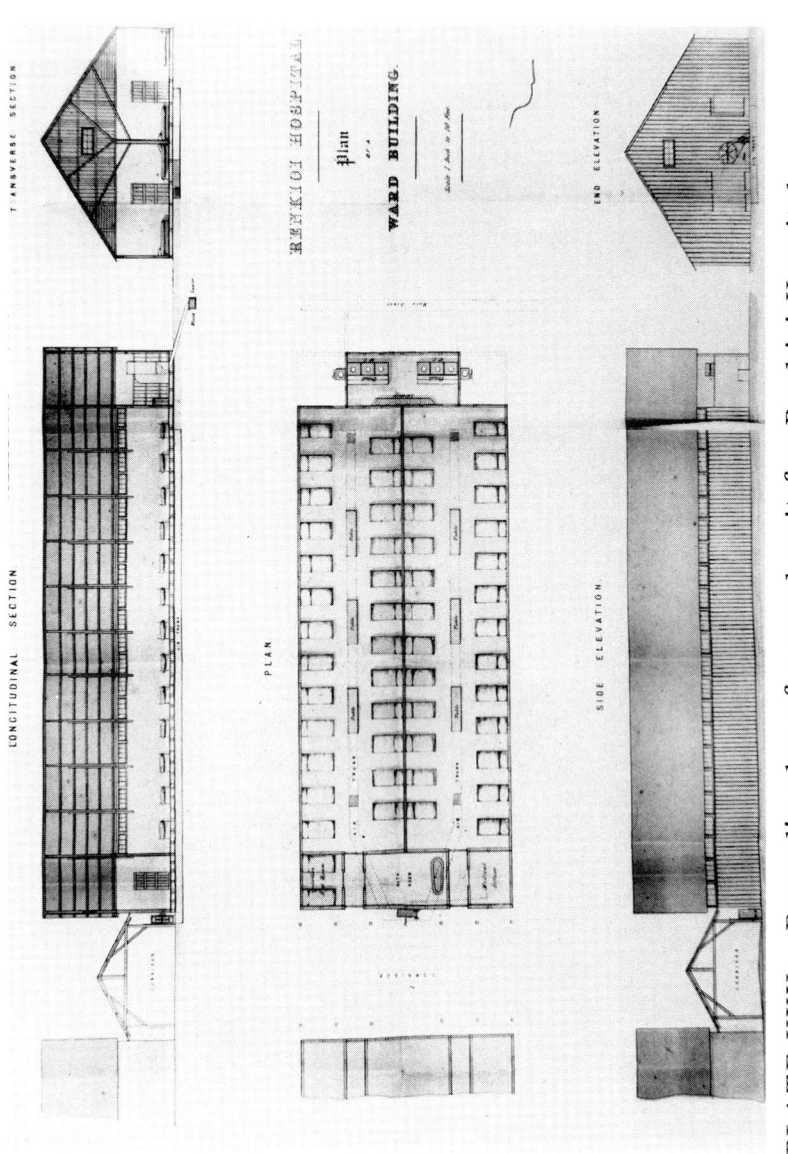

PLATE XXV: Brunel's plan of a ward unit for Renkioi Hospital.

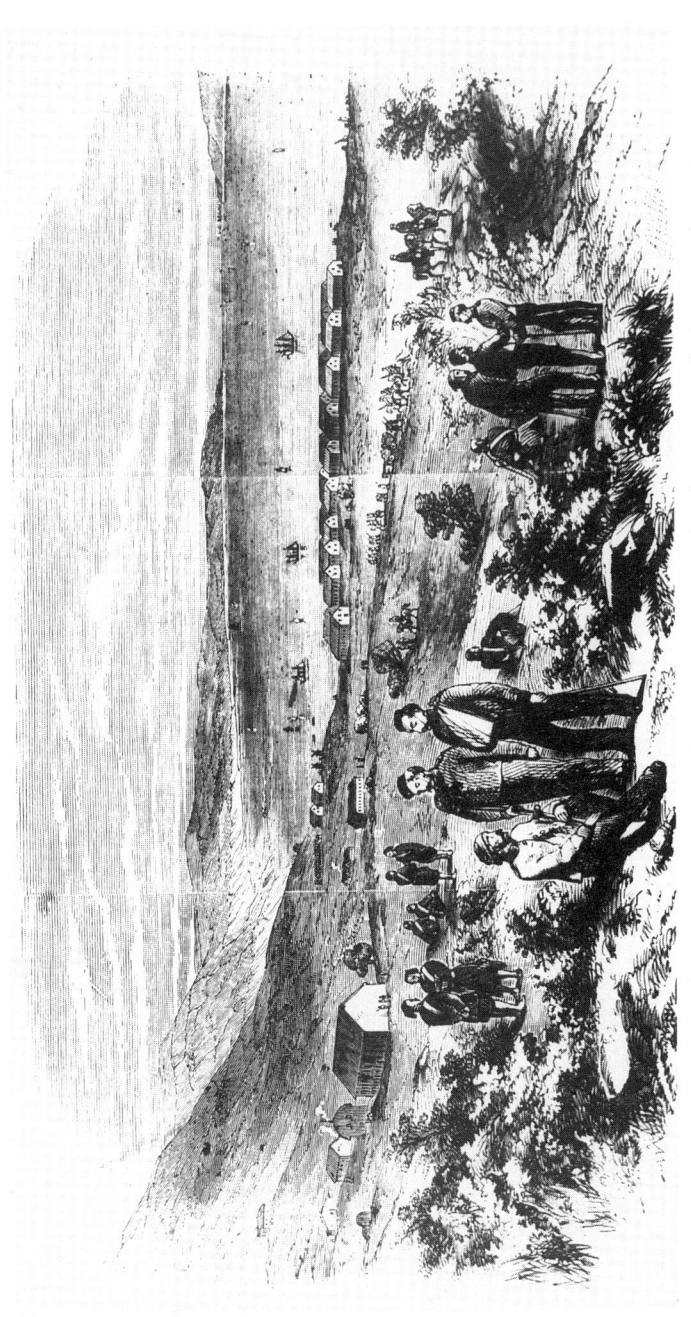

PLATE XXVI: Artist's impression of Renkioi Hospital, around September 1855.

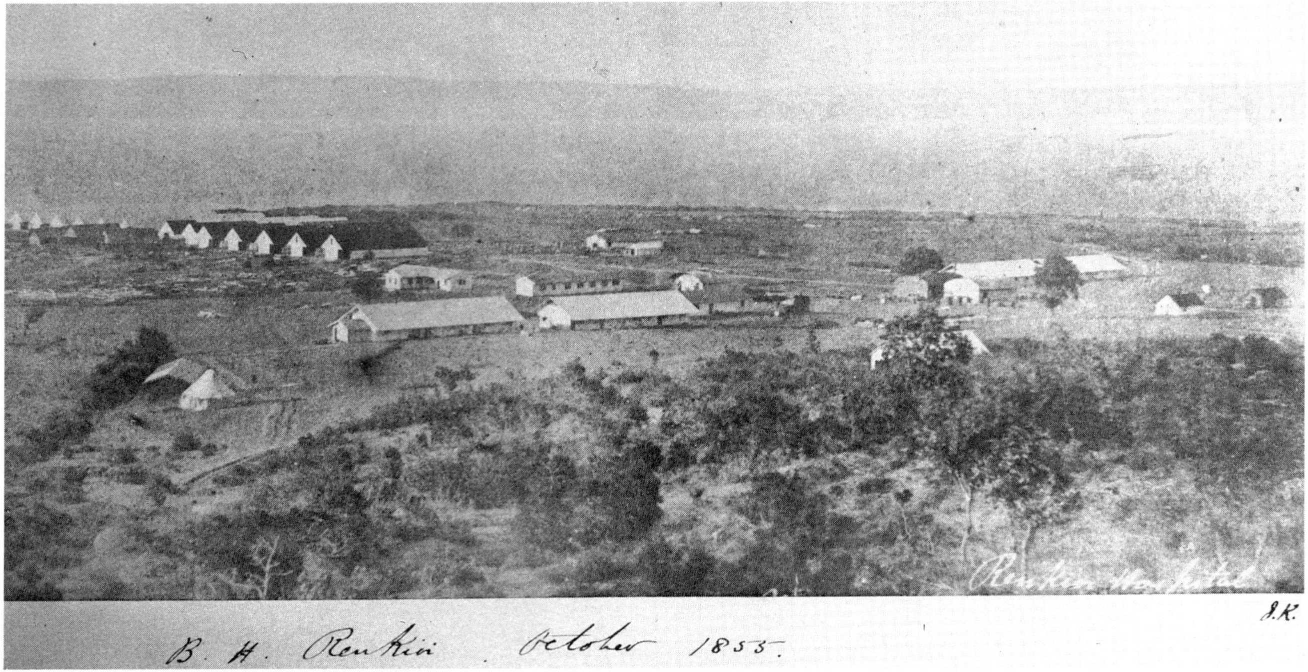

PLATE XXVII: Photograph of Renkioi Hospital.

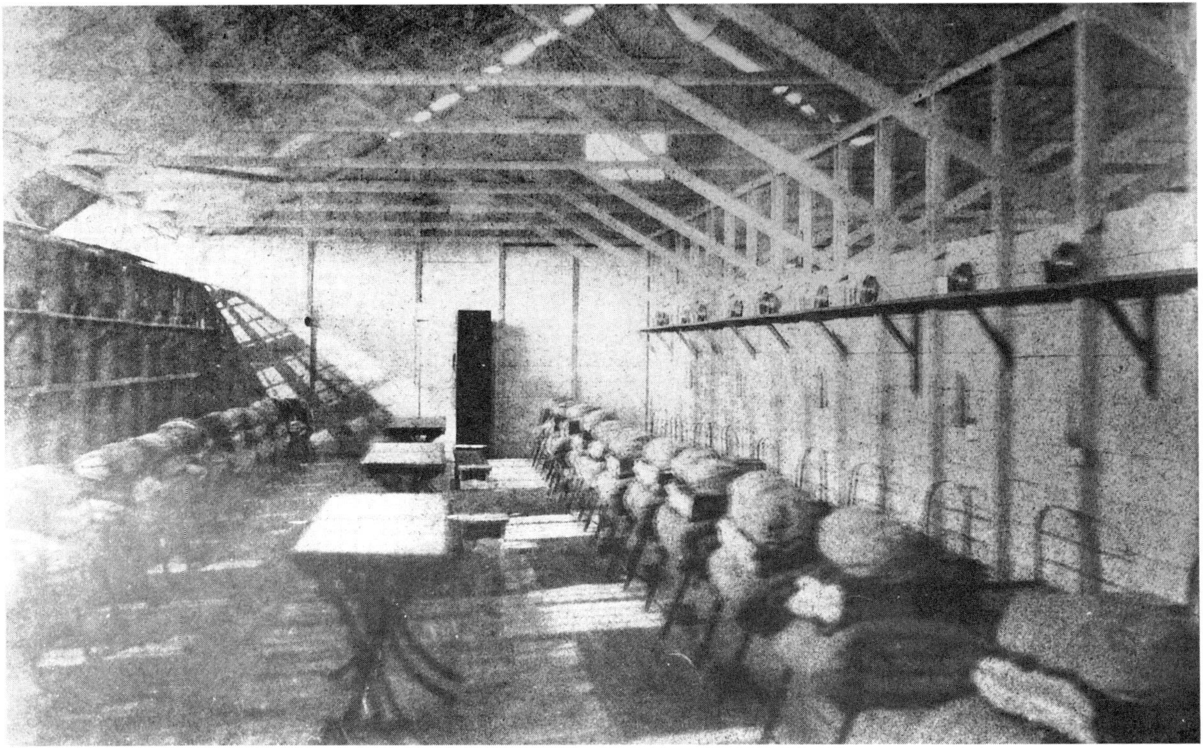

PLATE XXVIII: Photograph of the interior of a ward unit at Renkioi, about August 1855.

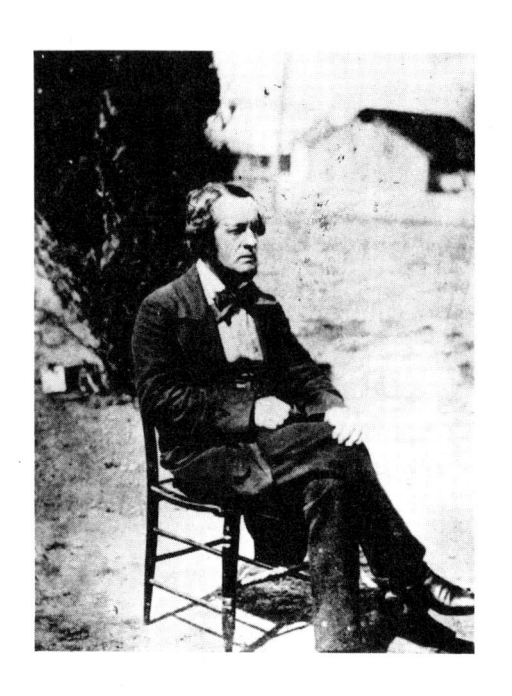

PLATE XXIX:
William Robertson
(1818-1882),
Physician,
Renkioi Hospital
(1855-1856).
Photograph taken
by himself.

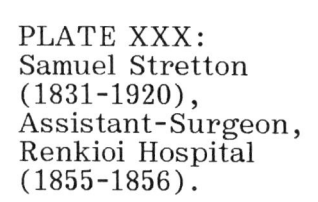

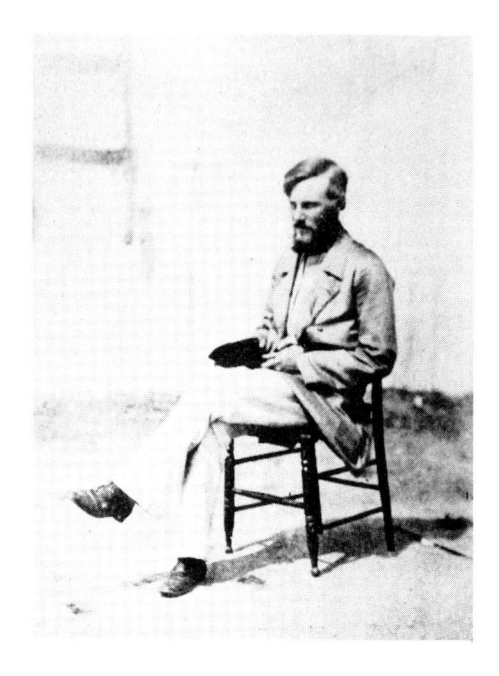

PLATE XXX:
Samuel Stretton
(1831-1920),
Assistant-Surgeon,
Renkioi Hospital
(1855-1856).

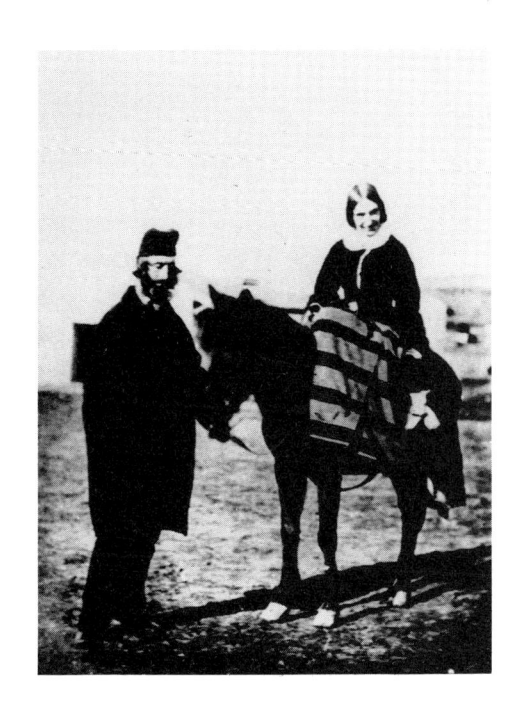

PLATE XXXI:
Dr. and Mrs. Parkes.
Edmund Parkes
(1819-1876),
Superintendent,
Renkioi Hospital
(1855-1856).

PLATE XXXII:
Dr. and Mrs. Goodeve.
Henry Goodeve
(1807-1884),
Physician,
Renkioi Hospital
(1855-1856)

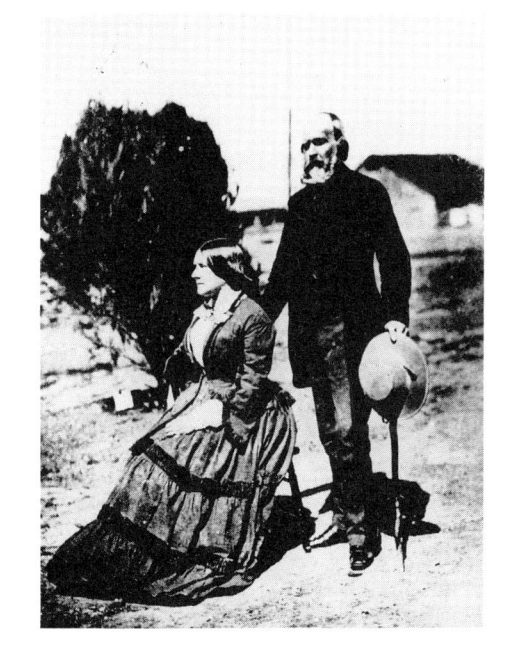

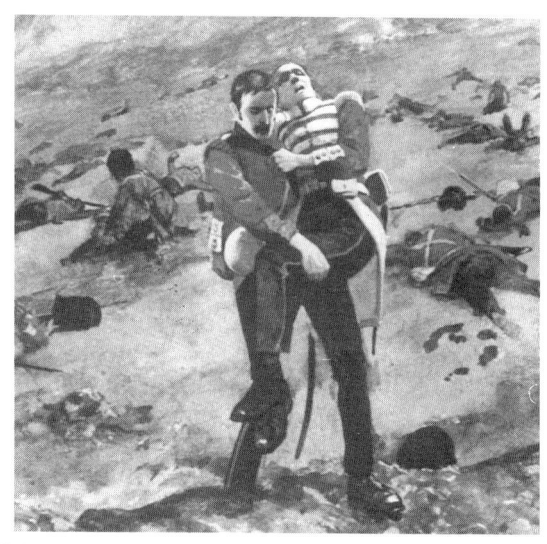

PLATE XXXIII: Assistant-Surgeon Thomas Hale (1832-1909). Awarded the Victoria Cross for heroism at the final assault on Sebastopol.

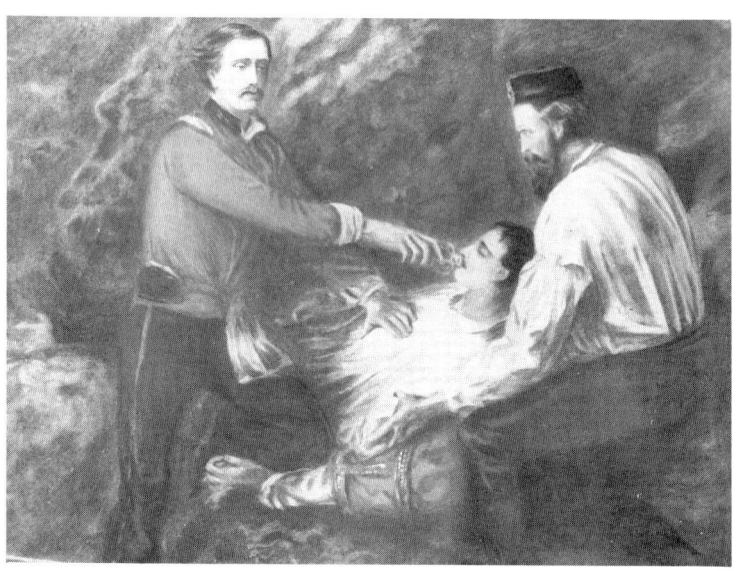

PLATE XXXIV: Assistant-Surgeon Henry Sylvester (1831-1920). Awarded the Victoria Cross for heroism at the final assault on Sebastopol.

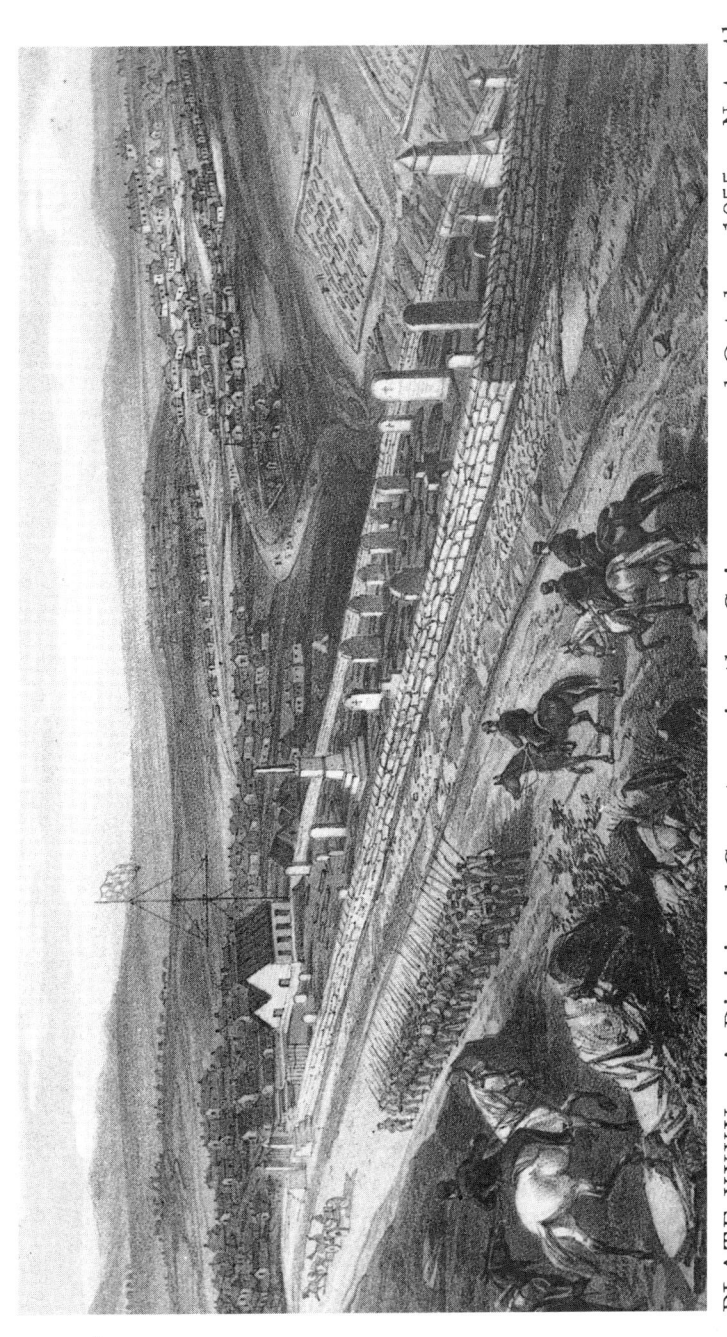

PLATE XXXV: A Divisional Cemetery in the Crimea, around October 1855. Note the almost total replacement of tents by huts in the adjacent regimental camp.

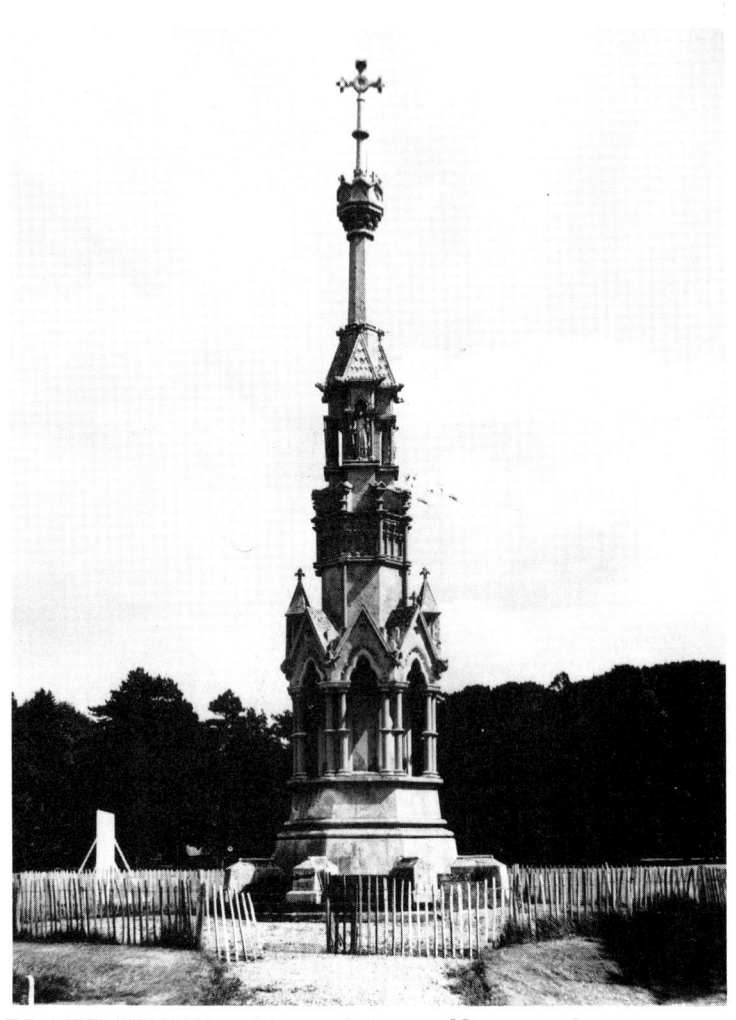

PLATE XXXVI: Memorial to officers of the Army Medical Service who died during the Crimean War. Formerly at Netley Hospital, but now demolished.

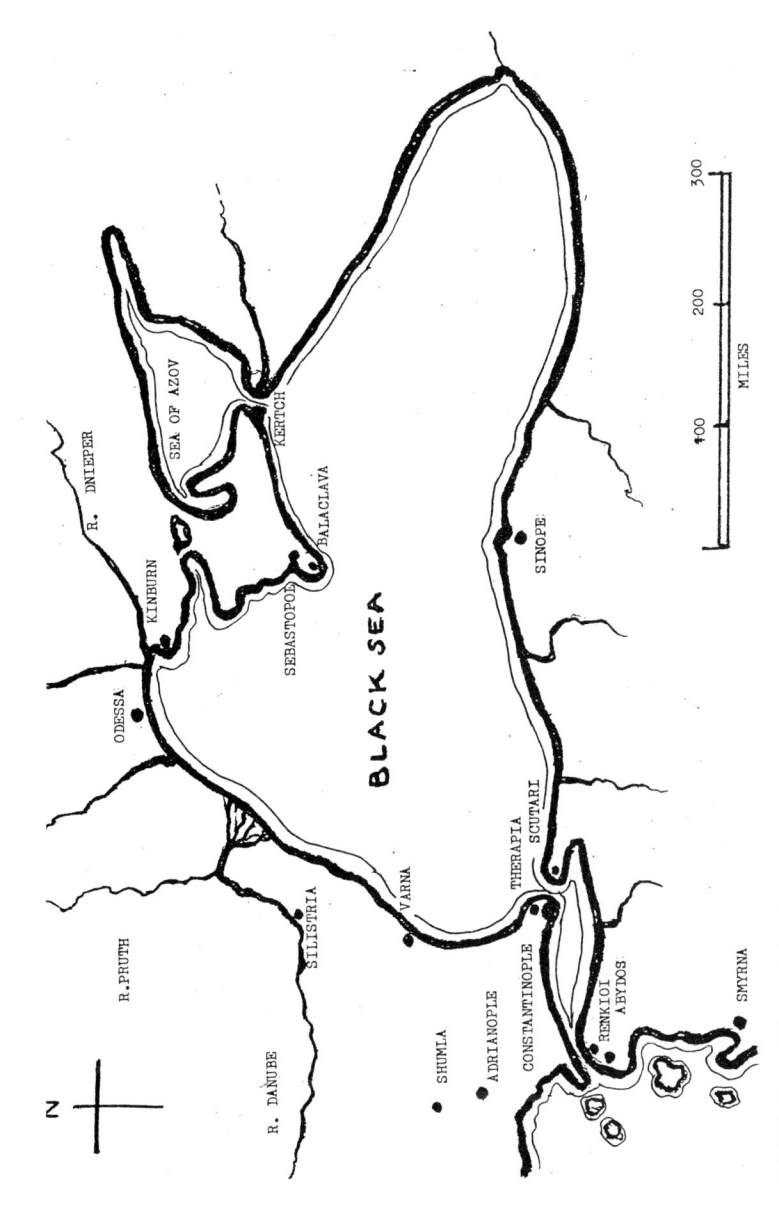

MAP I: The Black Sea

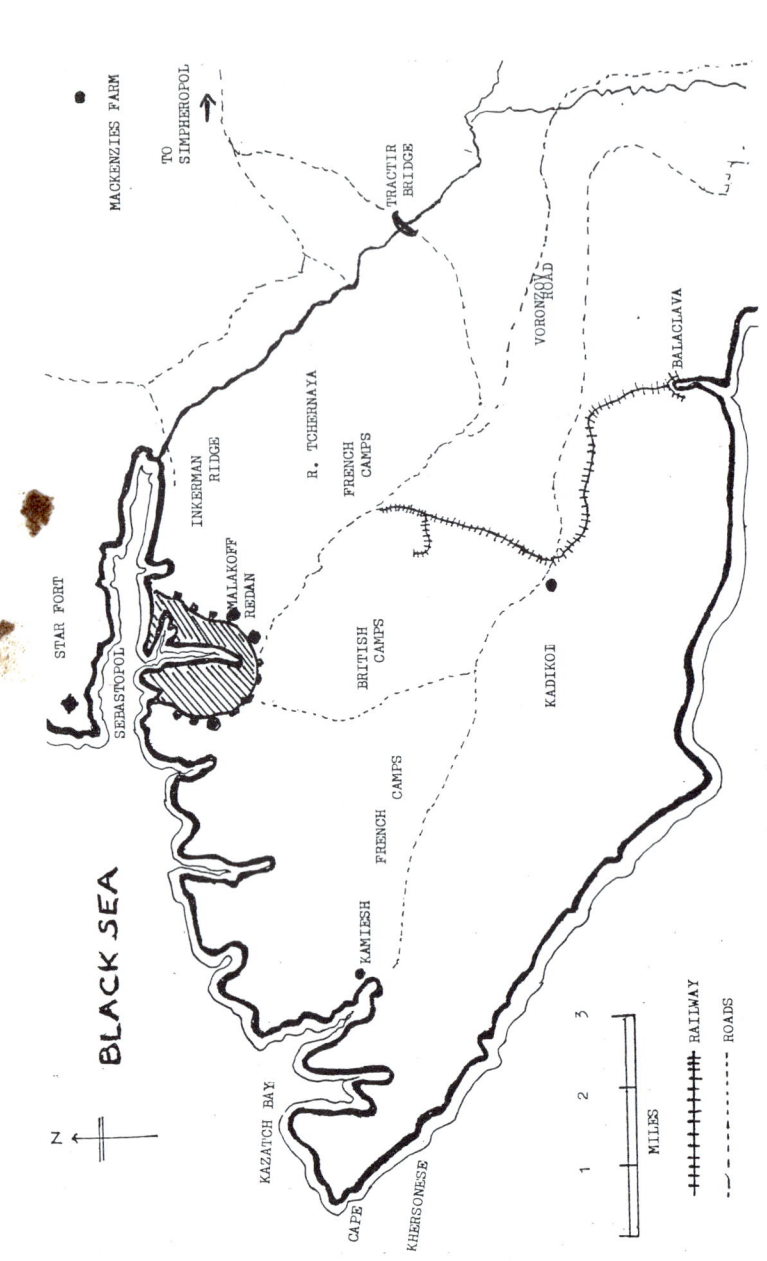

MAP II: The Crimean Peninsula